NURSING MANAGEMENT AND PROFESSIONAL CONCEPTS

OPEN RESOURCES FOR NURSING (OPEN RN)

Second Edition

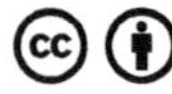

ISBN 4/C: 978-1-957068-17-6
ISBN B/W: 979-8-3851-6465-3

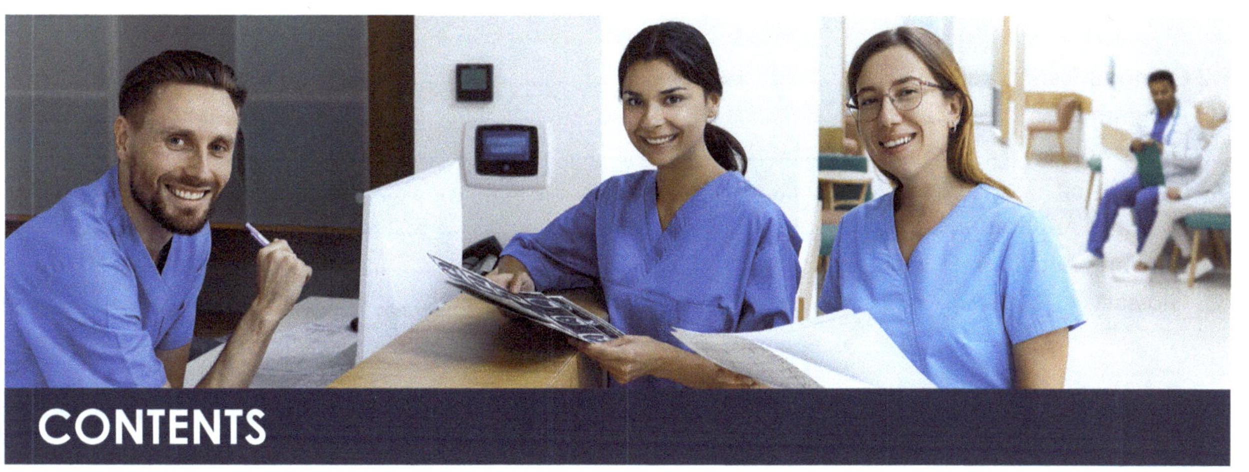

CONTENTS

CHAPTER 7: COLLABORATION WITHIN THE INTERPROFESSIONAL TEAM 155

CHAPTER 8: HEALTH CARE ECONOMICS 213

CHAPTER 9: QUALITY AND EVIDENCE-BASED PRACTICE...243

CHAPTER 10: ADVOCACY 271

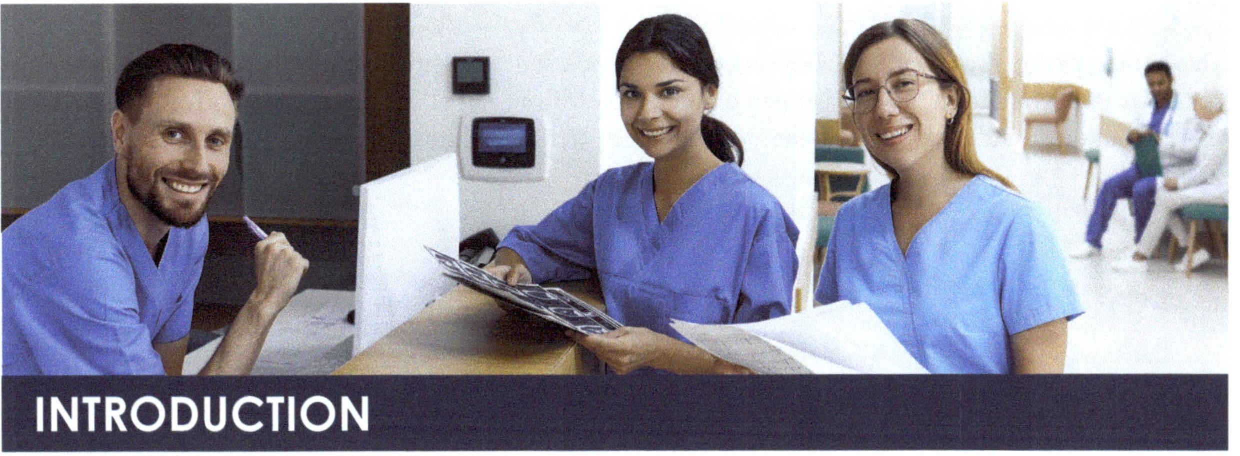

INTRODUCTION

This is the second edition of the *Nursing Management & Professional Concepts* nursing OER textbook that was developed specifically for prelicensure nursing students preparing to graduate and take the NCLEX-RN to obtain their nursing license. Content is based on the Wisconsin Technical College System (WTCS) statewide nursing curriculum for the Nursing Management & Professional Concepts course (543-114), the 2023 NCLEX-RN Test Plan,[1] and the Wisconsin Nurse Practice Act.[2] Here is a summary of updates made to the second edition.

This book introduces concepts related to nursing leadership and management, prioritization strategies, delegation and supervision, legal implications of nursing practice, ethical nursing practice, collaboration within the interprofessional team, health care economics, quality and evidence-based practice, advocacy, preparation for the RN role, and the avoidance of burnout with self-care. Several free, online, interactive learning activities are included in each chapter, including NCLEX Next Generation-style case studies that encourage students to develop clinical judgment while applying content to client-care situations. Additionally, the Appendix includes a "suite of patients" with suggested prompts for classroom discussion to assist students in applying concepts from the book to real client-care situations.

The ebook is free with CC BY 4.0 licensing and can be viewed using the QR code in the following textbox.

View the online book and associated interactive learning activities using this QR code.

1. NCSBN. (n.d.) *Test plans.* https://www.nclex.com/test-plans.page
2. Wisconsin State Legislature. (2024). *Chapter 6: Standards of practice for registered nurses and licensed practical nurses.* Board of Nursing. https://docs.legis.wisconsin.gov/statutes/statutes/441

This book is part of the Open RN© Nursing OER textbook series, originally funded by a $2.5 million Open Textbook Pilot grant from the Department of Education with sustainability funded by WisTech Open. Read more about other OER textbooks on the WisTech Open website at https://www.cvtc.edu/grants/wistech.

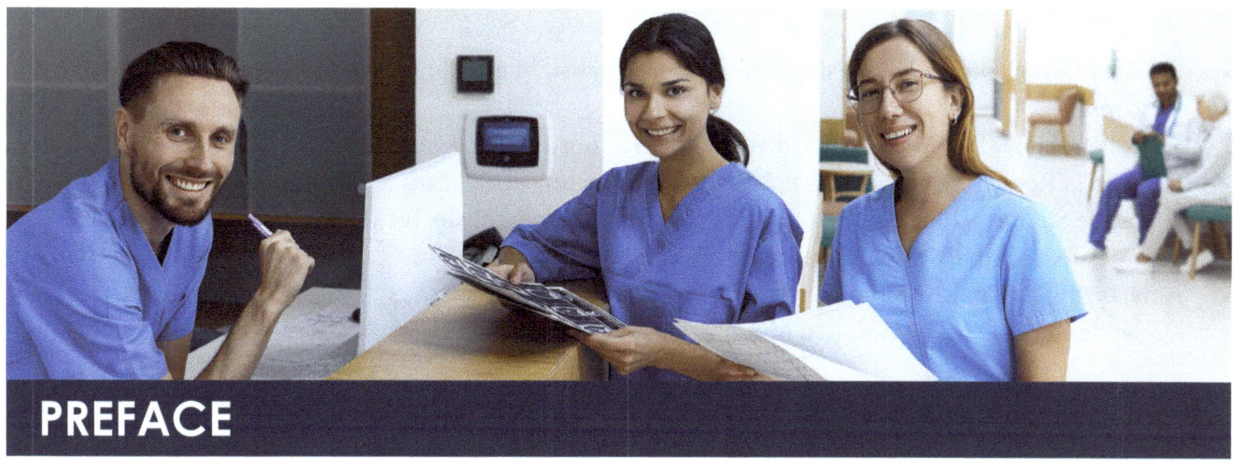

PREFACE

ABOUT THIS BOOK

Editors

- Kimberly Ernstmeyer, MSN, RN, CNE, CHSE, APNP-BC
- Dr. Elizabeth Christman, DNP, RN, CNE

Graphics Editor

- Nic Ashman, MLIS, Librarian, Chippewa Valley Technical College

Developing Authors

This second edition of this textbook was developed based on feedback received from WTCS nursing faculty, the 2023 NCLEX-RN and NCLEX-PN Test Plans, the updated WTCS statewide nursing curriculum, new evidence-based guidelines, and current industry practices. The developing author for the second edition was Dr. Elizabeth Christman, DNP, RN, CNE.

Developing authors for the first edition of this book included the following industry nurses and nursing faculty:

- Dr. Elizabeth Christman, DNP, RN, CNE
- Travis Christman, MSN, RN, Chief Nursing Officer, HSHS Sacred Heart and St. Joseph's Hospitals
- Vonni Demaster, MSN, RN, CNE, Lakeshore Technical College
- Kim Ernstmeyer, MSN, RN, CNE, CHSE, APNP-BC, Chippewa Valley Technical College
- Dr. Kerri Kliminski, EdD, MSN, RN, Madison Area Technical College

- Dr. Amy Olson, DNP, RN, Nursing Education Specialist, Mayo Clinic Health System Northwest Wisconsin
- Mary Pomietlo, MSN, RN, CNE, University of Wisconsin – Eau Claire
- Dr. Angela Roesler, DNP, MSN, RN, Northcentral Technical College
- Dr. Jackie Stewart, DNP, MS, RN, CPNP-PC, Northeast Wisconsin Technical College
- Dr. Julie Teeter, DNP, RN, CNE, Gateway Technical College
- Amy Tyznik, MSN, RN, Moraine Park Technical College
- Dr. Jamie Zwicky, EdD, MSN, RN, Moraine Park Technical College

Contributors

Contributors who assisted in creating the second edition of this textbook included:

- Kelly Carpenter, MLIS, Moraine Park Technical College
- Travis Christman, MSN, RN, Mayo Clinic Health System Northwest Wisconsin, Eau Claire, WI
- Jane Flesher, MST, Proofreader, Chippewa Valley Technical College
- Ashley Gilson, MSN, RN, Moraine Park Technical College
- Krista Polomis, MSN, RN, CNE, Nicolet College
- Wendy Suess, MSN, RN, Fox Valley Technical College
- Suzanne Williamson, MSN, RN, CHSE, Gateway Technical College

Contributors who assisted in the creation of the first edition of this textbook included:

- Kellea Ewen, MSN, RN, Lakeshore Technical College
- Jane Flesher, MST, Proofreader, Chippewa Valley Technical College
- Vince Mussehl, MLIS, Open RN Lead Librarian, Chippewa Valley Technical College
- Joshua Myers, Web Developer, Chippewa Valley Technical College
- Meredith Pomietlo, BA, Retail Design and Marketing, University of Wisconsin – Stout
- Jenna Raths, MSN, RN, Chippewa Valley Technical College
- Lauren Richards, Graphics Designer, Chippewa Valley Technical College
- Grace Rommelfanger, MSN, RN, Moraine Park Technical College
- Dominic Slauson, Instructional Technologist and Designer for the Open RN Project, California State University Northridge

Advisory Committee

The Open RN Advisory Committee consisted of the following individuals:

- Jenny Bauer, MSN, RN, NPD-BC, Mayo Clinic Health System Northwest Wisconsin, Eau Claire, WI
- Gina Bloczynski, MSN, RN, Dean of Nursing, Chippewa Valley Technical College
- Lisa Cannestra, Eastern Wisconsin Healthcare Alliance
- Travis Christman, MSN, RN, Chief Nursing Officer, HSHS Sacred Heart and St. Joseph's Hospitals
- Sheri Johnson, UW Population Health Institute
- Dr. Vicki Hulback, DNP, RN, Dean of Nursing, Gateway Technical College

- Jenna Julson, MSN, RN, NPD-BC, Nursing Education Specialist, Mayo Clinic Health System Northwest Wisconsin, Eau Claire, WI
- Brian Krogh, MSN, RN, Associate Dean – Health Sciences, Northeast Wisconsin Technical College
- Hugh Leasum, MBA, MSN, RN, Nurse Manager Cardiology/ICU, Marshfield Clinic Health System, Eau Claire, WI
- Pam Maxwell, SSM Health
- Mari Kay-Nobozny, NW Wisconsin Workforce Development Board
- Dr. Amy Olson, DNP, RN, Nursing Education Specialist, Mayo Clinic Health System Northwest Wisconsin, Eau Claire, WI
- Rorey Pritchard, EdS, MEd, MSN, RN-BC, CNOR(E), CNE, Senior RN Clinical Educator, Allevant Solutions, LLC
- Kelly Shafaie, MSN, RN, Associate Dean of Nursing, Moraine Park Technical College
- Dr. Ernise Watson, PhD, RN, Associate Dean of Nursing, Madison Area Technical College
- Sherry Willems, HSHS St. Vincent Hospital

Reviewers

Peer reviewers of the first edition of this textbook included the following:

- Dr. Kimberly A. Amos, PhD, RN, CNE, Isothermal Community College
- Sara Annunziato, RN, MSN, Rockland Community College
- Megan Baldwin, MSN, RN, CNOR, MercyOne Medical Center Des Moines
- Ginger Becker, Nursing Student, Portland Community College
- Dr. Kim Belcik, PhD, RN-BC, CNE, Texas State University, St. David's School of Nursing
- Nancy Bonard, MSN, RN-BC, St. Joseph's College of Maine
- Dr. Jessica Brown, DNP, AGPCNP-BC, CBCN
- Dr. Joan Buckley, PhD, RN, Nassau Community College
- Dr. Sarah Carlyle, DNP, RN, CCRN-K, Asante Health System
- Travis Christman, MSN, RN, HSHS Sacred Heart and St. Joseph's Hospitals
- Pasang Comfort, Nursing Student, Portland Community College
- Judith R. Corcoran, RN, MSN, CNE, Moraine Valley Community College
- Dr. Victoria Coyle, DNP, RN, CHSE, Gateway Technical College
- Tamara Davis, MSN, RN, Chippewa Valley Technical College
- Dr. Andrea Dobogai, DNP, RN, Moraine Park Technical College
- Stacy Svoma Doering, MAEd, BS, RDMS, RVT, Chippewa Valley Technical College
- Dr. Judith D. Dornbach, DNP, MSN, RN, NEA-BC, Southwestern Oregon Community College
- Jessica Dwork, RN, MSN-Ed, Maricopa Community College
- Dr. Rachael Farrell, EdD, MSN, CNE, Howard Community College
- Kathleen Fraley, MSN, RN, St. Clair County Community College
- Dr. Sharon Gebelein, DNP, RN, CMSRN, Mid-State Technical College
- Julia Harelstad, MSN, RN, NE-BC, Mayo Clinic Health System
- Deborah Harmon, BSN, RN, Pasco-Hernando State College
- Melissa Hauge, RN, MSN, Madison College
- Lexa Hosier, Nursing Student, St. Catherine University
- Katherine Howard, MS, RN-BC, CNE, Middlesex College

- Leslie A. Jackson, MSN/Ed, RN, Northcentral Technical College
- Susan Jepsen, MSN, RN, CNE, Lansing Community College
- Doris R. Jepson, MSN, RN, Clatsop Community College
- Jenna Julson, MSN, RN, NPD-BC, Mayo Clinic Health System
- Mary F. Kakenmaster, MSN, RN, CNE, Oakton Community College
- Maria Kindrai, MSN, RN, Southwest Wisconsin Technical College
- Lindsay Kuhlman, RN, BSN, Sacred Heart Hospital
- Dr. Coleen Kumar, PhD, RN, CNE, JFK University Medical Center Harold B. and
- Dorothy A. Snyder School of Nursing and Medical Imaging
- Dara Lanman, MSN, RN, CNE, Galen College of Nursing
- Kathy Loppnow, MSN, RN, Wisconsin Technical College System
- Dawn M. Lyon, MSN, RN, St. Clair County Community College
- Dr. Lydia Massias, EdD, MS, RN, Pasco-Hernando State College
- Dr. Marylou E. Mercado, EdD, MSN, RN, CNE, FNP-BC, Yavapai College, Prescott, AZ
- Dr. Jamie Murphy, PhD, RN, State University of New York, Delhi
- Angela Ngo-Bigge, RN, MSN, FNP-C, Grossmont College
- Dr. Tennille O'Connor, DNP, RN, CNE, Pasco-Hernando State College
- Dr. Amy Irene Olson, DNP, RN, Mayo Clinic Health System
- Amy Ortscheid, MSN, CNE, RN, Fox Valley Technical College
- Dr. Grace Paul, DNP, M.Phil, MSN, RN, CNE, Glendale Community College, Arizona
- Krista Polomis, RN, MSN, Nicolet College
- Mary Pomietlo, MSN, RN, CNE, University of Wisconsin – Eau Claire
- Cassandra Porter, MSN, RN, Lake Land College
- Angela Powell, MSN, RN, CEN, CPEN, TCRN, Mercy Medical Center
- Dr. Regina Prusinski, DNP, APRN, CPNP-AC, BC, FNP, Otterbein University
- Tyra Rideaux, MSN, RN, San Jacinto College North
- Kathleen S. Rizzo, MSN, RN, St. Louis Community College at Forest Park
- Ann K. Rosemeyer, MSN, RN, Chippewa Valley Technical College
- Callie Schlegel, Nursing Student, St. Catherine University
- Celee Schuch, Nursing Student, St. Catherine University
- Julie A. Sigler, MSN, RN, Chippewa Valley Technical College
- Dr. Jackie Stewart, DNP, MS, RN, CPNP-PC, Northeast Wisconsin Technical College
- Dr. Suzanne H. Tang, DNP, MSN, RN, FNP-BC, PHN, Rio Hondo College
- Jacquelyn Titus, MS, RN, Sun Lake High School
- Jane Trainis, MS, PMHCNS-BC, CNE, Community College of Baltimore County
- Jennie E. Ver Steeg, Mercy College of Health Sciences
- Devon Rice Weaver, MSN, BSN, RN, Clatsop Community College
- Dr. Nancy Whitehead, PhD, APNP, RN, Milwaukee Area Technical College
- Dr. Jamie Zwicky, EdD, MSN, RN, Moraine Park Technical College

Licensing/Terms of Use

Attribution

Some of the content for this textbook was adapted from the following open educational resources. For specific reference information about what was used and/or changed in this adaptation, please refer to the footnotes at the bottom of each page of the book.

- Ernstmeyer, K., & Christman, E. (Eds.). (2024). *Nursing fundamentals 2E.* Open RN | WisTech Open. https://wtcs.pressbooks.pub/nursingfundamentals/
- Wagner, J. (2018). *Leadership and Influencing Change in Nursing.* University of Regina Press. https://pressbooks.pub/leadershipandinfluencingchangeinnursing/
- World Health Organization. (2024). *Medication without harm: Policy brief.* WHO. https://www.who.int/publications/i/item/9789240062764
- Lowey, S. E. (2015). *Nursing care at the end of life.* Open Library. https://ecampusontario.pressbooks.pub/nursingcare/
- Steinmetz, J. (2019). *Politics, Power, and Purpose: An Orientation to Political Science.* FHSU Digital Press. https://fhsu.pressbooks.pub/orientationpolisci/
- Lapum, J., St-Amant, O., Hughes, M., Tan, A., Bogdan, A., Dimaranan, F., Frantzke, R., & Savicevic, N. (2019). *The scholarship of writing in nursing education: 1st Canadian edition.* Toronto LibreTexts. (2024). Anatomy and physiology (boundless). LibreTexts: Medicine.
- *StatPearls* [Internet]. (2025). StatPearls Publishing. https://www.ncbi.nlm.nih.gov/books/NBK430685/

Content that is not taken from the above OER or the public domain should include the following attribution statement:

Ernstmeyer, K., & Christman, E. (Eds.). (2024). *Nursing management and professional concepts 2e.* Open RN | WisTech Open. https://wtcs.pressbooks.pub/nursingmpc/

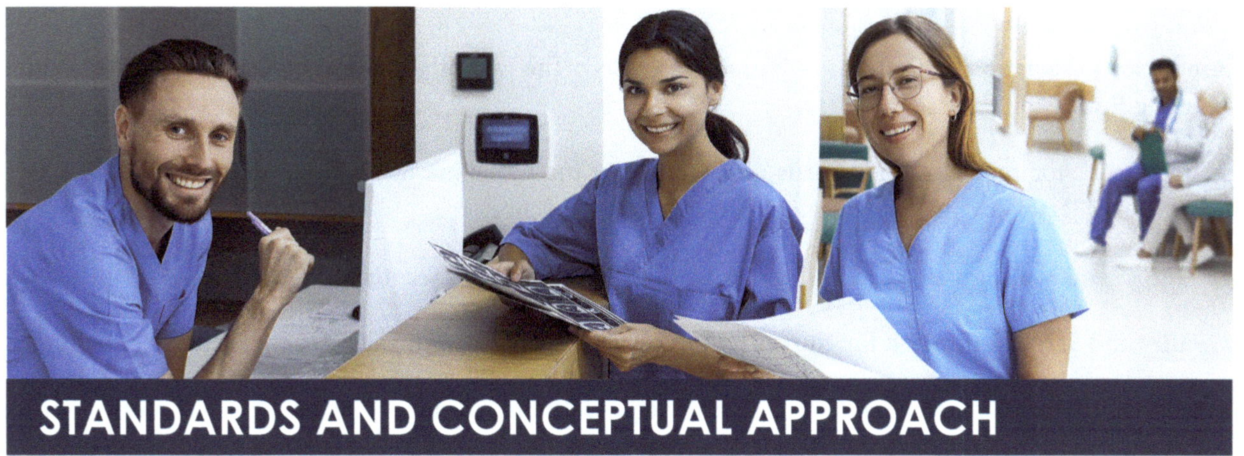

STANDARDS AND CONCEPTUAL APPROACH

The Open RN *Nursing Management and Professional Concepts, 2e* textbook is based on several external standards and uses a conceptual approach.

EXTERNAL STANDARDS

American Nurses Association (ANA)

The ANA establishes Standards for Professional Nursing Practice a Nursing Code of Ethics.[3,4]

- https://www.nursingworld.org/ana/about-ana/standards/

The National Council Licensure Examination for Registered Nurses: NCLEX-RN Test Plans

The NCLEX-RN test plans are updated every three years to reflect fair, comprehensive, current, and entry-level nursing competency.

- https://www.ncsbn.org/nclex.htm

The National League of Nursing (NLN): Competencies for Graduates of Nursing Programs

NLN competencies guide nursing curricula to position graduates in a dynamic health care arena with practice that is informed by a body of knowledge and ensures that all members of the public receive safe, quality care.

- https://www.nln.org/education/nursing-education-competencies/

---

3. American Nurses Association. (2021). *Nursing: Scope and standards of practice* (4th ed.). American Nurses Association.
4. American Nurses Association. (2015). *Code of ethics for nurses with interpretive statements*. American Nurses Association. https://www.nursingworld.org/practice-policy/nursing-excellence/ethics/code-of-ethics-for-nurses/competencies-for-graduates-of-nursing-programs

American Association of Colleges of Nursing (AACN): The Essentials: Competencies for Professional Nursing Education

A framework for preparing individuals as members of the discipline of nursing, reflecting expectations across the trajectory of nursing education and applied experience.

- https://www.aacnnursing.org/Portals/42/AcademicNursing/pdf/Essentials-2021.pdf

Quality and Safety Education for Nurses (QSEN) Institute: Pre-licensure Competencies

Quality and safety competencies include knowledge, skills, and attitudes to be developed in nursing pre-licensure programs. QSEN competencies include client-centered care, teamwork and collaboration, evidence-based practice, quality improvement, safety, and informatics.

- https://qsen.org/competencies/

Wisconsin State Legislature, Administrative Code Chapter N6

The Wisconsin Administrative Code governs the Registered Nursing and Practical Nursing professions in Wisconsin.

- https://docs.legis.wisconsin.gov/code/admin_code/n/6

Healthy People 2030

Healthy People 2030 envisions a society in which all people can achieve their full potential for health and well-being across the life span. Healthy People provides objectives based on national data and includes social determinants of health.

- https://health.gov/healthypeople

Conceptual Approach

The Open RN *Nursing Management and Professional Concepts, 2e* textbook incorporates the following concepts:

- **Holism.** Florence Nightingale taught nurses to focus on the principles of holism, including wellness and the interrelationship of human beings and their environment. This textbook encourages holistic nursing care by addressing the impact of social determinants of health (SDOH) and health care reimbursement models on client health.
- **Evidence-Based Practice (EBP).** Evidence-based practices are referenced by footnotes throughout the textbook. The Open RN textbooks will be updated as new EBP is established and after the release of updated NCLEX Test Plans every three years.

- **Clinical Judgment.** Associated unfolding case studies are written to reflect the NCSBN Clinical Judgment Measurement Model used on the NCLEX-RN. Formative assessments encourage students to recognize cues, analyze cues, prioritize hypotheses, generate solutions, take action, and evaluate outcomes.[5]
- **Cultural Competency.** Nurses have an ethical obligation to practice with cultural humility and provide culturally responsive care to the clients and communities they serve based on the ANA Code of Ethics[6] and the ANA Scope and Standards of Practice.[7]
- **Safe, Quality, Client-Centered Care.** Content reflects the priorities of safe, quality, client-centered care.
- **Clear and Inclusive Language.** Clear language is used based on preferences expressed by prelicensure nursing students to enhance understanding of complex concepts.[8] "They" is used as a singular pronoun to refer to a person whose gender is unknown or irrelevant to the context of the usage, as endorsed by APA style. It is inclusive of all people and helps writers avoid making assumptions about gender.[9]
- **Open Source Images and Fair Use.** Images are included to promote visual learning. Students and faculty can reuse open source images by following the terms of their associated Creative Commons licensing. Some images are included based on Fair Use as described in the "Code of Best Practices in Fair Use for Open Educational Resources" presented at the OpenEd 2020 conference. Refer to the footnotes of images for source and licensing information throughout the text.
- **Open Pedagogy.** Students are encouraged to contribute to the Open RN project in meaningful ways by reviewing content for clarity and assisting in the creation of open source images.[10]

Supplementary Material Provided

Several supplementary resources are provided with this textbook.

- Supplementary, free videos promote student understanding of concepts and procedures.
- Online, interactive, and written learning activities provide formative feedback. and promote the development of clinical judgment as students apply content to realistic client scenarios.
- Free NCLEX Next Generation-style case studies are provided in each chapter
- Free downloadable textbook versions are available for offline use.

---

5. Dickison, P., Haerling, K. A., & Lasater, K. (2019). Integrating the national council of state boards of nursing clinical judgment model into nursing educational frameworks.*Journal of Nursing Education. 58*(2), 72-78. https://doi.org/10.3928/01484834-20190122-03
6. American Nurses Association. (2015). *Code of ethics for nurses with interpretive statements.* American Nurses Association. https://www.nursingworld.org/practice-policy/nursing-excellence/ethics/code-of-ethics-for-nurses/
7. American Nurses Association. (2021). *Nursing: Scope and standards of practice* (4th ed.). American Nurses Association.
8. Verkuyl, M., Lapum, J., St-Amant, O., Bregstein, J., & Hughes, M. (2020). Healthcare students' use of an e-textbook open educational resource on vital sign measurement: A qualitative study. *Open Learning: The Journal of Open, Distance and e-Learning.* https://doi.org/10.1080/02680513.2020.1835623
9. American Psychological Association. (2021). *Singular "They."* https://apastyle.apa.org/style-grammar-guidelines/grammar/singular-they
10. Wagstaff, S. (2023). *Open Pedagogy Notebook.* https://openpedagogy.org/

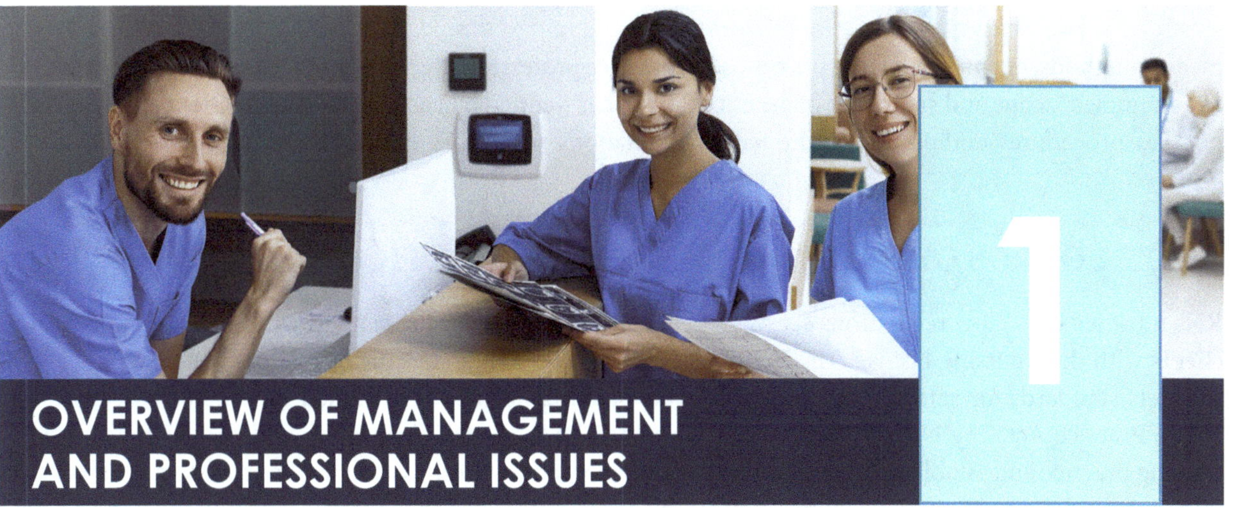

1 OVERVIEW OF MANAGEMENT AND PROFESSIONAL ISSUES

1.1 OVERVIEW

This textbook discusses professional and management concepts related to the role of a registered nurse (RN) as defined by the American Nurses Association (ANA). The ANA publishes two resources that set standards and guide professional nursing practice in the United States: The *Code of Ethics for Nurses With Interpretive Statements* and *Nursing: Scope and Standards of Practice*. The *Code of Ethics for Nurses With Interpretive Statements* establishes an ethical framework for nursing practice across all roles, levels, and settings and is discussed in greater detail in the "Ethical Practice" chapter of this book. The *Nursing: Scope and Standards of Practice* resource defines the "who, what, where, when, why, and how of nursing" and sets the standards for practice that all registered nurses are expected to perform competently.[1]

The ANA defines the "who" of nursing practice as the nurses who have been educated, titled, and maintain active licensure to practice nursing. The "what" of nursing is the recently revised ANA definition of nursing: "**Nursing** integrates the art and science of caring and focuses on the protection, promotion, and optimization of health and human functioning; prevention of illness and injury; facilitation of healing; and alleviation of suffering through compassionate presence. Nursing is the diagnosis and treatment of human responses and advocacy in the care of individuals, families, groups, communities, and populations in recognition of the connection of all humanity."[2] Simply put, nurses treat human responses to health problems and life processes and advocate for the care of others.

Nursing practice occurs "when" there is a need for nursing knowledge, wisdom, caring, leadership, practice, or education, anytime, anywhere. Nursing practice occurs in any environment "where" there is a health care consumer in need of care, information, or advocacy. The "why" of nursing practice is described as nursing's response to the changing needs of society to achieve positive health care consumer outcomes in keeping with nursing's social contract and obligation to society. The "how" of nursing practice is defined as the ways,

1. American Nurses Association. (2021). *Nursing: Scope and standards of practice* (4th ed.). American Nurses Association.
2. American Nurses Association. (2021). *Nursing: Scope and standards of practice* (4th ed.). American Nurses Association.

means, methods, and manners that nurses use to practice professionally.[3] The "how" of nursing, also referred to as a nurse's "scope and standards of practice," is further defined by each state's Nurse Practice Act; agency policies, procedures, and protocols; and federal regulations and ANA's Standards of Practice.

STATE BOARDS OF NURSING AND NURSE PRACTICE ACTS

RNs must legally follow regulations set by the Nurse Practice Act by the state in which they are caring for clients with their nursing license. The **Board of Nursing** is the state-specific licensing and regulatory body that sets standards for safe nursing care and issues nursing licenses to qualified candidates based on the Nurse Practice Act. The **Nurse Practice Act** is enacted by that state's legislature and defines the scope of nursing practice and establishes regulations for nursing practice within that state. If nurses do not follow the standards and scope of practice set forth by the Nurse Practice Act, they may be disciplined by the Board of Nursing in the form of reprimand, probation, suspension, or revocation of their nursing license. Investigations and discipline actions are reportable among states participating in the Nurse Licensure Compact (that allows nurses to practice across state lines) or when a nurse applies for licensure in a different state. The scope and standards of practice set forth in the Nurse Practice Act can also be used as evidence if a nurse is sued for malpractice.

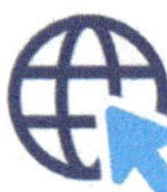

Find your state's Nurse Practice Act on the National Council of State Board of Nursing (NCSBN) website. Access supplementary digital content in the online book using this QR code.

Read more about malpractice and protecting your nursing license in the "Legal Implications" chapter of this book.

Read Wisconsin's Nurse Practice Act, Standards of Practice for Registered Nurses and Licensed Practical Nurses (Chapter N6) PDF, and Rules of Conduct (Chapter N7) PDF. Access supplementary digital content in the online book using this QR code.

3. American Nurses Association. (2021). *Nursing: Scope and standards of practice* (4th ed.). American Nurses Association.

AGENCY POLICIES, PROCEDURES, AND PROTOCOLS

In addition to practicing according to the Nurse Practice Act in the state they are employed, nurses must also practice according to agency policies, procedures, and protocols.

A **policy** is an expected course of action set by an agency. For example, hospitals set a policy requiring a thorough skin assessment to be completed when a client is admitted and then reassessed and documented daily.

Agencies also establish their own set of procedures. A **procedure** is the method or defined steps for completing a task. For example, each agency has specific procedural steps for inserting a urinary catheter.

A **protocol** is a detailed, written plan for performing a regimen of therapy. For example, agencies typically establish a hypoglycemia protocol that nurses can independently and quickly implement when a client's blood sugar falls below a specific number without first calling a provider. A hypoglycemia protocol typically includes actions such as providing orange juice and rechecking the blood sugar and then reporting the incident to the provider.

Agency-specific policies, procedures, and protocols supersede the information taught in nursing school, and nurses can be held legally liable if they don't follow them. It is vital for nurses to review and follow current agency-specific procedures, policies, and protocols while also practicing according to that state's nursing scope of practice. Malpractice cases have occurred when a nurse was asked by their employer to do something outside their legal scope of practice, impacting their nursing license. It is up to you to protect your nursing license and follow the Nurse Practice Act when providing client care. If you have a concern about an agency's policy, procedure, or protocol, follow the agency's chain of command to report your concern.

FEDERAL REGULATIONS

Nursing practice is impacted by regulations enacted by federal agencies. Two examples of federal agencies setting standards of care are The Joint Commission and the Centers for Medicare and Medicaid Services.

The Joint Commission accredits and certifies over 20,000 health care organizations in the United States. The Joint Commission's standards help health care organizations measure, assess, and improve performance on functions that are essential to providing safe, high-quality care. The standards are updated regularly to reflect the rapid advances in health care and address topics such as client rights and education, infection control, medication management, and prevention of medical errors. The annual National Patient Safety Goals are also set by The Joint Commission after reviewing emerging client safety issues.[4]

The Centers for Medicare & Medicaid Services (CMS) is an example of another federal agency that establishes regulations affecting nursing care. CMS is a part of the U.S. Department of Health and Human Services (HHS) that administers the Medicare program and works in partnership with state governments to administer Medicaid. The CMS establishes and enforces regulations to protect client safety in hospitals that receive Medicare and Medicaid funding. For example, one CMS regulation often referred to as "checking the rights of medication administration" requires nurses to confirm specific information several times before medication is administered to a client.[5]

4. The Joint Commission. (2025). *National Patient Safety Goals.* https://www.jointcommission.org/standards/national-patient-safety-goals/
5. Centers for Medicare & Medicaid Services. (2024). *Quality initiatives-general information.* U.S. Department of Health and Human Services. https://www.cms.gov/medicare/quality/initiatives

STANDARDS OF PRACTICE

The ANA defines **Standards of Professional Nursing Practice** as "authoritative statements of the actions and behaviors that all registered nurses, regardless of role, population, specialty, and setting, are expected to perform competently."[6] These standards are classified into two categories: Standards of Practice and Standards of Professional Performance.

The **ANA's Standards of Practice** describe a competent level of nursing practice as demonstrated by the critical thinking model known as the **nursing process**. The nursing process includes the components of assessment, diagnosis, outcomes identification, planning, implementation, and evaluation and forms the foundation of the nurse's decision-making, practice, and provision of care.[7]

Read more information about the nursing process in the "Nursing Process" chapter of Open RN *Nursing Fundamentals, 2e*.[8] Access supplementary digital content in the online book using this QR code.

The **ANA's Standards of Professional Performance** "describe a competent level of behavior in the professional role, including activities related to ethics, advocacy, respectful and equitable practice, communication, collaboration, leadership, education, scholarly inquiry, quality of practice, professional practice evaluation, resource stewardship, and environmental health. All registered nurses are expected to engage in professional role activities, including leadership, reflective of their education, position, and role."[9] This book discusses content related to these professional practice standards. Each professional practice standard is defined in the following subsections with information provided to related content in this book and the Open RN *Nursing Fundamentals, 2e* textbook.[10]

ETHICS

The ANA's *Ethics* standard states, "The registered nurse integrates ethics in all aspects of practice."[11]

6. American Nurses Association. (2021). *Nursing: Scope and standards of practice* (4th ed.). American Nurses Association.
7. American Nurses Association. (2021). *Nursing: Scope and standards of practice* (4th ed.). American Nurses Association.
8. Ernstmeyer, K., & Christman, E. (Eds.). (2024). *Nursing fundamentals 2E.* Open RN | WisTech Open. https://wtcs.pressbooks.pub/nursingfundamentals/
9. American Nurses Association. (2021). *Nursing: Scope and standards of practice* (4th ed.). American Nurses Association.
10. Ernstmeyer, K., & Christman, E. (Eds.). (2024). *Nursing fundamentals 2E.* Open RN | WisTech Open. https://wtcs.pressbooks.pub/nursingfundamentals/
11. American Nurses Association. (2021). *Nursing: Scope and standards of practice* (4th ed.). American Nurses Association.

Read about ethical nursing practice in the "Ethical Practice" chapter of this book.

ADVOCACY

The ANA's *Advocacy* standard states, "The registered nurse demonstrates advocacy in all roles and settings."[12]

Read about nurse advocacy in the "Advocacy" chapter of this book.

RESPECTFUL AND EQUITABLE PRACTICE

The ANA's *Respectful and Equitable Practice* standard states, "The registered nurse practices with cultural humility and inclusiveness."

Read about cultural humility and culturally responsive care in the "Diverse Patients" chapter in Open RN *Nursing Fundamentals, 2e.*[13] Access supplementary digital content in the online book using this QR code.

COMMUNICATION

The ANA's *Communication* standard states, "The registered nurse communicates effectively in all areas of professional practice."[14]

12. American Nurses Association. (2021). *Nursing: Scope and standards of practice* (4th ed.). American Nurses Association.
13. Ernstmeyer, K., & Christman, E. (Eds.). (2024). *Nursing fundamentals 2E.* Open RN | WisTech Open. https://wtcs.pressbooks.pub/nursingfundamentals/
14. American Nurses Association. (2021). *Nursing: Scope and standards of practice* (4th ed.). American Nurses Association.

Read about communicating with clients and team members in the "Communication" chapter in Open RN *Nursing Fundamentals, 2e.*[15] Access supplementary digital content in the online book using this QR code.

Read about interprofessional communication strategies that promote client safety in the "Collaboration Within the Interprofessional Team" chapter of this book.

COLLABORATION

The ANA's *Collaboration* standard states, "The registered nurse collaborates with the health care consumer and other key stakeholders."[16]

Read about strategies to enhance the performance of the interprofessional team and manage conflict in the "Collaboration Within the Interprofessional Team" chapter of this book.

LEADERSHIP

The ANA's *Leadership* standard states, "The registered nurse leads within the profession and practice setting."[17]

Read about leadership, management, and implementing change in the "Leadership and Management" chapter of this book.

15. Ernstmeyer, K., & Christman, E. (Eds.). (2024). *Nursing fundamentals 2E.* Open RN | WisTech Open. https://wtcs.pressbooks.pub/nursingfundamentals/
16. American Nurses Association. (2021). *Nursing: Scope and standards of practice* (4th ed.). American Nurses Association.
17. American Nurses Association. (2021). *Nursing: Scope and standards of practice* (4th ed.). American Nurses Association.

Read about assigning, delegating, and supervising client care in the "Delegation and Supervision" chapter of this book.

Read about tools for prioritizing client care and managing resources for the nursing team in the "Prioritization" chapter of this book.

EDUCATION

The ANA's *Education* standard states, "The registered nurse seeks knowledge and competence that reflects current nursing practice and promotes futuristic thinking."[18]

Read about professional development and specialty certification in the "Preparation for the RN Role" chapter of this book.

SCHOLARLY INQUIRY

The ANA's *Scholarly Inquiry* standard states, "The registered nurse integrates scholarship, evidence, and research findings into practice."[19]

Read about integrating evidence-based practice into one's nursing practice in the "Quality and Evidence-Based Practice" chapter of this book.

18. American Nurses Association. (2021). *Nursing: Scope and standards of practice* (4th ed.). American Nurses Association.
19. American Nurses Association. (2021). *Nursing: Scope and standards of practice* (4th ed.). American Nurses Association.

QUALITY OF PRACTICE

The ANA's *Quality of Practice* standard states, "The nurse contributes to quality nursing practice."[20]

Read about improving quality care and participating in quality improvement initiatives in the "Quality and Evidence-Based Practice" chapter of this book.

PROFESSIONAL PRACTICE EVALUATION

The ANA's *Professional Practice Evaluation* standard states, "The registered nurse evaluates one's own and others' nursing practice."[21]

Read about nursing practice within the legal framework of health care, negligence, malpractice, and protecting your nursing license in the "Legal Implications" chapter of this book.

Read about reviewing the interprofessional team's performance, providing constructive feedback, and advocating for client safety with assertive statements in the "Collaboration Within the Interprofessional Team" chapter of this book.

RESOURCE STEWARDSHIP

The ANA's *Resource Stewardship* standard states, "The registered nurse utilizes appropriate resources to plan, provide, and sustain evidence-based nursing services that are safe, effective, financially responsible, and used judiciously."[22]

Read more about health care funding, reimbursement models, budgets and staffing, and resource stewardship in the "Health Care Economics" chapter of this book.

20. American Nurses Association. (2021). *Nursing: Scope and standards of practice* (4th ed.). American Nurses Association.
21. American Nurses Association. (2021). *Nursing: Scope and standards of practice* (4th ed.). American Nurses Association.
22. American Nurses Association. (2021). *Nursing: Scope and standards of practice* (4th ed.). American Nurses Association.

ENVIRONMENTAL HEALTH

The ANA's *Environmental Health* standard states, "The registered nurse practices in a manner that advances environmental safety and health."[23]

Read about promoting workplace safety for nurses in the "Safety" chapter in Open RN *Nursing Fundamentals, 2e.*[24] Access supplementary digital content in the online book using this QR code.

Read about fostering a professional environment that does not tolerate abusive behaviors in the "Collaboration Within the Interprofessional Team" chapter of this book.

Read about addressing the impacts of social determinants of health in the "Advocacy" chapter of this book.

23. American Nurses Association. (2021). *Nursing: Scope and standards of practice* (4th ed.). American Nurses Association.
24. Ernstmeyer, K., & Christman, E. (Eds.). (2024). *Nursing fundamentals 2E.* Open RN | WisTech Open. https://wtcs.pressbooks.pub/nursingfundamentals/

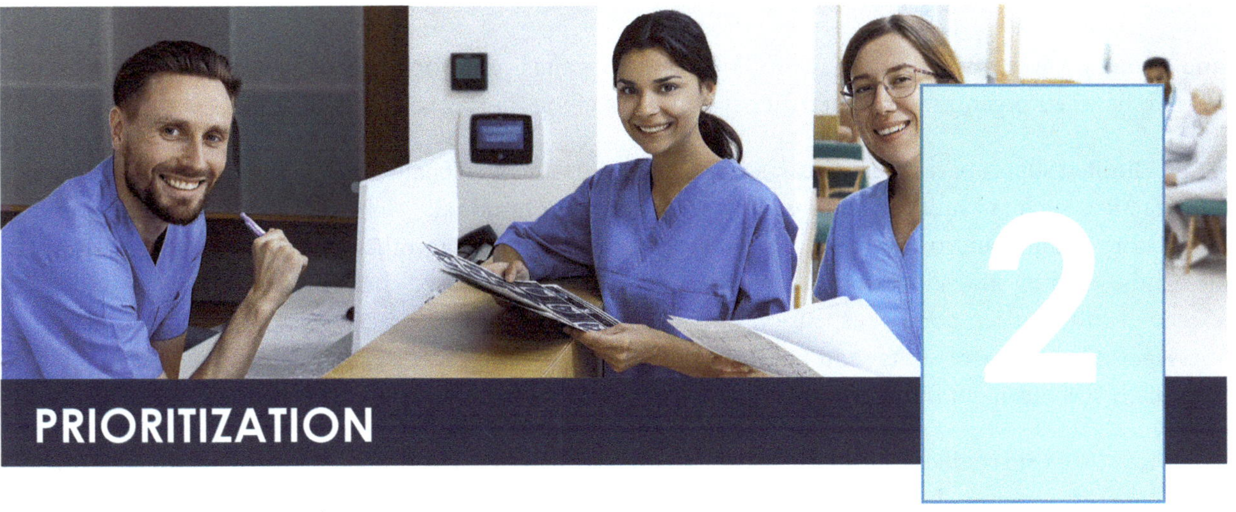

2.1 PRIORITIZATION INTRODUCTION

LEARNING OBJECTIVES

- Prioritize nursing care based on client acuity
- Use principles of time management to organize work
- Analyze effectiveness of time management strategies
- Incorporate clinical judgment to prioritize nursing care
- Apply a framework for prioritization

"So much to do, so little time." This is a common mantra of today's practicing nurse in various health care settings. Whether practicing in acute inpatient care, long-term care, clinics, home care, or other agencies, nurses may feel there is "not enough of them to go around."

The health care system faces a significant challenge in balancing the ever-expanding task of meeting client care needs with scarce nursing resources that has even worsened as a result of the COVID-19 pandemic. Many health care organizations have seen exacerbation in nurse turnover post-pandemic as nurses struggle with increasing stress, burnout, and feeling of uncertainty within the profession.[1] A recent nursing survey done by the American Nurses Foundation found that 60% of nurses reported extremely stressful, violent,

1. Kurtzman, E.T., Ghazal, L.V., Girouard,S., Ma, C., Martin, B., McGee, B.T., Pogue, C.A., Riman, K.A., Root, M.C., Schlak, A.E., Smith, J.M., Stolldorf, D.P., Townley, J.N., Turi, E., Germack, H.L. (2022). Nursing workforce challenges in the postpandemic world. *Journal of Nursing Regulation, 13*(2),49-60. https://doi.org/10.1016/S2155-8256(22)00061-8

and traumatic events as a result of the COVID-19 pandemic.[2] Additionally, a staggering 89% of nurses reported that their organizations experience significant staffing shortages.[3]

With a limited supply of registered nurses, nurse managers are often challenged to implement creative staffing practices such as sending staff to units where they do not normally work (i.e., floating), implementing mandatory staffing and/or overtime, utilizing travel nurses, or using other practices to meet client care demands.[4] Staffing strategies can result in nurses experiencing increased client assignments and workloads, extended shifts, or temporary suspension of paid time off. Nurses may receive a barrage of calls and text messages offering "extra shifts" and bonus pay, and although the extra pay may be welcomed, they often eventually feel burnt out trying to meet the ever-expanding demands of the client-care environment.

A novice nurse who is still learning how to navigate the complex health care environment and provide optimal client care may feel overwhelmed by these conditions. Novice nurses frequently report increased levels of stress and disillusionment as they transition to the reality of the nursing role.[5] How can we address this professional dilemma and enhance the novice nurse's successful role transition to practice? The novice nurse must enter the profession with purposeful tools and strategies to help prioritize tasks and manage time so they can confidently address client care needs, balance role demands, and manage day-to-day nursing activities.

Let's take a closer look at the foundational concepts related to prioritization and time management in the nursing profession.

2.2 TENETS OF PRIORITIZATION

Prioritization

As new nurses begin their career, they look forward to caring for others, promoting health, and saving lives. However, when entering the health care environment, they often discover there are numerous and competing demands for their time and attention. Client care is often interrupted by call lights, rounding physicians, and phone calls from the laboratory department or other interprofessional team members. Even individuals who are strategic and energized in their planning can feel frustrated as their task lists and planned client-care activities build into a long collection of "to dos."

Without utilization of appropriate prioritization strategies, nurses can experience **time scarcity**, a feeling of racing against a clock that is continually working against them. Functioning under the burden of time scarcity can cause feelings of frustration, inadequacy, and eventually burnout. Time scarcity can also impact client safety,

2. Kurtzman, E.T., Ghazal, L.V., Girouard,S., Ma, C., Martin, B., McGee, B.T., Pogue, C.A., Riman, K.A., Root, M.C., Schlak, A.E., Smith, J.M., Stolldorf, D.P., Townley, J.N., Turi, E., Germack, H.L. (2022). Nursing workforce challenges in the postpandemic world. *Journal of Nursing Regulation, 13*(2),49-60. https://doi.org/10.1016/S2155-8256(22)00061-8
3. Kurtzman, E.T., Ghazal, L.V., Girouard,S., Ma, C., Martin, B., McGee, B.T., Pogue, C.A., Riman, K.A., Root, M.C., Schlak, A.E., Smith, J.M., Stolldorf, D.P., Townley, J.N., Turi, E., Germack, H.L. (2022). Nursing workforce challenges in the postpandemic world. *Journal of Nursing Regulation, 13*(2),49-60. https://doi.org/10.1016/S2155-8256(22)00061-8
4. Rochefort, C. M., Abrahamowicz, M., Biron, A., Bourgault, P., Gaboury, I., Haggerty, J., & McCusker, J. (2021). Nurse staffing practices and adverse events in acute care hospitals: The research protocol of a multisite patient-level longitudinal study. *Journal of Advanced Nursing, 77*(3), 1567-1577. https://doi.org/10.1111/jan.14710
5. Hoeve, Y. T., Brouwer, J., Roodbol, P. F., & Kunnen, S. (2018). The importance of contextual, relational and cognitive factors for novice nurses' emotional state and affective commitment to the profession. A multilevel study. *Journal of Advanced Nursing, 74*(9), 2082-2093. https://doi.org/10.1111/jan.13709

resulting in adverse events and increased mortality.[6] Additionally, missed or rushed nursing activities can negatively impact client satisfaction scores that ultimately affect an institution's reimbursement levels.

It is vital for nurses to plan client care and implement their task lists while ensuring that critical interventions are safely implemented first. Identifying priority client problems and implementing priority interventions are skills that require ongoing cultivation as one gains experience in the practice environment.[7] To develop these skills, students must develop an understanding of organizing frameworks and prioritization processes for delineating care needs. These frameworks provide structure and guidance for meeting the multiple and ever-changing demands in the complex health care environment.

Let's consider a clinical scenario in the following box to better understand the implications of prioritization and outcomes.

Scenario A

Imagine you are beginning your shift on a busy medical-surgical unit. You receive a handoff report on four medical-surgical clients from the night shift nurse:

- Client A is a 34-year-old client post-op Day 1 from a total knee replacement who had an uneventful night. It is anticipated that she will be discharged today and needs health teaching for self-care at home.
- Client B is a 67-year-old male admitted with weakness, confusion, and a suspected urinary tract infection. He has been restless and attempting to get out of bed throughout the night. He has a bed alarm in place.
- Client C is a 49-year-old male, post-op Day 1 for a total hip replacement. He has been frequently using his patient-controlled analgesia (PCA) pump and last rated his pain as a "6."
- Client D is a 73-year-old male admitted for pneumonia. He has been hospitalized for three days and receiving intravenous (IV) antibiotics. His next dose is due in an hour. His oxygen requirements have decreased from 4 L/minute of oxygen by nasal cannula to 2 L/minute by nasal cannula.

Based on the handoff report you received, you ask the nursing assistant to check on Client B while you do an initial assessment on Client D. As you are assessing Client D's oxygenation status, you receive a phone call from the laboratory department relating a critical lab value on Client C, indicating his hemoglobin is low. The provider calls and orders a STAT blood transfusion for Client C. Client A rings the call light and states she and her husband have questions about her discharge and are ready to go home. The nursing assistant finds you and reports that Client B got out of bed and experienced a fall during the handoff reports.

It is common for nurses to manage multiple and ever-changing tasks and activities like this scenario, illustrating the importance of self-organization and priority setting. This chapter will further discuss the tools nurses can use for prioritization.

6. Cho, S., Lee, J., You, S. J., Song, K. J., & Hong, K. J. (2020). Nurse staffing, nurses prioritization, missed care, quality of nursing care, and nurse outcomes. *International Journal of Nursing Practice, 26*(1), e12803. https://doi.org/10.1111/ijn.12803

7. Jessee, M. A. (2019). Teaching prioritization: "Who, what, & why?" *Journal of Nursing Education, 58*(5), 302-305. https://doi.org/10.3928/01484834-20190422-10

2.3 TOOLS FOR PRIORITIZING

Prioritization of care for multiple clients while also performing daily nursing tasks can feel overwhelming in today's fast-paced health care system. Because of the rapid and ever-changing conditions of clients and the structure of one's workday, nurses must use organizational frameworks to prioritize actions and interventions. These frameworks can help ease anxiety, enhance personal organization and confidence, and ensure client safety.

Acuity

Acuity and intensity are foundational concepts for prioritizing nursing care and interventions. **Acuity** refers to the level of client care that is required based on the severity of a client's illness or condition. For example, acuity may include characteristics such as unstable vital signs, oxygenation therapy, high-risk IV medications, multiple drainage devices, or uncontrolled pain. A "high-acuity" client requires several nursing interventions and frequent nursing assessments.

Intensity addresses the time needed to complete nursing care and interventions such as providing assistance with activities of daily living (ADLs), performing wound care, or administering several medication passes. For example, a "high-intensity" client generally requires frequent or long periods of psychosocial, educational, or hygiene care from nursing staff members. High-intensity clients may also have increased needs for safety monitoring, familial support, or other needs.[8]

Many health care organizations structure their staffing assignments based on acuity and intensity ratings to help provide equity in staff assignments. Acuity helps to ensure that nursing care is strategically divided among nursing staff. An equitable assignment of clients benefits both the nurse and client by helping to ensure that client care needs do not overwhelm individual staff and safe care is provided.

Organizations use a variety of systems when determining client acuity with rating scales based on nursing care delivery, client stability, and care needs. See an example of a client acuity tool published in the *American Nurse* in Table 2.3.[9] In this example, ratings range from 1 to 4, with a rating of 1 indicating a relatively stable client requiring minimal individualized nursing care and intervention. A rating of 2 reflects a client with a moderate risk who may require more frequent intervention or assessment. A rating of 3 is attributed to a complex client who requires frequent intervention and assessment. This client might also be a new admission or someone who is confused and requires more direct observation. A rating of 4 reflects a high-risk client. For example, this individual may be experiencing frequent changes in vital signs, may require complex interventions such as the administration of blood transfusions, or may be experiencing significant uncontrolled pain. An individual with a rating of 4 requires more direct nursing care and intervention than a client with a rating of 1 or 2.[10]

---

8. Oregon Health Authority. (2024, April 29). *Hospital nurse staffing interpretive guidance on staffing for acuity & intensity.* Public Health Division, Center for Health Protection. https://www.oregon.gov/oha/ph/providerpartnerresources/healthcareprovidersfacilities/healthcarehealthcareregulationqualityimprovement/pages/nursestaffing.aspx

9. Ingram, A., & Powell, J. (2018). Patient acuity tool on a medical surgical unit. *American Nurse.* https://www.myamericannurse.com/patient-acuity-medical-surgical-unit/

10. Kidd, M., Grove, K., Kaiser, M., Swoboda, B., & Taylor, A. (2014). A new patient-acuity tool promotes equitable nurse-patient assignments. *American Nurse Today, 9*(3), 1-4. https://www.myamericannurse.com/a-new-patient-acuity-tool-promotes-equitable-nurse-patient-assignments/

TABLE 2.3. Example of a Client Acuity Tool[11]

	1: Stable Client	2: Moderate-Risk Client	3: Complex Client	4: High-Risk Client
Assessment	• Q8h VS • A & O X 4	• Q4h VS • CIWA < 8	• Q2h VS • Delirium • CIWA > 8	• Unstable VS
Respiratory	• Stable on RA	• O2 < 2L NC	• O2 > 2L NC	• O2 via mask
Cardiac	• VS	• Temp < 98.7 F • Pacemaker/AICD • HR > 130	• Change in BP • Temp > 100.3 F	• Unstable rhythm • Afib
Medications	• PO/IVPB	• TPN, heparin infusion, blood glucose, PICC for blood draws	• CBI • 1 unit blood transfusion • Fluid bolus	• > 1 unit blood transfusion •Chemotherapy
Drainage Devices	• < 2 JP, hemo-vac, neph tube	• Chest to water seal • NG tube	• Chest tube to suction • Drain measured Q2 hrs	• Drain measured Q1 hr • CT > 100 mL/2 hrs
Pain Management	• Pain well-managed with PO or IV meds Q4 hrs	• PCA, nerve block • Nausea/Vomiting	• Q2h pain management	• Uncontrolled pain with multiple pain devices
Admit/Transfer/ Discharge	• Stable transfer, routine discharge	• Discharge to outside facility	• New admission, discharge to hospice	• Complicated post-op
ADLs and Isolation	• Independent	• Assist with ADLs • Two-person assist out of bed • Isolation	• Turns Q2h • Bedrest • Respiratory isolation	• Paraplegic • Total care
Client Score	**Most = 1**	**Two or > = 2**	**Any = 3**	**Any = 4**

Rating scales may vary among institutions, but the principles of the rating system remain the same. Organizations include various client care elements when constructing their staffing plans for each unit. Read more information about staffing models and acuity in the following box.

11. Ingram, A., & Powell, J. (2018). Patient acuity tool on a medical surgical unit. *American Nurse*. https://www.myamericannurse.com/patient-acuity-medical-surgical-unit/

Read more about using a client acuity tool on a medical-surgical unit. Access supplementary digital content in the online book using this QR code.

Staffing Models and Acuity

Organizations that base staffing on acuity systems attempt to evenly staff client assignments according to their acuity ratings. This means that when comparing client assignments across nurses on a unit, similar acuity team scores should be seen with the goal of achieving equitable and safe division of workload across the nursing team. For example, one nurse should not have a total acuity score of 6 for their client assignments while another nurse has a score of 15. If this situation occurred, the variation in scoring reflects a discrepancy in workload balance and would likely be perceived by nursing peers as unfair. Using **acuity-rating staffing models** is helpful to reflect the individualized nursing care required by different clients.

Alternatively, nurse staffing models may be determined by staffing ratio. **Ratio-based staffing models** are more straightforward in nature, where each nurse is assigned care for a set number of clients during their shift. Ratio-based staffing models may be useful for administrators creating budget requests based on the number of staff required for client care, but can lead to an inequitable division of work across the nursing team when client acuity is not considered. Increasingly complex clients require more time and interventions than others, so a blend of both ratio and acuity-based staffing is helpful when determining staffing assignments.[12]

As a practicing nurse, you will be oriented to the elements of acuity ratings within your health care organization, but it is also important to understand how you can use these acuity ratings for your own prioritization and task delineation. Let's consider the Scenario B in the following box to better understand how acuity ratings can be useful for prioritizing nursing care.

12. Welton, J. M. (2017). Measuring patient acuity. *JONA: The Journal of Nursing Administration, 47*(10), 471. https://doi.org/10.1097/nna.0000000000000516

Scenario B

You report to work at 6 a.m. for your nursing shift on a busy medical-surgical unit. Prior to receiving the handoff report from your night shift nursing colleagues, you review the unit staffing grid and see that you have been assigned to four clients to start your day. The clients have the following acuity ratings:

Client A: 45-year-old client with paraplegia admitted for an infected sacral wound, with an acuity rating of 4.

Client B: 87-year-old client with pneumonia with a low-grade fever of 99.7 F and receiving oxygen at 2 L/minute via nasal cannula, with an acuity rating of 2.

Client C: 63-year-old client who is postoperative Day 1 from a right total hip replacement and is receiving pain management via a PCA pump, with an acuity rating of 2.

Client D: 83-year-old client admitted with a UTI who is finishing an IV antibiotic cycle and will be discharged home today, with an acuity rating of 1.

Based on the acuity rating system, your client assignment load receives an overall acuity score of 9. Consider how you might use their acuity ratings to help you prioritize your care. Based on what is known about the clients related to their acuity rating, whom might you identify as your care priority? Although this can feel like a challenging question to answer because of the many unknown elements in the situation using acuity numbers alone, Client A with an acuity rating of 4 would be identified as the care priority requiring assessment early in your shift.

Although acuity can a useful tool for determining care priorities, it is important to recognize the limitations of this tool and consider how other client needs impact prioritization.

Maslow's Hierarchy of Needs

When thinking back to your first nursing or psychology course, you may recall a historical theory of human motivation based on various levels of human needs called Maslow's Hierarchy of Needs. **Maslow's Hierarchy of Needs** reflects foundational human needs with progressive steps moving towards higher levels of achievement. This hierarchy of needs is traditionally represented as a pyramid with the base of the pyramid serving as essential needs that must be addressed before one can progress to another area of need.[13] See Figure 2.1[14] for an illustration of Maslow's Hierarchy of Needs.

13. Maslow, A. H. (1943). A theory of human motivation. *Psychological Review, 50*(4), 370–396. https://doi.org/10.1037/h0054346
14. "Maslow's_hierarchy_of_needs.svg" by J. Finkelstein is licensed under CC BY-SA 3.0

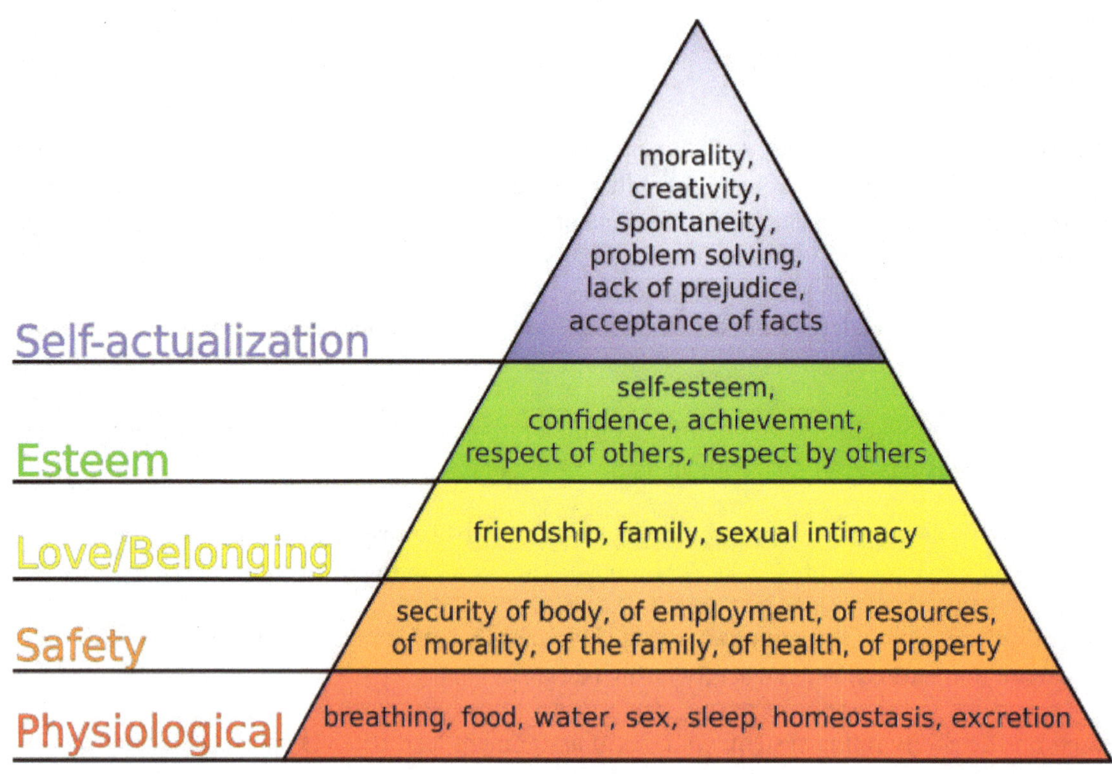

FIGURE 2.1 Maslow's Hierarchy of Needs

Maslow's Hierarchy of Needs places physiological needs as the foundational base of the pyramid.[15] Physiological needs include oxygen, food, water, sex, sleep, homeostasis, and excretion. The second level of Maslow's hierarchy reflects safety needs. Safety needs include elements that keep individuals safe from harm. Examples of safety needs in health care include fall precautions. The third level of Maslow's hierarchy reflects emotional needs such as love and a sense of belonging. These needs are often reflected in an individual's relationships with family members and friends. The top two levels of Maslow's hierarchy include esteem and self-actualization. An example of addressing these needs in a health care setting is helping an individual build self-confidence in performing blood glucose checks that leads to improved self-management of their diabetes.

So how does Maslow's theory impact prioritization? To better understand the application of Maslow's theory to prioritization, consider Scenario C in the following box.

15. Stoyanov, S. (2017). *An analysis of Abraham Maslow's A Theory of Human Motivation* (1st ed.). Routledge. https://doi.org/10.4324/9781912282517

Scenario C

You are an emergency response nurse working at a local shelter in a community that has suffered a devastating hurricane. Many individuals have relocated to the shelter for safety in the aftermath of the hurricane. Much of the community is still without electricity and clean water, and many homes have been destroyed. You approach a young woman who has a laceration on her scalp that is bleeding through her gauze dressing. The woman is weeping as she describes the loss of her home stating, "I have lost everything! I just don't know what I am going to do now. It has been a day since I have had water or anything to drink. I don't know where my sister is, and I can't reach any of my family to find out if they are okay!"

Despite this relatively brief interaction, this woman has shared with you a variety of needs. She has demonstrated a need for food, water, shelter, homeostasis, and family. As the nurse caring for her, it might be challenging to think about where to begin her care. These thoughts could be racing through your mind:

Should I begin to make phone calls to try and find her family? Maybe then she would be able to calm down.

Should I get her on the list for the homeless shelter so she wouldn't have to worry about where she will sleep tonight?

She hasn't eaten in a while; I should probably find her something to eat.

All these needs are important and should be addressed at some point, but Maslow's hierarchy provides guidance on what needs must be addressed first. Use the foundational level of Maslow's pyramid of physiological needs as the top priority for care. The woman is bleeding heavily from a head wound and has had limited fluid intake. As the nurse caring for this client, it is important to immediately intervene to stop the bleeding and restore fluid volume. Stabilizing the client by addressing her physiological needs is required before undertaking additional measures such as contacting her family. Imagine if instead you made phone calls to find the client's family and didn't address the bleeding or dehydration – you might return to a severely hypovolemic client who has deteriorated and may be near death. In this example, prioritizing emotional needs above physiological needs can lead to significant harm to the client.

Although this is a relatively straightforward example, the principles behind the application of Maslow's hierarchy are essential. Addressing physiological needs before progressing toward additional need categories concentrates efforts on the most vital elements to enhance client well-being. Maslow's hierarchy provides the nurse with a helpful framework for identifying and prioritizing critical client care needs.

ABCs

Airway, breathing, and circulation, otherwise known by the mnemonic "ABCs," are another foundational element to assist the nurse in prioritization. Like Maslow's hierarchy, using the ABCs to guide decision-making concentrates on the most critical needs for preserving human life. If a client does not have a patent airway, is unable to breathe, or has inadequate circulation, very little of what else we do matters. The client's **ABCs** are reflected in Maslow's foundational level of physiological needs and direct critical nursing actions and timely interventions. Let's consider Scenario D in the following box regarding prioritization using the ABCs and the physiological base of Maslow's hierarchy.

Scenario D

You are a nurse on a busy cardiac floor charting your morning assessments on a computer at the nurses' station. Down the hall from where you are charting, two of your assigned clients are resting comfortably in Room 504 and Room 506. Suddenly, both call lights ring from the rooms, and you answer them via the intercom at the nurses' station.

Room 504 has an 87-year-old male who has been admitted with heart failure, weakness, and confusion. He has a bed alarm for safety and has been ringing his call bell for assistance appropriately throughout the shift. He requires assistance to get out of bed to use the bathroom. He received his morning medications, which included a diuretic about 30 minutes previously, and now reports significant urge to void and needs assistance to the bathroom.

Room 506 has a 47-year-old woman who was hospitalized with new onset atrial fibrillation with rapid ventricular response. The client underwent a cardioversion procedure yesterday that resulted in successful conversion of her heart back into normal sinus rhythm. She is reporting via the intercom that her "heart feels like it is doing that fluttering thing again" and she is having chest pain with breathlessness.

Based upon these two client scenarios, it might be difficult to determine whom you should see first. Both clients are demonstrating needs in the foundational physiological level of Maslow's hierarchy and require assistance. To prioritize between these clients' physiological needs, the nurse can apply the principles of the ABCs to determine intervention. The client in Room 506 reports both breathing and circulation issues, warning indicators that action is needed immediately. Although the client in Room 504 also has an urgent physiological elimination need, it does not overtake the critical one experienced by the client in Room 506. The nurse should immediately assess the client in Room 506 while also calling for assistance from a team member to assist the client in Room 504.

CURE

Prioritizing what should be done and when it can be done can be a challenging task when several clients all have physiological needs. Recently, there has been professional acknowledgement of the cognitive challenge for novice nurses in differentiating physiological needs. To expand on the principles of prioritizing using the ABCs, the CURE hierarchy has been introduced to help novice nurses better understand how to manage competing client needs. The CURE hierarchy uses the acronym "CURE" to guide prioritization based on identifying the differences among Critical needs, Urgent needs, Routine needs, and Extras.[16]

"Critical" client needs require immediate action. Examples of critical needs align with the ABCs and Maslow's physiological needs, such as symptoms of respiratory distress, chest pain, and airway compromise. No matter the complexity of their shift, nurses can be assured that addressing clients' critical needs is the correct prioritization of their time and energies.

After critical client care needs have been addressed, nurses can then address "urgent" needs. Urgent needs are characterized as needs that cause client discomfort or place the client at a significant safety risk.[17]

The third part of the CURE hierarchy reflects "routine" client needs. Routine client needs can also be characterized as "typical daily nursing care" because the majority of a standard nursing shift is spent addressing routine client needs. Examples of routine daily nursing care include actions such as administering medication and performing physical assessments.[18] Although a nurse's typical shift in a hospital setting includes these routine client needs, they do not supersede critical or urgent client needs.

The final component of the CURE hierarchy is known as "extras." Extras refer to activities performed in the care setting to facilitate client comfort but are not essential.[19] Examples of extra activities include providing a massage for comfort or washing a client's hair. If a nurse has sufficient time to perform extra activities, they contribute to a client's feeling of satisfaction regarding their care, but these activities are not essential to achieve client outcomes.

Let's apply the CURE mnemonic to client care in the following box.

> If we return to Scenario D regarding clients in Room 504 and 506, we can see the client in Room 504 is having urgent needs. He is experiencing a physiological need to urgently use the restroom and may also have safety concerns if he does not receive assistance and attempts to get up on his own because of weakness. He is on a bed alarm, which reflects safety considerations related to his potential to get out of bed without assistance. Despite these urgent indicators, the client in Room 506 is experiencing a critical need and takes priority. Recall that critical needs require immediate nursing action to prevent client deterioration. The client in Room 506 with a rapid, fluttering heartbeat and shortness of breath has a critical need because without prompt assessment and intervention, their condition could rapidly decline and become fatal.

16. Kohtz, C., Gowda, C., & Guede, P. (2017). Cognitive stacking: Strategies for the busy RN. *Nursing, 47*(1), 18-20. https://doi.org/10.1097/01.nurse.0000510758.31326.92
17. Kohtz, C., Gowda, C., & Guede, P. (2017). Cognitive stacking: Strategies for the busy RN. *Nursing, 47*(1), 18-20. https://doi.org/10.1097/01.nurse.0000510758.31326.92
18. Kohtz, C., Gowda, C., & Guede, P. (2017). Cognitive stacking: Strategies for the busy RN. *Nursing, 47*(1), 18-20. https://doi.org/10.1097/01.nurse.0000510758.31326.92
19. Kohtz, C., Gowda, C., & Guede, P. (2017). Cognitive stacking: Strategies for the busy RN. *Nursing, 47*(1), 18-20. https://doi.org/10.1097/01.nurse.0000510758.31326.92

DATA CUES

In addition to using the identified frameworks and tools to assist with priority setting, nurses must also look at their clients' data cues to help them identify care priorities. **Data cues** are pieces of significant clinical information that direct the nurse toward a potential clinical concern or a change in condition. For example, have the client's vital signs worsened over the last few hours? Is there a new laboratory result that is concerning? Data cues are used in conjunction with prioritization frameworks to help the nurse holistically understand the client's current status and where nursing interventions should be directed. Common categories of data clues include acute versus chronic conditions, actual versus potential problems, unexpected versus expected conditions, information obtained from the review of a client's chart, and diagnostic information.

Acute Versus Chronic Conditions

A common data cue that nurses use to prioritize care is considering if a condition or symptom is acute or chronic. **Acute conditions** have a sudden and severe onset. These conditions occur due to a sudden illness or injury, and the body often has a significant response as it attempts to adapt. **Chronic conditions** have a slow onset and may gradually worsen over time. The difference between an acute versus a chronic condition relates to the body's adaptation response. Individuals with chronic conditions often experience less symptom exacerbation because their body has had time to adjust to the illness or injury. Let's consider an example of two clients admitted to the medical-surgical unit complaining of pain in Scenario E in the following box.

Scenario E

As part of your client assignment on a medical-surgical unit, you are caring for two clients who both ring the call light and report pain at the start of the shift. Client A was recently admitted with acute appendicitis, and Client B was admitted for observation due to weakness. Not knowing any additional details about the clients' conditions or current symptoms, which client would receive priority in your assessment? Based on using the data cue of acute versus chronic conditions, Client A with a diagnosis of acute appendicitis would receive top priority for assessment over a client with chronic pain due to osteoarthritis. Clients experiencing acute pain require immediate nursing assessment and intervention because it can indicate a change in condition. Acute pain also elicits physiological effects related to the stress response, such as elevated heart rate, blood pressure, and respiratory rate, and should be addressed quickly.

Actual Versus Potential Problems

Nursing diagnoses and the nursing care plan have significant roles in directing prioritization when interpreting assessment data cues. **Actual problems** refer to a clinical problem that is actively occurring with the client. A **risk problem** indicates the client may potentially experience a problem but they do not have current signs or symptoms of the problem actively occurring.

Consider an example of prioritizing actual and potential problems in Scenario F in the following box.

Scenario F

A 74-year-old woman with a previous history of chronic obstructive pulmonary disease (COPD) is admitted to the hospital for pneumonia. She has generalized weakness, a weak cough, and crackles in the bases of her lungs. She is receiving IV antibiotics, fluids, and oxygen therapy. The client can sit at the side of the bed and ambulate with the assistance of staff, although she requires significant encouragement to ambulate.

Nursing diagnoses are established for this client as part of the care planning process. One nursing diagnosis for this client is *Ineffective Airway Clearance.* This nursing diagnosis is an actual problem because the client is currently exhibiting signs of poor airway clearance with an ineffective cough and crackles in the lungs. Nursing interventions related to this diagnosis include coughing and deep breathing, administering nebulizer treatment, and evaluating the effectiveness of oxygen therapy. The client also has the nursing diagnosis *Risk for Skin Breakdown* based on her weakness and lack of motivation to ambulate. Nursing interventions related to this diagnosis include repositioning every two hours and assisting with ambulation twice daily.

The established nursing diagnoses provide cues for prioritizing care. For example, if the nurse enters the client's room and discovers the client is experiencing increased shortness of breath, nursing interventions to improve the client's respiratory status receive top priority before attempting to get the client to ambulate.

Although there may be times when risk problems may supersede actual problems, looking to the "actual" nursing problems can provide clues to assist with prioritization.

Unexpected Versus Expected Conditions

In a similar manner to using acute versus chronic conditions as a cue for prioritization, it is also important to consider if a client's signs and symptoms are "expected" or "unexpected" based on their overall condition. **Unexpected conditions** are findings that are not likely to occur in the normal progression of an illness, disease, or injury. **Expected conditions** are findings that are likely to occur or are anticipated in the course of an illness, disease, or injury. Unexpected findings often require immediate action by the nurse.

Let's apply this tool to the two clients previously discussed in Scenario E. As you recall, both Client A (with acute appendicitis) and Client B (with weakness and diagnosed with osteoarthritis) are reporting pain. Acute pain typically receives priority over chronic pain. But what if both clients are also reporting nausea and have an elevated temperature? Although these symptoms must be addressed in both clients, they are "expected" symptoms with acute appendicitis (and typically addressed in the treatment plan) but are "unexpected" for the client with osteoarthritis. Critical thinking alerts you to the unexpected nature of these symptoms in Client B, so they receive priority for assessment and nursing interventions.

Handoff Report/Chart Review

Additional data cues that are helpful in guiding prioritization come from information obtained during a handoff nursing report and review of the client chart. These data cues can be used to establish a client's baseline status and prioritize new clinical concerns based on abnormal assessment findings. Let's consider Scenario G in the following box based on cues from a handoff report and how it might be used to help prioritize nursing care.

Scenario G

Imagine you are receiving the following handoff report from the night shift nurse for a client admitted to the medical-surgical unit with pneumonia:

> *At the beginning of my shift, the client was on room air with an oxygen saturation of 93%. She had slight crackles in both bases of her posterior lungs. At 0530, the client rang the call light to go to the bathroom. As I escorted her to the bathroom, she appeared slightly short of breath. Upon returning the client to bed, I rechecked her vital signs and found her oxygen saturation at 88% on room air and respiratory rate of 20. I listened to her lung sounds and noticed more persistent crackles and coarseness than at bedtime. I placed the client on 2 L/minute of oxygen via nasal cannula. Within five minutes, her oxygen saturation increased to 92%, and she reported increased ease in respiration.*

Based on the handoff report, the night shift nurse provided substantial clinical evidence that the client may be experiencing a change in condition. Although these changes could be attributed to lack of lung expansion that occurred while the client was sleeping, there is enough information to indicate to the oncoming nurse that follow-up assessment and interventions should be prioritized for this client because of potentially worsening respiratory status. In this manner, identifying data cues from a handoff report can assist with prioritization.

Now imagine the night shift nurse had not reported this information during the handoff report. Is there another method for identifying potential changes in client condition? Many nurses develop a habit of reviewing their clients' charts at the start of every shift to identify trends and "baselines" in client condition. For example, a chart review reveals a client's heart rate on admission was 105 beats per minute. If the client continues to have a heart rate in the low 100s, the nurse is not likely to be concerned if today's vital signs reveal a heart rate in the low 100s. Conversely, if a client's heart rate on admission was in the 60s and has remained in the 60s throughout their hospitalization, but it is now in the 100s, this finding is an important cue requiring prioritized assessment and intervention.

Diagnostic Information

Diagnostic results are also important when prioritizing care. In fact, the National Patient Safety Goals from The Joint Commission include prompt reporting of important test results. New abnormal laboratory results are typically flagged in a client's chart or are reported directly by phone to the nurse by the laboratory as they become available. Newly reported abnormal results, such as elevated blood levels or changes on a chest

X-ray, may indicate a client's change in condition and require additional interventions. For example, consider Scenario H in which you are the nurse providing care for five medical-surgical clients.

Scenario H

You completed morning assessments on your assigned five clients. Client A previously underwent a total right knee replacement and will be discharged home today. You are about to enter Client A's room to begin discharge teaching when you receive a phone call from the laboratory department, reporting a critical hemoglobin of 6.9 gm/dL on Client B. Rather than enter Client A's room to perform discharge teaching, you immediately reprioritize your care. You call the primary provider to report Client B's critical hemoglobin level and determine if additional intervention, such as a blood transfusion, is required.

Prioritization Principles & Staffing Considerations[20]

With the complexity of different staffing variables in health care settings, it can be challenging to identify a method and solution that will offer a resolution to every challenge. The American Nurses Association has identified five critical principles that should be considered for nurse staffing. These principles are as follows:

1. **Health Care Consumer:** Nurse staffing decisions are influenced by the specific number and needs of the health care consumer. The health care consumer includes not only the client, but also families, groups, and populations served. Staffing guidelines must always consider the client safety indicators and clinical and operational outcomes that are specific to a practice setting. What is appropriate for the consumer in one setting, may be quite different in another. Additionally, it is important to ensure that there is resource allocation for care coordination and health education in each setting.
2. **Interprofessional Teams:** As organizations identify what constitutes appropriate staffing in various settings, they must also consider the appropriate credentials and qualifications of the nursing staff within a specific setting. This involves utilizing an interprofessional care team that allows each individual to practice to the full extent of their educational, training, and scope of practice as defined by their state Nurse Practice Act, and licensure. Staffing plans must include an appropriate skill mix and acknowledge the impact of more experienced nurses to help serve in mentoring and precepting roles.

20. American Nurses Association. (2024). *Principles for nurse staffing.* ANA. https://www.nursingworld.org/practice-policy/nurse-staffing/staffing-principles/

3. **Workplace culture:** Staffing considerations must also account for the importance of balance between costs associated with best practice and the optimization of care outcomes. Health care leaders and organizations must strive to ensure a balance between quality, safety, and health care cost. Organizations are responsible for creating work environments, which develop policies allowing for nurses to practice to the full extent of their licensure in accordance with their documented competence. Leaders must foster a culture of trust, collaboration, and respect among all members of the health care team, which will create environments that engage and retain health care staff.
4. **Practice environment:** Staffing structures must be founded in a culture of safety where appropriate staffing is integral to achieve client safety and quality goals. An optimal practice environment encourages nurses to report unsafe conditions or poor staffing that may impact safe care. Organizations should ensure that nurses have autonomy in reporting any concerns and may do so without threat of retaliation. The ANA has also taken the position to state that mandatory overtime is an unacceptable solution to achieve appropriate staffing. Organizations must ensure that they have clear policies delineating length of shifts, meal breaks, and rest period to help ensure safety in client care.
5. **Evaluation:** Staffing plans should be consistently evaluated and changed based upon evidence and client outcomes. Environmental factors and issues such as work-related illness, injury, and turnover are important elements of determining the success of need for modification within a staffing plan.[21]

2.4 CRITICAL THINKING AND CLINICAL REASONING

Prioritization of client care should be grounded in critical thinking rather than just a checklist of items to be done. **Critical thinking** is a broad term used in nursing that includes "reasoning about clinical issues such as teamwork, collaboration, and streamlining workflow."[22] Certainly, there are many actions that nurses must complete during their shift, but nursing requires adaptation and flexibility to meet emerging client needs. It can be challenging for a novice nurse to change their mindset regarding their established "plan" for the day, but the sooner a nurse recognizes prioritization is dictated by their clients' needs, the less frustration the nurse might experience. Prioritization strategies include collection of information and utilization of clinical reasoning to determine the best course of action. **Clinical reasoning** is defined as, "A complex cognitive process that uses formal and informal thinking strategies to gather and analyze client information, evaluate the significance of this information, and weigh alternative actions."[23] Clinical reasoning is fostered within nurses when they are challenged to integrate data in various contexts. The clinical reasoning cycle begins when nurses first consider a client situation and progress to collecting cues and information. As nurses pro-

21. American Nurses Association. (2024). *Principles for nurse staffing.* ANA. https://www.nursingworld.org/practice-policy/nurse-staffing/staffing-principles/
22. Klenke-Borgmann, L., Cantrell, M. A., & Mariani, B. (2020). Nurse educator's guide to clinical judgment: A review of conceptualization, measurement, and development. *Nursing Education Perspectives, 41*(4), 215-221. https://doi.org/10.1097/01.nep.0000000000000669
23. Klenke-Borgmann, L., Cantrell, M. A., & Mariani, B. (2020). Nurse educator's guide to clinical judgment: A review of conceptualization, measurement, and development. *Nursing Education Perspectives, 41*(4), 215-221. https://doi.org/10.1097/01.nep.0000000000000669

cess the information, they begin to identify problems and establish realistic goals. They then take appropriate actions and evaluate outcomes. Finally, they reflect upon the process and the learning that has occurred. The reflection piece is critical for solidifying or changing future actions and developing knowledge.

When nurses use critical thinking and clinical reasoning skills, they set forth on a purposeful course of intervention to best meet client-care needs. Rather than focusing on one's own priorities, nurses utilizing critical thinking and reasoning skills recognize their actions must be responsive to their clients. For example, a nurse using critical thinking skills understands that scheduled morning medications for their clients may be late if one of the clients on their care team suddenly develops chest pain. Many actions may be added or removed from planned activities throughout the shift based on what is occurring holistically on the client-care team.

Additionally, in today's complex health care environment, it is important for the novice nurse to recognize the realities of the current health care environment. Clients have become increasingly complex in their health care needs, and organizations are often challenged to meet these care needs with limited staffing resources. It can become easy to slip into the mindset of disenchantment with the nursing profession when first assuming the reality of client-care assignments as a novice nurse. The workload of a nurse in practice often looks and feels quite different than that experienced as a nursing student. As a nursing student, there may have been time for lengthy conversations with clients and their family members, ample time to chart, and opportunities to offer personal cares, such as a massage or hair wash. Unfortunately, in the time-constrained realities of today's health care environment, novice nurses should recognize that even though these "extra" tasks are not always possible, they can still provide quality, safe client care using the "CURE" prioritization framework. Rather than feeling frustrated about "extras" that cannot be accomplished in time-constrained environments, it is vital to use prioritization strategies to ensure appropriate actions are taken to complete what must be done. With increased clinical experience, a novice nurse typically becomes more comfortable with prioritizing and reprioritizing care.

2.5 TIME MANAGEMENT

Time management is not an unfamiliar concept to nursing students because many students are balancing time demands related to work, family, and school obligations. To determine where time should be allocated, prioritization processes emerge. Although the prioritization frameworks of nursing may be different than those used as a student, the concept of prioritization remains the same. Despite the context, prioritization is essentially using a structure to organize tasks to ensure the most critical tasks are completed first and then identify what to move onto next. To truly maximize time management, in addition to prioritization, individuals should be organized, strive for accuracy, minimize waste, mobilize resources, and delegate when appropriate.

Time management is one of the greatest challenges that nurses face in their busy workday. As novice nurses develop their practice, it is important to identify organizational strategies to ensure priority tasks are completed and time is optimized. Each nurse develops a personal process for organizing information and structuring the timing of their assessments, documentation, medication administration, interventions, and client education. However, one must always remember that this process and structure must be flexible because in a moment's time, a client's condition can change, requiring a reprioritization of care. An organizational tool is important to guide a nurse's daily task progression. Organizational tools may be developed individually by the nurse or may be recommended by the organization. Tools can be rudimentary in nature, such as a simple time column format outlining care activities planned throughout the shift, or more complex and integrated within an organization's electronic medical record. No matter the format, an organizational tool is helpful to provide structure and guide progression toward task achievement.

See examples of organizational tools that can be helpful for structuring nursing task progression. These tools can be modified to align with individual nursing preference, shift, unit needs, etc.

- Organizational Tool Sample 1
- Organizational Tool Sample 2
- Organizational Tool Sample 3
- Organizational Tool Sample 4

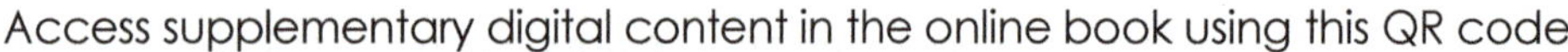

Access supplementary digital content in the online book using this QR code.

In addition to using an organizational tool, novice nurses should utilize other time management strategies to optimize their time. For example, assessments can start during bedside handoff report, such as what fluids and medications are running and what will need to be replaced soon. Take a moment after handoff reports to prioritize which clients you will see first during your shift. Other strategies such as grouping tasks, gathering appropriate equipment prior to initiating nursing procedures, and gathering assessment information while performing tasks are helpful in minimizing redundancy and increasing efficiency. For example, observe an experienced nurse providing care and note the efficient processes they use. They may conduct an assessment, bring in morning medications, flush an IV line, collect a morning blood glucose level, and provide health teaching about medications all during one client encounter. Efficiency becomes especially important if the client has transmission-based precautions and the time spent donning and doffing PPE are considered. The realities of the time-constrained health care environments often necessitate clustering tasks to ensure that all client-care tasks are completed. Furthermore, nurses who do not manage their time effectively may inadvertently place their clients at risk as a result of delayed care.[24] Effective time management benefits both the client and the nursing staff.

Time estimation is an additional helpful strategy to facilitate time management. **Time estimation** involves the review of planned tasks for the day and allocating time estimated to complete the task. Time estimation is especially helpful for novice nurses as they begin to structure and prioritize their shift based on the list of tasks that are required.[25] For example, estimating the time it will take to perform an assessment and administer morning medications to one client allows the nurse to better plan when to complete the dressing change on another client. Without using time estimation, the nurse may attempt to group all care tasks with the morning assessments and not leave themselves enough time to administer morning medications within the desired administration time window. Additionally, working in a time-constrained environment without

24. Nayak, S. G. (2018). Time management in nursing –hour of need. *International Journal of Caring Sciences, 11*(3), 1997-2000. http://www.internationaljournalofcaringsciences.org/docs/72_nayak_special_11_3_2.pdf
25. Nayak, S. G. (2018). Time management in nursing–Hour of need. *International Journal of Caring Sciences, 11*(3), 1997-2000. http://www.internationaljournalofcaringsciences.org/docs/72_nayak_special_11_3_2.pdf

using time estimation strategies increases the likelihood of performing tasks "in a rush" and subsequently increasing the potential for error.

Who's On My Team?

One of the most critical strategies to enhance time management is to mobilize the resources of the nursing team. The nursing care team includes advanced practice registered nurses (APRN), registered nurses (RN), licensed practical/vocational nurses (LPN/VN), and unlicensed assistive personnel (UAP). UAP include, but are not limited to, certified nursing assistants or aides (CNA), patient-care technicians (PCT), certified medical assistants (CMA), certified medication aides, and home health aides.[26] Each care environment may have a blend of staff, and it is important to understand the legalities associated with the scope and role of each member and what can be safely and appropriately delegated to other members of the team. For example, assistive personnel may be able to assist with ambulating a client in the hallway, but they would not be able to help administer morning medications. Dividing tasks appropriately among nursing team members can help ensure that the required tasks are completed and individual energies are best allocated to meet client needs.

The nursing care team and requirements around the process of delegation are explored in detail in the "Delegation and Supervision" chapter.

2.6 SPOTLIGHT APPLICATION

Sam is a novice nurse who is reporting to work for his 0600 shift on the medical telemetry/progressive care floor. He is waiting to receive handoff report from the night shift nurse for his assigned clients. The information that he has received thus far regarding his client assignment includes the following:

- **Room 501:** 64-year-old client admitted last night with heart failure exacerbation. Client received furosemide 80mg IV push at 2000 with 1600 mL urine output. He is receiving oxygen via nasal cannula at 2L/minute. According to the night shift aide, he has been resting comfortably overnight.
- **Room 507:** 74-year-old client admitted yesterday for possible cardioversion due to new onset of atrial fibrillation with rapid ventricular response and is scheduled for transesophageal echocardiogram and possible cardioversion at 1000.
- **Room 512:** 82-year-old client who is scheduled for coronary artery bypass graft (CABG) surgery today at 0700 and is receiving an insulin infusion.
- **Room 536:** 72-year-old client who had a negative heart catheterization yesterday but experienced a groin bleed; plans for discharge this morning.

Based on the limited information Sam has thus far, he begins to prioritize his activities for the morning. With what is known thus far regarding his client assignment, whom might Sam plan to see first and why? What principles of prioritization might be applied?

26. American Nurses Association and NCSBN. (2019). *National guidelines for nursing delegation.* https://www.ncsbn.org/NGND-PosPaper_06.pdf

Although Sam would benefit from hearing a full report on his clients and reviewing the clients' charts, he can already begin to engage in strategies for prioritization. Based on the information that has been shared thus far, Sam determines that none of the clients assigned to him are experiencing critical or urgent needs. All the clients' basic physiological needs are being met, but many have actual clinical concerns. Based on the time constraint with scheduled surgery and the insulin infusion for the client in Room 512, this client should take priority in Sam's assessments. It is important for Sam to ensure that this client's pre-op checklist is complete, and he is stable with the infusion prior to transferring him for surgery. Although Sam may later receive information that alters this priority setting, based on the information he has thus far, he has utilized prioritization principles to make an informed decision.

2.7 LEARNING ACTIVITIES

Learning Activities

(Answers to "Learning Activities" can be found in the "Answer Key" at the end of the book. Answers to interactive activities are provided as immediate feedback.)

1. The nurse is conducting an assessment on a 70-year-old male client who was admitted with atrial fibrillation. The client has a history of hypertension and Stage 2 chronic kidney disease. The nurse begins the head-to-toe assessment and notes the client is having difficulty breathing and is complaining about chest discomfort. The client states, "It feels as if my heart is going to pound out of my chest and I feel dizzy." The nurse begins the head-to-toe assessment and documents the findings. Client assessment findings are presented in the table below. Select the assessment findings requiring immediate follow-up by the nurse.

Temperature	98.9 °F (37.2°C)
Heart Rate	182 beats/min
Respirations	36 breaths/min
Blood Pressure	152/90 mm Hg
Oxygen Saturation	88% on room air
Capillary Refill Time	>3
Pain	9/10 chest discomfort
Physical Assessment Findings	
Glasgow Coma Scale Score	14
Level of Consciousness	Alert
Heart Sounds	Irregularly regular
Lung Sounds	Clear bilaterally anterior/posterior
Pulses-Radial	Rapid/bounding

Pulses-Pedal	Weak
Bowel Sounds	Present and active x 4
Edema	Trace bilateral lower extremities
Skin	Cool, clammy

2. The following nursing actions may or may not be required at this time based on the assessment findings. Indicate whether the actions are "Indicated" (i.e., appropriate or necessary), "Contraindicated" (i.e., could be harmful), or "Nonessential" (i.e., makes no difference or are not necessary).

Nursing Action	Indicated	Contraindicated	Nonessential
Apply oxygen at 2 liters per nasal cannula.			
Call imaging for a STAT lung CT.			
Perform the National Institutes of Health (NIH) Stroke Scale Neurologic Exam.			
Obtain a comprehensive metabolic panel (CMP).			
Obtain a STAT EKG.			
Raise the head-of-bed to less than 10 degrees.			
Establish patent IV access.			
Administer potassium 20 mEq IV push STAT.			

3. The CURE hierarchy has been introduced to help novice nurses better understand how to manage competing client needs. The CURE hierarchy uses the acronym "CURE" to help guide prioritization based on identifying the differences among **C**ritical needs, **U**rgent needs, **R**outine needs, and **E**xtras.

   You are the nurse caring for the clients in the following table. For each client, indicate if this is a "critical," "urgent," "routine," or "extra" need.

	Critical	Urgent	Routine	Extra
Client exhibits new left-sided facial droop				
Client reports 9/10 acute pain and requests PRN pain medication				

Client with BP 120/80 and regular heart rate of 68 has scheduled dose of oral amlodipine				
Client with insomnia requests a back rub before bedtime				
Client has a scheduled dressing change for a pressure ulcer on their coccyx				
Client is exhibiting new shortness of breath and altered mental status				
Client with fall risk precautions ringing call light for assistance to the restroom for a bowel movement				

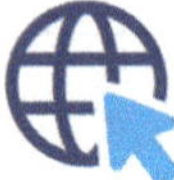

Interactive learning activities have been excluded from the print version of the text. Access free online learning activities in the online book using this QR code.

2.8 GLOSSARY

ABCs: Airway, breathing, and circulation.

Actual problems: Nursing problems currently occurring with the client.

Acuity: The level of client care that is required based on the severity of a client's illness or condition.

Acuity-rating staffing models: A staffing model used to make client assignments that reflects the individualized nursing care required for different types of clients.

Acute conditions: Conditions having a sudden onset.

Chronic conditions: Conditions that have a slow onset and may gradually worsen over time.

Clinical reasoning: "A complex cognitive process that uses formal and informal thinking strategies to gather and analyze client information, evaluate the significance of this information, and weigh alternative actions."[27]

Critical thinking: A broad term used in nursing that includes "reasoning about clinical issues such as teamwork, collaboration, and streamlining workflow."[28]

CURE hierarchy: A strategy for prioritization based on identifying "critical" needs, "urgent" needs, "routine" needs, and "extras."

Data cues: Pieces of significant clinical information that direct the nurse toward a potential clinical concern or a change in condition.

Expected conditions: Conditions that are likely to occur or anticipated in the course of an illness, disease, or injury.

Maslow's Hierarchy of Needs: Prioritization strategies often reflect the foundational elements of physiological needs and safety and progress toward higher levels.

Ratio-based staffing models: A staffing model used to make client assignments in terms of one nurse caring for a set number of clients.

Risk problem: A nursing problem that reflects that a client may experience a problem but does not currently have signs reflecting the problem is actively occurring.

Time estimation: A prioritization strategy, including the review of planned tasks and allocation of time believed to be required to complete each task.

Time scarcity: A feeling of racing against a clock that is continually working against you.

Unexpected conditions: Conditions that are not likely to occur in the normal progression of an illness, disease, or injury.

27. Klenke-Borgmann, L., Cantrell, M. A., & Mariani, B. (2020). Nurse educator's guide to clinical judgment: A review of conceptualization, measurement, and development. *Nursing Education Perspectives, 41*(4), 215-221. https://doi.org/10.1097/01.nep.0000000000000669

28. Klenke-Borgmann, L., Cantrell, M. A., & Mariani, B. (2020). Nurse educator's guide to clinical judgment: A review of conceptualization, measurement, and development. *Nursing Education Perspectives, 41*(4), 215-221. https://doi.org/10.1097/01.nep.0000000000000669

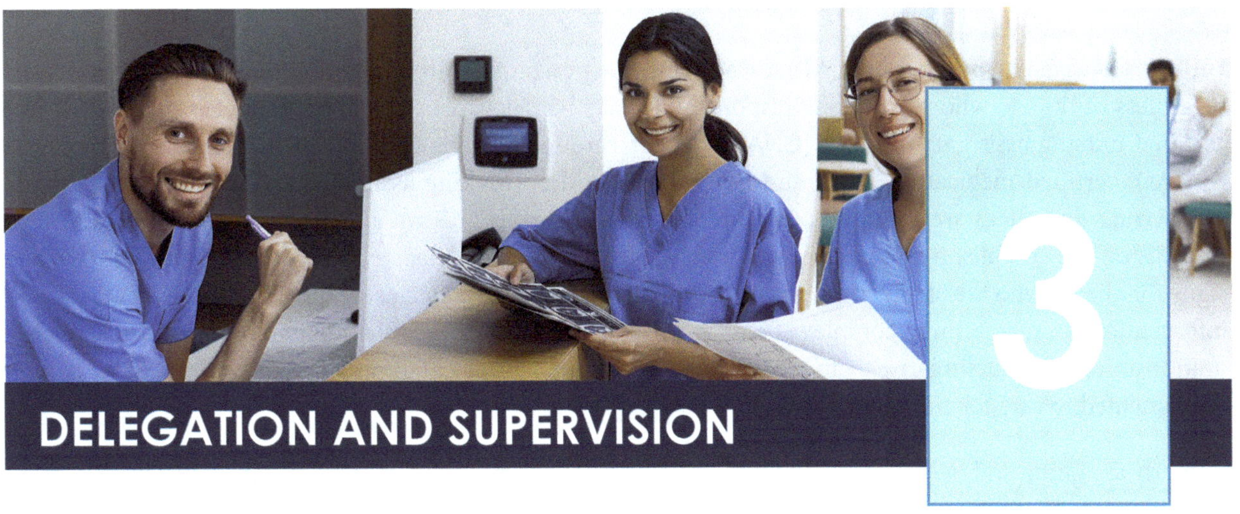

3.1 DELEGATION & SUPERVISION INTRODUCTION

LEARNING OBJECTIVES

- Explain principles of delegation
- Evaluate the criteria used for delegation
- Apply effective communication techniques when delegating care
- Determine specific barriers to delegation
- Evaluate team members' performance based on delegation and supervision principles
- Incorporate principles of supervision and evaluation in the delegation process
- Identify scope of practice of the RN, LPN/VN, and unlicensed assistive personnel roles
- Identify tasks that can and cannot be delegated to members of the nursing team

As health care technology continues to advance, clients require increasingly complex nursing care, and as staffing becomes more challenging, health care agencies respond with an evolving variety of nursing and assistive personnel roles and responsibilities to meet these demands. As an RN, you are on the front lines caring for ill or injured clients and their families, advocating for clients' rights, creating nursing care plans, educating clients on how to self-manage their health, and providing leadership throughout the complex health care system. Delivering safe, effective, quality client care requires the RN to coordinate care by the nursing team as tasks are assigned, delegated, and supervised. **Nursing team members** include advanced practice registered nurses (APRN), registered nurses (RN), licensed practical/vocational nurses (LPN/VN), and unlicensed assistive personnel (UAP).[1]

1. American Nurses Association and NCSBN. (2019). *National guidelines for nursing delegation.* https://www.ncsbn.org/public-files/NGND-PosPaper_06.pdf

Unlicensed assistive personnel (UAP) are any assistive personnel trained to function in a supportive role, regardless of title, to whom a nursing responsibility may be delegated. This includes, but is not limited to, certified nursing assistants or aides (CNAs), patient-care technicians (PCTs), certified medical assistants (CMAs), certified medication aides, and home health aides.[2] Making assignments, delegating tasks, and supervising delegatees are essential components of the RN role and can also provide the RN more time to focus on the complex needs of clients. For example, an RN may delegate to UAP the attainment of vital signs for clients who are stable, thus providing the nurse more time to closely monitor the effectiveness of interventions in maintaining complex clients' hemodynamics, thermoregulation, and oxygenation. Collaboration among the nursing care team members allows for the delivery of optimal care as various skill sets are implemented to care for the client.

Properly assigning and delegating tasks to nursing team members can promote efficient client care. However, inappropriate assignments or delegation can compromise client safety and produce unsatisfactory client outcomes that may result in legal issues. How does the RN know what tasks can be assigned or delegated to nursing team members and assistive personnel? What steps should the RN follow when determining if care can be delegated? After assignments and delegations are established, what is the role and responsibility of the RN in supervising client care? This chapter will explore and define the fundamental concepts involved in assigning, delegating, and supervising client care according to the most recent joint national delegation guidelines published by the National Council of State Boards of Nursing (NCSBN) and the American Nurses Association (ANA).[3]

3.2 COMMUNICATION

Effective communication is a vital component of proper assignment, delegation, and supervision. It is also one of the Standards of Professional Performance established by the American Nurses Association (ANA).[4] Research has identified that new graduate nurses are more susceptible to stress and isolation within their job roles due to poor communication and teamwork within the interdisciplinary team.[5] Strong communication skills foster a supportive work environment and colleagial relationships that benefit both clients and nursing staff.

Consider the fundamentals of good communication practices. Effective communication requires each interaction to include a sender of the message, a clear and concise message, and a receiver who can decode and interpret that message. The receiver also provides a feedback message back to the sender in response to the received message. See Figure 3.1[6] for an image of effective communication between a sender and receiver. This feedback message is referred to as **closed-loop communication** in health care settings. Closed-loop communication enables the person giving the instructions to hear what they said reflected back and to

2. American Nurses Association and NCSBN. (2019). *National guidelines for nursing delegation.* https://www.ncsbn.org/NGND-PosPaper_06.pdf

3. American Nurses Association and NCSBN. (2019). *National guidelines for nursing delegation.* https://www.ncsbn.org/NGND-PosPaper_06.pdf

4. American Nurses Association. (2021). *Nursing: Scope and standards of practice* (4th ed.). American Nurses Association.

5. Leonard, J.C., Whiteman, K., Stephens, K., Henry, C., Swanson-Bieaman, B. (2022). Imporving communication and collaboration skills in graduate nurses: An evidence-based approach. *The Online Journal of Issues in Nursing, 27*(2), 3. https://www.doi.org/10.3912/OJIN.Vol27No02Man03

6. "Osgood-Schramm-model-of-communication.jpg" by Jordan Smith at eCampus Ontario is licensed under CC BY 4.0. Access for free at https://ecampusontario.pressbooks.pub/communicationatwork/chapter/1-3-the-communication-process/

confirm that their message was received correctly. It also allows the person receiving the instructions to verify and confirm the actions to be taken. If closed-loop communication is not used, the receiver may nod or say "OK," and the sender may assume the message has been effectively transmitted, but this may not be the case and can lead to errors and client harm.

An example of closed-loop communication can be found in the following exchange:

- **RN:** "Jane, can you get a set of vitals on Mr. Smith and let me know if the results are outside of normal range?"
- **Jane, CNA:** "OK, I'll get a set of vitals on Mr. Smith and let you know if they are out of range."

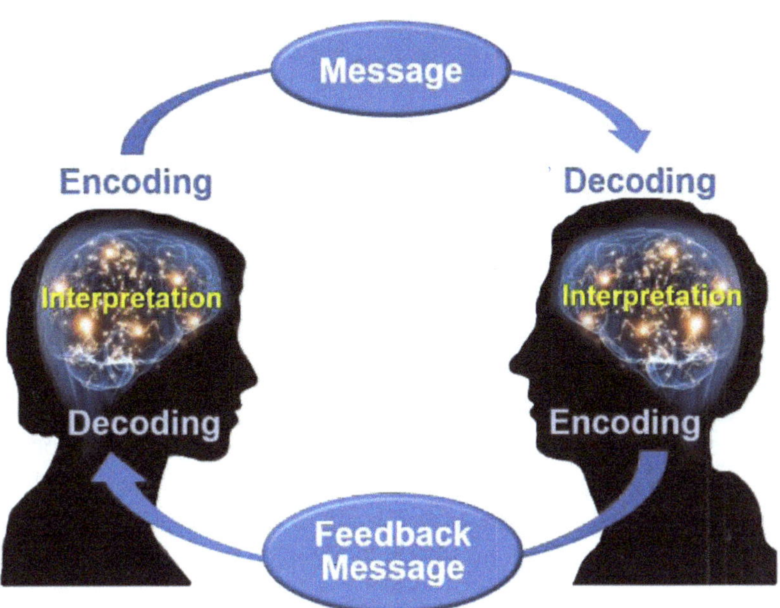

FIGURE 3.1 Effective Communication Between Sender and Receiver

Closed-loop communication is vital for communication among health care team members to avoid misunderstandings that can cause unsafe client care. According to the *HIPAA Journal*, poor communication leads to a "reduction in the quality of care, poor client outcomes, wastage of resources, and high health care costs."[7] Parameters for reporting results and the results that should be expected are often left unsaid rather than spelled out in sufficient detail. It is imperative for the RN to provide clear, complete, concise instructions when delegating. A lack of clarity can lead to misunderstanding, unfinished tasks, incomplete care, and/or medical errors.[8]

Effective communication is at the core of proper assignment, delegation, and supervision. With effective communication at the beginning of every shift, each nursing team member should have a clear plan for their shift, what to do and why, and what and when to report to the RN or team leader. Communication should

7. Alder, S. (2025). *Effects of poor communication in healthcare.* HIPPAA Journal. https://www.hipaajournal.com/effects-of-poor-communication-in-healthcare/

8. Alder, S. (2025). *Effects of poor communication in healthcare.* HIPPAA Journal. https://www.hipaajournal.com/effects-of-poor-communication-in-healthcare/

continue throughout the shift as tasks are accomplished and clients' needs change. Effective communication improves client outcomes and satisfaction scores, as well as improving team morale by enhancing the collaborative relationships of the health care team.

The RN is accountable for clear, concise, correct, and complete communication when making assignments and delegating, both initially and throughout the shift. These communication characteristics can be remembered by using the mnemonic the "4 Cs":

- **Clear:** Information is understood by the listener. Asking the listener to restate the instructions and the plan can be helpful to determine whether the communication is clear.
- **Concise:** Sufficient information should be provided to accurately perform the task, but excessive or irrelevant information should be avoided because it can confuse the listener and waste precious time.
- **Correct:** Correct communication is not vague or confusing. Accurate information is also aligned with agency policy and the team member's scope of practice as defined by their state's Nurse Practice Act and other state regulations.
- **Complete:** Complete instructions leave no room for doubt. Always ask if further information or clarification is needed, especially regarding tasks that are infrequently performed or include unique instructions.[9]

The use of closed-loop communication is the best method to achieve clear, concise, correct, and complete information exchanged among team members. Closed-loop communication allows team members the opportunity to verify and validate the exchange of information. By repeating back information, members confirm the exchange has occurred, understanding is clear, and expectations are heard.

Closed-loop communication should also be used when the RN is receiving a verbal order from a provider. For example, when the resuscitation team leader gives a verbal order of "Epinephrine 1 mg/mL IV push now," the RN confirms correct understanding of the order by repeating back, "I will prepare Epinephrine 1 mg/mL to be given IV push now." After the provider confirms the verbal order and the task is completed, the nurse confirms completion of the task by stating, "Epinephrine 1 mg/mL IV push was administered."

In addition to using closed-loop communication, a common format used by health care team members to exchange client information is ISBARR, a mnemonic for the components of **I**ntroduction, **S**ituation, **B**ackground, **A**ssessment, **R**equest/Recommendations, and **R**epeat Back.

ISBARR and other communication strategies are discussed in more detail in the "Interprofessional Communication" section of the "Collaboration Within the Interprofessional Team" chapter.

3.3 ASSIGNMENT

Nursing team members working in inpatient or long-term care settings receive client assignments at the start of their shift. **Assignment** refers to routine care, activities, and procedures that are within the legal scope of practice of registered nurses (RN), licensed practical/vocational nurses (LPN/VN), or unlicensed

9. LaCharity, L. A., Kumagai, C. K., & Bartz, B. (2019). *Prioritization, delegation and assignment* (4th ed.). Mosby, p. 6.

assistive personnel (UAP).[10] Scope of practice for RNs and LPNs is described in each state's Nurse Practice Act. Care tasks for UAP vary by state; regulations are typically listed on sites for the state's Board of Nursing, Department of Health, Department of Aging, Department of Health Professions, Department of Commerce, or Office of Long-Term Care.[11]

See Table 3.3a for common tasks performed by members of the nursing team based on their scope of practice. These tasks are within the traditional role and training the team member has acquired through a basic educational program. They are also within the expectations of the health care agency during a shift of work. Agency policy can be more restrictive than federal or state regulations, but it cannot be less restrictive.

Client assignments are typically made by the charge nurse (or nurse supervisor) from the previous shift. A charge nurse is an RN who provides leadership on a client-care unit within a health care facility during their shift. Charge nurses perform many of the tasks that general nurses do, but also have some supervisory duties such as making assignments, delegating tasks, preparing schedules, monitoring admissions and discharges, and serving as a staff member resource.[12]

TABLE 3.3A. Nursing Team Members' Scope of Practice and Common Tasks[13]

Nursing Team Member	Scope of Practice	Common Tasks
RN	• Create and implement individualized nursing care plans and revise as needed • Review prescribed medications for safety concerns, administer medications, and titrate medications based on protocols or standing orders • Plan and provide client education • Admit and discharge clients • Make referrals, such as to a caseworker, dietician, or chaplain, according to agency policy. (Many referrals to interprofessional team members require a provider order.) • Delegate appropriate tasks to LPN/VNs and UAPs	• Assess clients • Initiate administration of blood products to a client • Administer high-risk medications, including heparin and chemotherapeutic agents • Establish intravenous (IV) access • Initiate IV fluids and IV medications • Administer IV push medications • Titrate medications per provider order • Perform any tasks that may be performed by a LPN/VN or UAP

10. American Nurses Association and NCSBN. (2019). *National guidelines for nursing delegation.* https://www.ncsbn.org/public-files/NGND-PosPaper_06.pdf

11. McMullen, T. L., Resnick, B., Chin-Hansen, J., Geiger-Brown, J. M., Miller, N., & Rubenstein, R. (2015). Certified nurse aide scope of practice: State-by-state differences in allowable delegated activities. *Journal of the American Medical Directors Association, 16*(1), 20–24. https://doi.org/10.1016/j.jamda.2014.07.003

12. RegisteredNursing.org. (2025, April 13). *What is a charge nurse?* https://www.registerednursing.org/specialty/charge-nurse/

13. RegisteredNursing.org. (2024, January 27). *Assignment, delegation and supervision: NCLEX-RN.* https://www.registerednursing.org/nclex/assignment-delegation-supervision/

TABLE 3.3A. Continued...

LPN/VN	• Assist the RN by performing routine, basic nursing care with predictable outcomes • Assist the RN with collecting data and monitoring client findings on stable clients • Implement interventions outlined in the nursing care plan, as appropriate • Reinforce client education as outlined in the nursing care plan • Delegate tasks to UAP	• Provide basic nursing care • Assist with the collection of client assessment data • Assist the RN with the development and revision of a nursing care plan • Reinforce teaching provided by an RN • Administer medications that are not high-risk • Administer enteral feeding • Perform routine dressing changes • Perform tracheostomy care on stable clients • Perform suctioning on stable or routine clients • Insert a urinary catheter • Perform any of the tasks that UAPs are permitted to perform Tasks That Potentially Can Be Delegated According to the Five Rights of Delegation: • Monitor the administration of blood products after they have been initiated by an RN and report findings to the RN • Assist with the administration of IV fluids and medications after they have been initiated by an RN and under the supervision of an RN; cannot hang the first dose or change medications
UAP	• Assist clients with activities of daily living (ADLs), including: – Eating – Bathing – Toileting – Ambulating • Perform routine data collection that does not require clinical assessment or critical thinking, such as: – Measuring vital signs, weight, and height – Measuring intake and output (e.g., food and drink, urine, bowel movements)	• Assist stable clients with eating (although clients with dysphagia or at an aspiration risk require qualified health care members with specific training in this area) • Assist with personal hygiene, grooming, bathing, positioning, transfers, range-of-motion exercises, toileting, and making beds • Obtain vital signs on stable clients • Transport clients • Collect and transport routine urine specimens • Restock supplies • Report to the RN if a change in client's status is observed. Example, "Client is now complaining of pain at 9/10 when repositioned. Last time client was repositioned, no pain was reported."

An example of a client assignment is when an RN assigns an LPN/VN to care for a client with stable heart failure. The LPN/VN collects assessment data, monitors intake/output throughout the shift, and administers routine oral medication. The LPN/VN documents this information and reports information back to the RN. This is considered the LPN/VN's "assignment" because the skills are taught within an LPN educational program and are consistent with the state's Nurse Practice Act for LPN/VN scope of practice. They are also included in the unit's job description for an LPN/VN. The RN may also assign some care for this client to UAP. These tasks may include assistance with personal hygiene, toileting, and ambulation. The UAP documents these tasks as they are completed and reports information back to the RN or LPN/VN. These tasks are considered the UAP's assignment because they are taught within a nursing aide's educational program, are consistent with the UAP's scope of practice for that state, and are included in the job description for the nursing aide's role in this unit. The RN continues to be accountable for the care provided to this client despite the assignments made to other nursing team members.

Special consideration is required for UAP with additional training. With increased staffing needs, skills such as administering medications, inserting Foley catheters, or performing injections are included in specialized training programs for UAP. Due to the impact these skills can have on the outcome and safety of the client, the National Council of State Board of Nursing (NCSBN) recommends these activities be considered delegated tasks by the RN or nurse leader. By delegating these advanced skills when appropriate, the nurse validates competency, provides supervision, and maintains accountability for client outcomes. Read more about delegation in the "Delegation" section of this chapter.

When making assignments to other nursing team members, it is essential for the RN to keep in mind specific tasks that cannot be delegated to other nursing team members based on federal and/or state regulations. These tasks include, but are not limited to, those tasks described in Table 3.3b.

TABLE 3.3B. Examples of Tasks Outside the Scope of Practice of Nursing Assistive Personnel

Nursing Team Member	Tasks That Cannot Be Delegated
LPN/VN	• Cannot create nursing care plans, analyze client assessment data, establish nursing diagnoses or expected outcomes, or evaluate the effectiveness of a nursing care plan. (However, LPN/VNs can collect data and contribute to the development and revision of a client's nursing care plan in collaboration with the RN.) • Cannot administer high-risk medications (such as heparin and chemotherapeutic medications). • Cannot titrate medications. (**Titrate** refers to adjusting the dosage of medication until the desired effects are achieved.) • Cannot independently provide client education. (However, they can implement client education that has been planned by the RN.) • Cannot perform admission assessments or initial postoperative assessments. • Cannot discharge clients.

TABLE 3.3B. Continued...

Unlicensed Assistive Personnel (UAP)	• Cannot complete tasks requiring clinical judgement and/or professional knowledge. For example, a nursing assessment of a client's skin cannot be delegated to UAP. However, UAP are encouraged to report concerns about skin breakdown and other potential signs and symptoms to a licensed nurse. • Cannot delegate tasks. • Cannot provide client education but can reinforce education previously provided. For example, UAP can encourage a client to keep their nasal cannula in place while eating. • Cannot complete tasks that require clinical expertise unless advanced training has been received and written agency policy allows, such as: – Administering medications and injections – Inserting Foley catheters – Administering tube feedings – Performing wound care or dressing changes[14]

As always, refer to each state's Nurse Practice Act and other state regulations for specific details about nursing team members' scope of practice when providing care in that state.

Find and review Nurse Practice Acts by state at https://www.ncsbn.org/policy/npa.page. Access supplementary digital content in the online book using this QR code.

Read more about the Wisconsin's Nurse Practice Act and the standards and scope of practice for RNs and LPNs at Wisconsin's Legislative Code Chapter N6. Access supplementary digital content in the online book using this QR code.

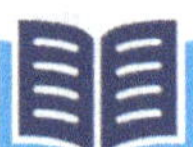

Read more about scope of practice, skills, and practices of nurse aides in Wisconsin at DHS 129.07 Standards for Nurse Aide Training Programs. Access supplementary digital content in the online book using this QR code.

14. State of Wisconsin Department of Health Services. (2018). *Medication administration by unlicensed assistive personnel (UAP): Guidelines for registered nurses delegating medication administration to unlicensed assistive personnel.* https://www.dhs.wisconsin.gov/publications/p01908.pdf

3.4 DELEGATION

There has been significant national debate over the difference between assignment and delegation over the past few decades. In 2019 the National Council of State Boards of Nursing (NCSBN) and the American Nurses Association (ANA) published updated joint National Guidelines on Nursing Delegation (NGND).[15] These guidelines apply to all levels of nursing licensure (advanced practice registered nurses [APRN], registered nurses [RN], and licensed practical/vocational nurses [LPN/VN]) when delegating when there is no specific guidance provided by the state's Nurse Practice Act (NPA).[16] It is important to note that states have different laws and rules/regulations regarding delegation, so it is the responsibility of all licensed nurses to know what is permitted in their jurisdiction.

The NGND defines a **delegatee** as an RN, LPN/VN, or UAP who is delegated a nursing responsibility by either an APRN, RN, or LPN/VN, is competent to perform the task, and verbally accepts the responsibility.[17] **Delegation** is allowing a delegatee to perform a specific nursing activity, skill, or procedure that is beyond the delegatee's traditional role and not routinely performed, but the individual has obtained additional training and validated their competence to perform the delegated responsibility.[18] However, the licensed nurse still maintains accountability for overall client care. **Delegated responsibility** is a nursing activity, skill, or procedure that is transferred from a licensed nurse to a delegatee.[19] **Accountability** is defined as being answerable to oneself and others for one's own choices, decisions, and actions as measured against a standard. Therefore, if a nurse does not feel it is appropriate to delegate a certain responsibility to a delegatee, the delegating nurse should perform the activity themselves.[20]

Delegation is summarized in the NGND as the following[21]:

- A delegatee is allowed to perform a specific nursing activity, skill, or procedure that is outside the traditional role and basic responsibilities of the delegatee's current job.
- The delegatee has obtained the additional education and training and validated competence to perform the care/delegated responsibility. The context and processes associated with competency validation will be different for each activity, skill, or procedure being delegated. Competency validation should be specific to the knowledge and skill needed to safely perform the delegated responsibility, as well as to the level of the practitioner (e.g., RN, LPN/VN, UAP) to whom the activity, skill, or procedure has been delegated. The licensed nurse who delegates the "responsibility" maintains overall accountability for the client, but the delegatee bears the responsibility for completing the delegated activity, skill, or procedure.

15. American Nurses Association and NCSBN. (2019). *National guidelines for nursing delegation.* https://www.ncsbn.org/public-files/NGND-PosPaper_06.pdf
16. American Nurses Association and NCSBN. (2019). *National guidelines for nursing delegation.* https://www.ncsbn.org/public-files/NGND-PosPaper_06.pdf
17. American Nurses Association and NCSBN. (2019). *National guidelines for nursing delegation.* https://www.ncsbn.org/public-files/NGND-PosPaper_06.pdf
18. American Nurses Association and NCSBN. (2019). *National guidelines for nursing delegation.* https://www.ncsbn.org/public-files/NGND-PosPaper_06.pdf
19. American Nurses Association and NCSBN. (2019). *National guidelines for nursing delegation.* https://www.ncsbn.org/public-files/NGND-PosPaper_06.pdf
20. American Nurses Association and NCSBN. (2019). *National guidelines for nursing delegation.* https://www.ncsbn.org/public-files/NGND-PosPaper_06.pdf
21. American Nurses Association and NCSBN. (2019). *National guidelines for nursing delegation.* https://www.ncsbn.org/public-files/NGND-PosPaper_06.pdf

- The licensed nurse cannot delegate nursing clinical judgment or any activity that will involve nursing clinical judgment or critical decision-making to UAP.
- Nursing responsibilities are delegated by a licensed nurse who has the authority to delegate and the delegated responsibility is within the delegator's scope of practice.

An example of delegation is medication administration that is delegated by a licensed nurse to UAP with additional training in some agencies, according to agency policy. This task is outside the traditional role of UAP, but the delegatee has received additional training for this delegated responsibility and has completed competency validation in completing this task accurately.

An example illustrating the difference between assignment and delegation is assisting clients with eating. Feeding clients is typically part of the routine role of UAP. However, if a client has recently experienced a stroke (i.e., cerebrovascular accident) or is otherwise experiencing swallowing difficulties (e.g., dysphagia), this task cannot be assigned to UAP because it is not considered routine care. Instead, the RN should perform this task themselves or delegate it to a UAP who has received additional training on feeding assistance.

The delegation process is multifaceted. See Figure 3.2[22] for an illustration of the intersecting responsibilities of the employer/nurse leader, licensed nurse, and delegatee with two-way communication that protects the safety of the public. "Delegation begins at the administrative/nurse leader level of the organization and includes determining nursing responsibilities that can be delegated, to whom, and under what circumstances; developing delegation policies and procedures; periodically evaluating delegation processes; and promoting a positive culture/work environment. The licensed nurse is responsible for determining client needs and when to delegate, ensuring availability to the delegatee, evaluating outcomes, and maintaining accountability for delegated responsibility. Finally, the delegatee must accept activities based on their competency level, maintain competence for delegated responsibility, and maintain accountability for delegated activity."[23]

Five Rights of Delegation

How does the RN determine what tasks can be delegated, when, and to whom? According to the National Council of State Boards of Nursing (NCSBN), RNs should use the five rights of delegation to ensure proper and appropriate delegation: right task, right circumstance, right person, right directions and communication, and right supervision and evaluation[24]:

- **Right task:** The activity falls within the delegatee's job description or is included as part of the established policies and procedures of the nursing practice setting. The facility needs to ensure the policies and procedures describe the expectations and limits of the activity and provide any necessary competency training.
- **Right circumstance:** The health condition of the client must be stable. If the client's condition changes, the delegatee must communicate this to the licensed nurse, and the licensed nurse must reassess the situation and the appropriateness of the delegation.[25]

22. "Delegation.png" by Meredith Pomietlo for Chippewa Valley Technical College is licensed under CC BY 4.0
23. American Nurses Association and NCSBN. (2019). *National guidelines for nursing delegation.* https://www.ncsbn.org/public-files/NGND-PosPaper_06.pdf
24. American Nurses Association and NCSBN. (2019). *National guidelines for nursing delegation.* https://www.ncsbn.org/public-files/NGND-PosPaper_06.pdf
25. American Nurses Association and NCSBN. (2019). *National guidelines for nursing delegation.* https://www.ncsbn.org/public-files/NGND-PosPaper_06.pdf

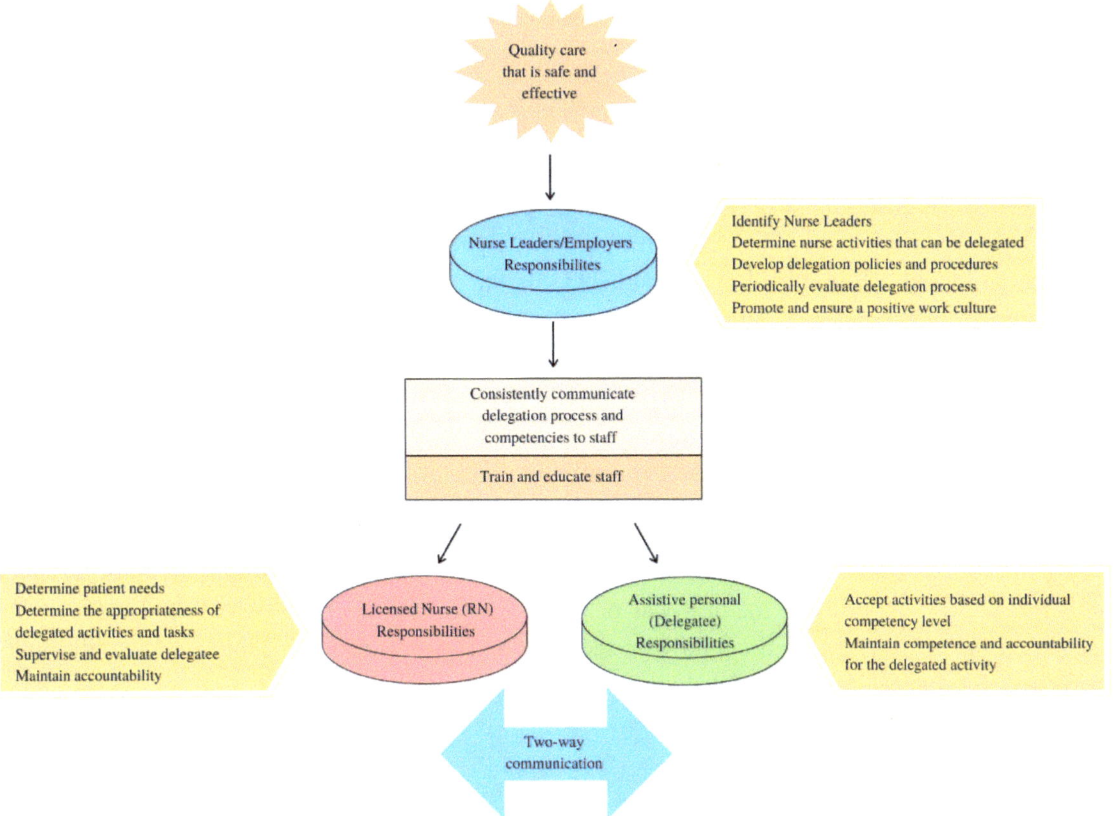

FIGURE 3.2 Multifaceted Delegation Process

- **Right person:** The licensed nurse, along with the employer and the delegatee, is responsible for ensuring that the delegatee possesses the appropriate skills and knowledge to perform the activity.[26]
- **Right directions and communication:** Each delegation situation should be specific to the client, the nurse, and the delegatee. The licensed nurse is expected to communicate specific instructions for the delegated activity to the delegatee; the delegatee, as part of two-way communication, should ask any clarifying questions. This communication includes any data that need to be collected, the method for collecting the data, the time frame for reporting the results to the licensed nurse, and additional information pertinent to the situation. The delegatee must understand the terms of the delegation and must agree to accept the delegated activity. The licensed nurse should ensure the delegatee understands they cannot make any decisions or modifications in carrying out the activity without first consulting the licensed nurse.[27]

26. American Nurses Association and NCSBN. (2019). *National guidelines for nursing delegation.* https://www.ncsbn.org/public-files/NGND-PosPaper_06.pdf
27. American Nurses Association and NCSBN. (2019). *National guidelines for nursing delegation.* https://www.ncsbn.org/public-files/NGND-PosPaper_06.pdf

- **Right supervision and evaluation:** The licensed nurse is responsible for monitoring the delegated activity, following up with the delegatee at the completion of the activity, and evaluating client outcomes. The delegatee is responsible for communicating client information to the licensed nurse during the delegation situation. The licensed nurse should be ready and available to intervene as necessary. The licensed nurse should ensure appropriate documentation of the activity is completed.[28]

Simply stated, the licensed nurse determines the right person is assigned the right tasks for the right clients under the right circumstances. When determining what aspects of care can be delegated, the licensed nurse uses clinical judgment while considering the client's current clinical condition, as well as the abilities of the health care team member. The RN must also consider if the circumstances are appropriate for delegation. For example, although obtaining routine vital signs on stable clients may be appropriate to delegate to assistive personnel, obtaining vital signs on an unstable client is not appropriate to delegate.

After the decision has been made to delegate, the nurse assigning the tasks must communicate appropriately with the delegatee and provide the right directions and supervision. Communication is key to successful delegation. Clear, concise, and closed-loop communication is essential to ensure successful completion of the delegated task in a safe manner. During the final step of delegation, also referred to as **supervision**, the nurse verifies and evaluates that the task was performed correctly, appropriately, safely, and competently. Read more about supervision in the following section on "Supervision." See Table 3.4 for additional questions to consider for each "right" of delegation.

TABLE 3.4. Rights of Delegation[29]

Rights of Delegation	Description	Questions to Consider When Delegating
Right Task	A task that can be transferred to a member of the nursing team for a specific client.	• Is this task legally appropriate to delegate to this team member according to the state's Nurse Practice Act and written agency policy and procedures? • Has the team member been trained and demonstrated competency in performing this task? • Does the team member feel comfortable and willing to perform the task?
Right Circumstances	The client is stable.	• Is there enough staffing to support delegation in this circumstance? • What is the client's current status? • What are the client's current needs?

28. American Nurses Association and NCSBN. (2019). *National guidelines for nursing delegation.* https://www.ncsbn.org/public-files/NGND-PosPaper_06.pdf

29. NCSBN. (n.d.). *Delegation.* https://www.ncsbn.org/1625.htm

TABLE 3.4. Continued...

Right Person	The person delegating the task has the appropriate scope of practice to do so. The task is also appropriate for this delegatee's skills and knowledge.	• Is the delegatee suitable to meet the client's needs? • Is the delegatee willing to accept the delegated task? • Has the delegatee demonstrated competence to perform the task?
Right Directions and Communication	The task or activity is clearly defined and described.	• Have clear communication and instructions been given regarding the task? • Did the instructions include data that need to be collected, the method for collecting the data, the time frame for reporting the results to the licensed nurse, and additional information pertinent to the situation? • Does the delegatee understand what needs to be done? • Is the delegatee aware of what should be reported and when it needs to be reported? • Has the delegatee accepted the delegated task? • Has the time frame to complete the task been defined? • Does the delegatee understand they cannot make any decisions or modifications in carrying out the activity without first consulting the licensed nurse? • Was closed-loop communication used?
Right Supervision and Evaluation	The RN appropriately monitors the delegated activity, evaluates client outcomes, and follows up with the delegatee at the completion of the activity.	• When and how will the RN connect with the delegatee to discuss the completion of the activity and communication of client information? • How often should the RN directly or indirectly observe the team member's performance? • When will the RN evaluate client outcomes? • When will the RN provide feedback to the team member? • Has documentation of the activity been completed?

Keep in mind that any nursing intervention that requires specific nursing knowledge, clinical judgment, or use of the nursing process can only be delegated to another RN. Examples of these types of tasks include initial preoperative or admission assessments, client teaching, and creation and evaluation of a nursing care plan. See Figure 3.3[30] for an algorithm based on the 2019 National Guidelines for Nursing Delegation that can be used when deciding if a nursing task can be delegated.[31]

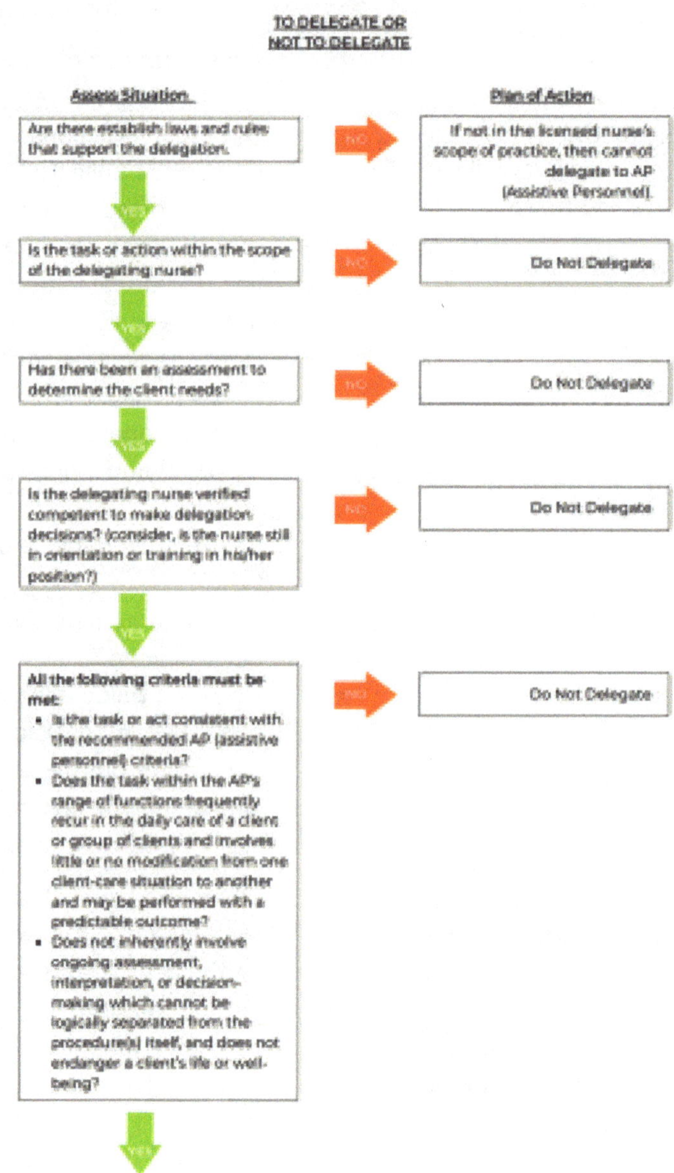

FIGURE 3.3 Delegation Algorithm

30. "Delegation Decision Tree.png" by Meredith Pomietlo for Chippewa Valley Technical College is licensed under CC BY 4.0
31. American Nurses Association and NCSBN. (2019). *National guidelines for nursing delegation*. https://www.ncsbn.org/public-files/NGND-PosPaper_06.pdf

Responsibilities of the Licensed Nurse

The licensed nurse has several responsibilities as part of the delegation process. According to the NGND, any decision to delegate a nursing responsibility must be based on the needs of the client or population, the stability and predictability of the client's condition, the documented training and competence of the delegatee, and the ability of the licensed nurse to supervise the delegated responsibility and its outcome with consideration to the available staff mix and client acuity. Additionally, the licensed nurse must consider the state Nurse Practice Act regarding delegation and the employer's policies and procedures prior to making a final decision to delegate. Licensed nurses must be aware that delegation is at the nurse's discretion, with consideration of the particular situation. The licensed nurse maintains accountability for the client, while the delegatee is responsible for the delegated activity, skill, or procedure. If, under the circumstances, a nurse does not feel it is appropriate to delegate a certain responsibility to a delegatee, the delegating nurse should perform the activity.[32]

1. The licensed nurse must determine when and what to delegate based on the practice setting, the client's needs and condition, the state's/jurisdiction's provisions for delegation, and the employer's policies and procedures regarding delegating a specific responsibility. The licensed nurse must determine the needs of the client and whether those needs are matched by the knowledge, skills, and abilities of the delegatee and can be performed safely by the delegatee. The licensed nurse cannot delegate any activity that requires clinical reasoning, nursing judgment, or critical decision-making. The licensed nurse must ultimately make the final decision whether an activity is appropriate to delegate to the delegatee based on the "Five Rights of Delegation."

- **Rationale:** The licensed nurse, who is present at the point of care, is in the best position to assess the needs of the client and what can or cannot be delegated in specific situations.[33]

2. The licensed nurse must communicate with the delegatee who will be assisting in providing client care. This should include reviewing the delegatee's assignment and discussing delegated responsibilities, including information on the client's condition/stability, any specific information pertaining to a certain client (e.g., no blood draws in the right arm), and any specific information about the client's condition that should be communicated back to the licensed nurse by the delegatee.

- **Rationale:** Communication must be a two-way process involving both the licensed nurse delegating the activity and the delegatee being delegated the responsibility. Evidence shows that the better the communication between the nurse and the delegatee, the more optimal the outcome. The licensed nurse must provide information about the client and care requirements. This includes any specific issues related to any delegated responsibilities. These instructions should include any unique client requirements. The licensed nurse must instruct the delegatee to regularly communicate the status of the client.[34]

32. American Nurses Association and NCSBN. (2019). *National guidelines for nursing delegation.* https://www.ncsbn.org/public-files/NGND-PosPaper_06.pdf
33. American Nurses Association and NCSBN. (2019). *National guidelines for nursing delegation.* https://www.ncsbn.org/public-files/NGND-PosPaper_06.pdf
34. American Nurses Association and NCSBN. (2019). *National guidelines for nursing delegation.* https://www.ncsbn.org/public-files/NGND-PosPaper_06.pdf

3. The licensed nurse must be available to the delegatee for guidance and questions, including assisting with the delegated responsibility, if necessary, or performing it themselves if the client's condition or other circumstances warrant doing so.

- **Rationale:** Delegation calls for nursing judgment throughout the process. The final decision to delegate rests in the hands of the licensed nurse as they have overall accountability for the client.[35]

4. The licensed nurse must follow up with the delegatee and the client after the delegated responsibility has been completed.

- **Rationale:** The licensed nurse who delegates the "responsibility" maintains overall accountability for the client, while the delegatee is responsible for the delegated activity, skill, or procedure.[36]

5. The licensed nurse must provide feedback information about the delegation process and any issues regarding delegatee competence level to the nurse leader. Licensed nurses in the facility need to communicate to the nurse leader responsible for delegation any issues arising related to delegation and any individual whom they identify as not being competent in a specific responsibility or unable to use good judgment and decision-making.

- **Rationale:** This will allow the nurse leader responsible for delegation to develop a plan to address the situation.[37]

The decision of whether or not to delegate or assign is based on the RN's judgment concerning the condition of the client, the competence of the nursing team member, and the degree of supervision that will be required of the RN if a task is delegated.[38]

Responsibilities of the Delegatee

Everyone is responsible for the well-being of clients. While the nurse is ultimately accountable for the overall care provided to a client, the delegatee shares the responsibility for the client and is fully responsible for the delegated activity, skill, or procedure.[39] The delegatee has the following responsibilities:

1. The delegatee must accept only the delegated responsibilities that they are appropriately trained and educated to perform and feel comfortable doing given the specific circumstances in the health care setting and client's condition. The delegatee should confirm acceptance of the responsibility to carry out the delegated activity. If the delegatee does not believe they have the appropriate competency to complete the delegated responsibility, then the delegatee should not accept the delegated responsibility. This includes informing the nursing leadership if they do not feel they have received adequate training to perform the

35. American Nurses Association and NCSBN. (2019). *National guidelines for nursing delegation.* https://www.ncsbn.org/public-files/NGND-PosPaper_06.pdf
36. American Nurses Association and NCSBN. (2019). *National guidelines for nursing delegation.* https://www.ncsbn.org/public-files/NGND-PosPaper_06.pdf
37. American Nurses Association and NCSBN. (2019). *National guidelines for nursing delegation.* https://www.ncsbn.org/public-files/NGND-PosPaper_06.pdf
38. American Nurses Association and NCSBN. (2019). *National guidelines for nursing delegation.* https://www.ncsbn.org/public-files/NGND-PosPaper_06.pdf
39. American Nurses Association and NCSBN. (2019). *National guidelines for nursing delegation.* https://www.ncsbn.org/public-files/NGND-PosPaper_06.pdf

delegated responsibility, do not perform the procedure frequently enough to do it safely, or their knowledge and skills need updating.

- **Rationale:** The delegatee shares the responsibility to keep clients safe, and this includes only performing activities, skills, or procedures in which they are competent and comfortable doing.[40]

2. The delegatee must maintain competency for the delegated responsibility.

- **Rationale:** Competency is an ongoing process. Even if properly taught, the delegatee may become less competent if they do not frequently perform the procedure. Given that the delegatee shares the responsibility for the client, the delegatee also has a responsibility to maintain competency.[41]

3. The delegatee must communicate with the licensed nurse in charge of the client. This includes any questions related to the delegated responsibility and follow-up on any unusual incidents that may have occurred while the delegatee was performing the delegated responsibility, any concerns about a client's condition, and any other information important to the client's care.

- **Rationale:** The delegatee is a partner in providing client care. They are interacting with the client/family and caring for the client. This information and two-way communication are important for successful delegation and optimal outcomes for the client.[42]

4. Once the delegatee verifies acceptance of the delegated responsibility, the delegatee is accountable for carrying out the delegated responsibility correctly and completing timely and accurate documentation per facility policy.

- **Rationale:** The delegatee cannot delegate to another individual. If the delegatee is unable to complete the responsibility or feels as though they need assistance, the delegatee should inform the licensed nurse immediately so the licensed nurse can assess the situation and provide support. Only the licensed nurse can determine if it is appropriate to delegate the activity to another individual. If at any time the licensed nurse determines they need to perform the delegated responsibility, the delegatee must relinquish responsibility upon request of the licensed nurse.[43]

Responsibilities of the Employer/Nurse Leader

The employer and nurse leaders also have responsibilities related to safe delegation of client care:

1. The employer must identify a nurse leader responsible for oversight of delegated responsibilities for the facility. If there is only one licensed nurse within the practice setting, that licensed nurse must be responsible for oversight of delegated responsibilities for the facility.

40. American Nurses Association and NCSBN. (2019). *National guidelines for nursing delegation.* https://www.ncsbn.org/public-files/NGND-PosPaper_06.pdf
41. American Nurses Association and NCSBN. (2019). *National guidelines for nursing delegation.* https://www.ncsbn.org/public-files/NGND-PosPaper_06.pdf
42. American Nurses Association and NCSBN. (2019). *National guidelines for nursing delegation.* https://www.ncsbn.org/public-files/NGND-PosPaper_06.pdf
43. American Nurses Association and NCSBN. (2019). *National guidelines for nursing delegation.* https://www.ncsbn.org/public-files/NGND-PosPaper_06.pdf

- **Rationale:** The nurse leader has the ability to assess the needs of the facility, understand the type of knowledge and skill needed to perform a specific nursing responsibility, and be accountable for maintaining a safe environment for clients. They are also aware of the knowledge, skill level, and limitations of the licensed nurses and UAP. Additionally, the nurse leader is positioned to develop appropriate staffing models that take into consideration the need for delegation. Therefore, the decision to delegate begins with a thorough assessment by a nurse leader designated by the institution to oversee the process.[44]

2. The designated nurse leader responsible for delegation, ideally with a committee (consisting of other nurse leaders) formed for the purposes of addressing delegation, must determine which nursing responsibilities may be delegated, to whom, and under what circumstances. The nurse leader must be aware of the state Nurse Practice Act and the laws/rules and regulations that affect the delegation process and ensure all institutional policies are in accordance with the law.

- **Rationale:** A systematic approach to the delegation process fosters communication and consistency of the process throughout the facility.[45]

3. Policies and procedures for delegation must be developed. The employer/nurse leader must outline specific responsibilities that can be delegated and to whom these responsibilities can be delegated. The policies and procedures should also indicate what may not be delegated. The employer must periodically review the policies and procedures for delegation to ensure they remain consistent with current nursing practice trends and that they are consistent with the state Nurse Practice Act. (Institution/employer policies can be more restrictive, but not less restrictive.)

- **Rationale:** Policies and procedures standardize the appropriate method of care and ensure safe practices. Having a policy and procedure specific to delegation and delegated responsibilities eliminates questions from licensed nurses and UAP about what can be delegated and how they should be performed.[46]

4. The employer/nurse leader must communicate information about delegation to the licensed nurses and UAP and educate them about what responsibilities can be delegated. This information should include the competencies of delegatees who can safely perform a specific nursing responsibility.

- **Rationale:** Licensed nurses must be aware of the competence level of staff and expectations for delegation (as described within the policies and procedures) to make informed decisions on whether or not delegation is appropriate for the given situation. Licensed nurses maintain accountability for the client. However, the delegatee has responsibility for the delegated activity, skill, or procedure.

In summary, delegation is the transfer of the nurse's responsibility for a task while retaining professional accountability for the client's overall outcome. The decision to delegate is based on the nurse's judgment, the act of delegation must be clearly defined by the nurse, and the outcomes of delegation are an extension of the nurse's guidance and supervision. Delegation, when rooted in mutual respect and trust, is a key component to an effective health care team.

---

44. American Nurses Association and NCSBN. (2019). *National guidelines for nursing delegation.* https://www.ncsbn.org/public-files/NGND-PosPaper_06.pdf
45. American Nurses Association and NCSBN. (2019). *National guidelines for nursing delegation.* https://www.ncsbn.org/public-files/NGND-PosPaper_06.pdf
46. American Nurses Association and NCSBN. (2019). *National guidelines for nursing delegation.* https://www.ncsbn.org/public-files/NGND-PosPaper_06.pdf

Delegation is an integral skill in the nursing profession to help manage the complexities of the dynamic and ever-changing health care environment. Delegation in nursing has been found to increase employee empowerment, decrease burnout, increase role commitment, and improve job satisfaction.[47] Cultivating delegation skills helps nurses better manage the complexities of their client care role, ensuring that their clients are safely cared for and outcomes are optimized. Delegation skills, like other nursing skills, require purposeful development and do not necessarily come easily when first transitioning into the nursing role. It is important that the new graduate nurse does not mistake delegation for pompous or arrogant behavior. Delegation requires mutual respect between the delegator and delegatee. Delegation is not seen as a sign or weakness and does not reflect one's desire to shirk their work responsibilities. Instead, delegation reflects strong leadership and organizational skills in which the nurse leader demonstrates that they understand how to leverage their team's strengths in order to achieve optimal care outcomes.

To help avoid any perception of arrogance in the delegation of an activity, it is important that the new graduate nurse approaches the task of delegation with humility. Clarity in the communication of the delegated responsibility is critical, and the rationale behind the delegation should be communicated to the delegatee. Within the task of delegation, the delegator should express appreciation for the delegatee and their contributions in the collaborative health care environment. Additionally, it is important to understand that no specific nurse delegated task is outside of the "nurse" role. For example, ambulating a client does not need to delegated to an unlicensed assistive personnel simply because that individual is able to perform that task. Rather, nurses must be willing to perform delegated tasks themselves when necessary. This reflects a team-oriented mindset and helps to reinforce among the care team that all roles are critical to optimizing client care. For new graduate nurses who first transition into a specific health care setting, having the opportunity to shadow individuals in various work roles helps to foster a team mindset. Asking questions of various team members regarding their work role can help a new graduate nurse demonstrate respect and value for other roles.

Examples of helpful questions may include the following:

- "What is the biggest challenge in your typical workday?"
- "What do you most enjoy about your job?"
- "How is it best to communicate with you when the unit is busy?"
- "What do you think people misunderstand most about your role?"

It is important to ensure that the team understands that care is optimized when they function as one collective unit and not in siloed roles. Each team member must feel valued and competent in their role. By understanding and practicing strategic delegation, new graduate nurses can overcome any misconceptions of arrogance and contribute positively to the healthcare team.

Review the example below to consider variation in approach to task delegation.

47. American Nurses Association. (2023). *Delegation in nursing: How to build a stronger team.* https://www.nursingworld.org/content-hub/resources/nursing-leadership/delegation-in-nursing/

Scenario A: Nurse June, a newly graduated nurse, is working in a busy hospital unit. She needs an unlicensed assistive personnel (UAP), Alex, to take vital signs of a client. Nurse June approaches Alex in the hallway and says in an abrupt tone, "Alex, I need you to take Mr. Smith's vital signs right now. I'm too busy to do it myself, and besides, that's what you're here for. Just get it done quickly."

Analysis: June's tone and words suggest she sees Alex's role as less important and purely as a means to offload her tasks. June does not explain the urgency or importance of the task. June doesn't acknowledge Alex's effort or capability, making the request seem like a command rather than a collaborative effort.

Scenario B: Nurse June, a newly graduated nurse, is working in a busy hospital unit. She needs an unlicensed assistive personnel (UAP), Alex, to take vital signs of a client. Nurse June approaches Alex and says, "Hi Alex, could you please help me by taking Mr. Smith's vital signs? I'm handling a few urgent matters right now, and it would really help to have your support. I know you're great at this, and your thoroughness really makes a difference in our client care. Thank you so much!"

Analysis: June speaks to Alex with courtesy and acknowledges the value of his role. June clearly explains why she needs Alex's help and the importance of the task. June acknowledges Alex's competence and expresses gratitude, fostering feelings of value and respect.

3.5 SUPERVISION

The licensed nurse has the responsibility to supervise, monitor, and evaluate the nursing team members who have received delegated tasks, activities, or procedures. As previously noted, the act of supervision requires the nurse to assess the staff member's ability, competency, and experience prior to delegating. After the nurse has made the decision to delegate, supervision continues in terms of coaching, supporting, assisting, and educating as needed throughout the task to assure appropriate care is provided.

The nurse is accountable for client care delegated to other team members. Communication and supervision should be ongoing processes throughout the shift within the nursing care team. The nurse must ensure quality of care, appropriateness, timeliness, and completeness through direct and indirect supervision. For example, an RN may directly observe the UAP reposition a client or assist them to the bathroom to assure both client and staff safety are maintained. An RN may also indirectly evaluate an LPN's administration of medication by reviewing documentation in the client's medical record for timeliness and accuracy. Through direct and indirect supervision of delegation, quality client care and compliance with standards of practice and facility policies can be assured.

Supervision also includes providing constructive feedback to the nursing team member. **Constructive feedback** is supportive and identifies solutions to areas needing improvement. It is provided with positive intentions to address specific issues or concerns as the person learns and grows in their role. Constructive feedback includes several key points:

- Was the task, activity, care, or procedure performed correctly?
- Were the expected outcomes involving delegation for that client achieved?
- Did the team member utilize effective and timely communication?
- What were the challenges of the activity and what aspects went well?
- Were there any problems or specific concerns that occurred and how were they managed?

After these questions have been addressed, the RN creates a plan for future delegation with the nursing team member. This plan typically includes the following:

- Recognizing difficulty of the nursing team member in initiating or completing the delegated activities.
- Observing the client's responses to actions performed by the nursing team member.
- Following up in a timely manner on any problems, incidents, or concerns that arose.
- Creating a plan for providing additional training and monitoring outcomes of future delegated tasks, activities, or procedures.
- Consulting with appropriate nursing administrators per agency policy if the client's safety was compromised.

Please review the following example regarding constructive feedback and task supervision

Nurse Sarah, an experienced RN, delegated a task to Peter, an unlicensed assistive personnel (UAP), to take the vital signs of a post-operative client, Mrs. Johnson, and report any abnormalities immediately.

Sarah: "Hi Peter, I wanted to discuss the task you completed earlier with Mrs. Johnson's vital signs. Thank you for your help with that. Let's review how it went."

Was the task, activity, care, or procedure performed correctly?

Sarah: "First, I noticed you recorded the vital signs accurately. Good job on that. However, there was a delay in reporting Mrs. Johnson's elevated blood pressure to me. Can you walk me through what happened?"

Peter: "I took her vital signs, and her blood pressure was high. I was going to inform you, but I got called to assist with another client immediately after."

Were the expected outcomes involving delegation for that client achieved?

Sarah: "Ultimately, we did address the elevated blood pressure, but the delay could have impacted her care. It's crucial to report such abnormalities immediately."

Did the team member utilize effective and timely communication?

Sarah: "While you communicated the vital signs correctly, the timing was off. In future, if you can't find me immediately, please inform any available nurse or use the intercom system."

What were the challenges of the activity and what aspects went well?

Peter: "The challenge was managing multiple tasks at once. I did feel confident in taking and recording the vital signs accurately, though."

Sarah: "It sounds like you're balancing a lot of responsibilities well, but prioritizing urgent communications is key. You handled the technical part perfectly."

Were there any problems or specific concerns that occurred and how were they managed?

Sarah: "The main concern was the delay in reporting the elevated blood pressure. Fortunately, there were no serious consequences, but it's a potential risk we need to manage better. Let's create a plan to support you moving forward."

Recognizing difficulty of the nursing team member in initiating or completing the delegated activities:

Sarah: "I recognize that you were busy with multiple tasks. It's important to prioritize client safety over other duties."

Observing the client's responses to actions performed by the nursing team member:

Sarah: "I will check on Mrs. Johnson's response to ensure there are no ongoing issues, and I'll keep exploring how we can improve this process."

Following up in a timely manner on any problems, incidents, or concerns that arose:

Sarah: "I'll follow up with you soon to see how you're managing your other tasks, and we can address any challenges you're facing."

Creating a plan for providing additional training and monitoring outcomes of future delegated tasks, activities, or procedures:

Sarah: "We'll arrange some additional training on prioritizing tasks and urgent communication. Let's monitor the outcomes of your delegated tasks over the next few weeks to ensure you're supported."

Consulting with appropriate nursing administrators per agency policy if the client's safety was compromised:

Sarah: "Fortunately, Mrs. Johnson is fine, but if there were any safety concerns, we'd need to report it according to our policy. Keep this in mind for the future."

Sarah: "Peter, you're doing a great job with your responsibilities, and with a bit more focus on communication priorities, I'm confident you'll excel even more. Let's touch base again in a week to see how things are going. Feel free to come to me with any questions or concerns in the meantime."

Peter: "Thank you, Sarah. I appreciate the feedback and will work on prioritizing urgent communications."

Sarah: "Great. Keep up the good work, and let's keep improving together."

3.6 SPOTLIGHT APPLICATION

You are an RN and are reporting to work on a 16-bed medical/renal unit in a county hospital for the 0700 – 1500 shift today. The client population is primarily socioeconomically disadvantaged. Staff for the shift includes four RNs, one LPN/VN, and two UAP.

You are a new RN graduate on the unit, and your orientation was completed two weeks ago. The LPN/VN has been working on the unit for ten years. Both UAP have been on the unit for six months and are certified nursing assistants after completing basic nurse aide training. You, as one of four RNs on the unit, have been assigned four clients. You share the LPN with the other RNs, and there is one UAP for every two RNs.

The charge nurse has assigned you the following four clients. Scheduled morning medications are due at 0800 and all four require some assistance with their ADLs.

- **Client A:** An obese 52-year-old male with hypertension and diabetes requiring insulin therapy. He has been depressed since recently being diagnosed with end-stage renal disease requiring hemodialysis. He needs his morning medications and assistance getting dressed for transport to hemodialysis in 30 minutes.
- **Client B:** A 83-year-old female client with acute pyelonephritis admitted two days ago. She has a PICC line in place and is receiving IV vancomycin every 12 hours. The next dose is due at 0830 after a trough level is drawn.
- **Client C:** A 78-year-old male recently diagnosed with bladder cancer. He has bright red urine today but reports it is painless. He has surgery scheduled at 0900 and the pre-op checklist has not yet been completed.
- **Client D:** A malnourished 80-year-old male client admitted with dehydration and imbalanced electrolyte levels. He is being discharged home today and requires health teaching.

Reflective Questions

1. At the start of the shift, you determine which tasks, cares, activities, and/or procedures you will delegate to the LPN and UAP. What factors must you consider prior to delegation?
2. What tasks will you delegate to the LPN/VN?
3. What tasks will you delegate to the UAP?

3.7 LEARNING ACTIVITIES

Learning Activities

(Answers to "Learning Activities" can be found in the "Answer Key" at the end of the book. Answers to interactive activities are provided as immediate feedback.)

1. Review the following case studies regarding nurse liability associated with inappropriate delegation:

    - Nurse Case Study: Wrongful delegation of patient care to unlicensed assistive personnel
    - Nurse Video Case Study: Failure to assess and monitor

Reflective Questions: What delegation errors occurred in each of these scenarios and what were the repercussions of these errors for the nurses involved?

Access free online learning activities in the online book using this QR code.

2. The RN is delegating tasks to the LPN/VN and UAP on a medical-surgical unit. Using the columns as reference, indicate where delegation errors occurred using the 5 Rs of delegation.

	Right Person	Right Task	Right Circumstance	Right Direction and Communication	Right Supervision and Evaluation
Directs the UAP to assess the pain level of a client who is post-op Day 3 after a hip replacement and report back the finding.					
Directs the LPN to give 1 mg IV push morphine to a client who is 2-hours post total left knee replacement and ensure documentation.					

Assigns the UAP to collect blood pressures on all clients on the unit by 0800. Assumes the UAP will report back any abnormal blood pressures.					
Directs a new UAP to ambulate a client who is post-op Day 2 from a shoulder replacement who needs the assistance of one person and an adaptive walker. The UAP voices concerns about never having used an adaptive walker before. The RN directs the UAP to get another UAP to help.					

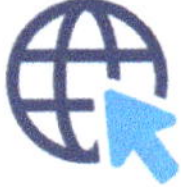

Interactive learning activities have been excluded from the print version of the text. Access free online learning activities in the online book using this QR code.

3.8 GLOSSARY

Accountability: Being answerable to oneself and others for one's own choices, decisions, and actions as measured against a standard.

Assignment: Routine care, activities, and procedures that are within the authorized scope of practice of the RN, LPN/VN, or routine functions of the assistive personnel.

Closed-loop communication: A process that enables the person giving the instructions to hear what they said reflected back and to confirm that their message was, in fact, received correctly.

Constructive feedback: Supportive feedback that offers solutions to areas of weakness.

Delegated responsibility: A nursing activity, skill, or procedure that is transferred from a license nurse to a delegatee.

Delegatee: An RN, LPN/VN, or AP who is delegated a nursing responsibility by either an APRN, RN, or LPN/VN who is competent to perform the task and verbally accepts the responsibility.

Delegation: Allowing a delegatee to perform a specific nursing activity, skill, or procedure that is beyond the delegatee's traditional role but in which they have received additional training.

Delegator: An APRN, RN, or LPN/VN who requests a specially trained delegatee to perform a specific nursing activity, skill, or procedure that is beyond the delegatee's traditional role.

Five rights of delegation: Right task, right circumstance, right person, right directions and communication, and right supervision and evaluation.

Nursing team members: Advanced practice registered nurses (APRN), registered nurses (RN), licensed practical/vocational nurses (LPN/VN), and assistive personnel (AP).

Scope of practice: Procedures, actions, and processes that a health care practitioner is permitted to undertake in keeping with the terms of their professional license.

Supervision: Appropriate monitoring of the delegated activity, evaluation of patient outcomes, and follow-up with the delegatee at the completion of the activity.

Titrate: Making adjustments to medication dosage per an established protocol to obtain a desired therapeutic outcome.

Unlicensed Assistive Personnel (UAP): Any assistive personnel trained to function in a supportive role, regardless of title, to whom a nursing responsibility may be delegated. This includes, but is not limited to, certified nursing assistants or aides (CNAs), patient-care technicians (PCTs), certified medical assistants (CMAs), certified medication aides, and home health aides.[48]

48. American Nurses Association and NCSBN. (2019). *National guidelines for nursing delegation*. https://www.ncsbn.org/NGND-PosPaper_06.pdf

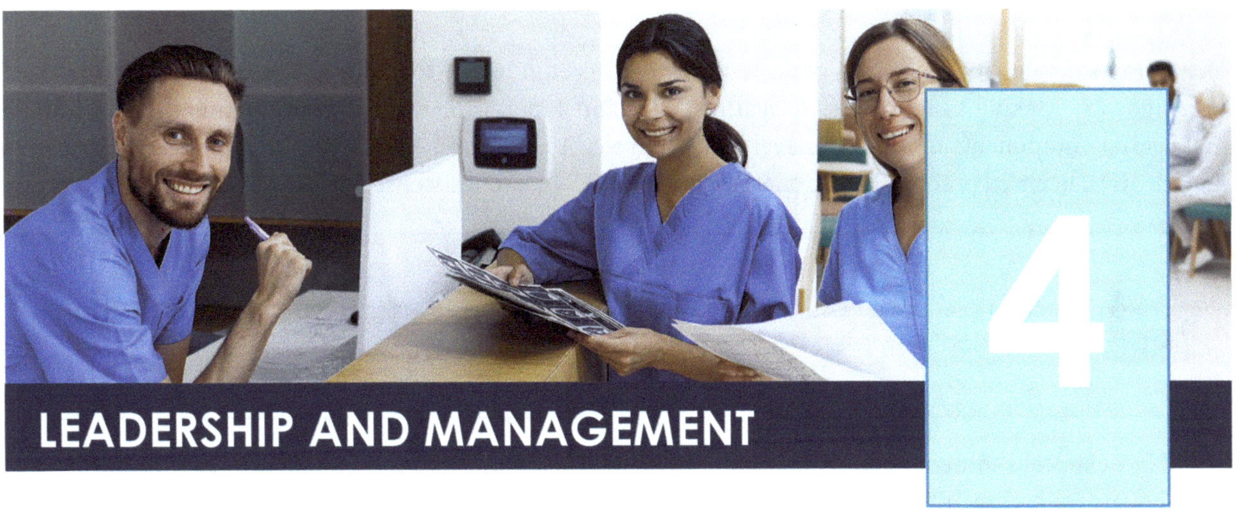

4.1 LEADERSHIP & MANAGEMENT INTRODUCTION

LEARNING OBJECTIVES

- Differentiate the role of leader and manager
- Examine the roles of team members
- Identify steps in the management process and activities that managers perform
- Describe the role of the RN as a leader and change agent
- Discuss effects of power, empowerment, and motivation in leading and managing a nursing team

As a nursing student preparing to graduate, you have spent countless hours on developing clinical skills, analyzing disease processes, creating care plans, and cultivating clinical judgment. In comparison, you have likely spent much less time on developing management and leadership skills. Yet, soon after beginning your first job as a registered nurse, you will become involved in numerous situations requiring nursing leadership and management skills. Some of these situations include the following:

- Prioritizing care for a group of assigned clients
- Collaborating with interprofessional team members regarding client care
- Participating in an interdisciplinary team conference
- Acting as a liaison when establishing community resources for a client being discharged home
- Serving on a unit committee
- Investigating and implementing a new evidence-based best practice
- Mentoring nursing students

Delivering safe, quality client care often requires registered nurses (RN) to manage care provided by the nursing team. Making assignments, delegating tasks, and supervising nursing team members are essential managerial components of an entry-level staff RN role. As previously discussed, nursing team members include RNs, licensed practical/vocational nurses (LPN/VN), and unlicensed assistive personnel (UAP).[1]

Read more about assigning, delegating, and supervising in the "Delegation and Supervision" chapter.

An RN is expected to demonstrate leadership and management skills in many facets of the role. Nurses manage care for high-acuity clients as they are admitted, transferred, and discharged; coordinate care among a variety of diverse health professionals; advocate for clients' needs; and manage limited resources with shrinking budgets.[2]

Read more about collaborating and communicating with the interprofessional team; advocating for clients; and admitting, transferring, and discharging clients in the "Collaboration Within the Interprofessional Team" chapter.

An article published in the *Online Journal of Issues in Nursing* states, "With the growing complexity of health-care practice environments and pending nurse leader retirements, the development of future nurse leaders is increasingly important."[3] This chapter will explore leadership and management responsibilities of an RN. Leadership styles are introduced, and change theories are discussed as a means for implementing change in the health care system.

4.2 BASIC CONCEPTS

Organizational Culture

The formal leaders of an organization provide a sense of direction and overall guidance for their employees by establishing organizational vision, mission, and values statements. An organization's **vision statement** defines why the organization exists, describes how the organization is unique from similar organizations, and specifies what the organization is striving to be. The **mission statement** describes how the organization

1. American Nurses Association & NCSBN. (2019). *National guidelines for nursing delegation.* https://www.ncsbn.org/public-files/NGND-PosPaper_06.pdf
2. Cherry, B., & Jacob, S. R. (2017). Nursing leadership and management. In Cherry, B. & Jacob, S. (Eds.), *Contemporary nursing: Issues, trends, and management* (8th ed.). Elsevier, pp. 294-314.
3. Dyess, S. M., Sherman, R. O., Pratt, B. A., & Chiang-Hanisko, L. (2016). Growing nurse leaders: Their perspectives on nursing leadership and today's practice environment. *OJIN: The Online Journal of Issues in Nursing, 21*(1). https://ojin.nursingworld.org/MainMenuCategories/ANAMarketplace/ANAPeriodicals/OJIN/TableofContents/Vol-21-2016/No1-Jan-2016/Articles-Previous-Topics/Growing-Nurse-Leaders.html

will fulfill its vision and establishes a common course of action for future endeavors. See Figure 4.1[4] for an illustration of a mission statement. A **values statement** establishes the values of an organization that assist with the achievement of its vision and mission. A values statement also provides strategic guidelines for decision-making, both internally and externally, by members of the organization. A values statement may also be reflected as the organization's "**core values**," which are the foundational ideals that guide the organization's actions and decision-making processes. The vision, mission, and values statements are expressed in a concise and clear manner that is easily understood by members of the organization and the public.[5]

Mission Statement
Our company is committed to providing quality
products and unsurpassed customer service

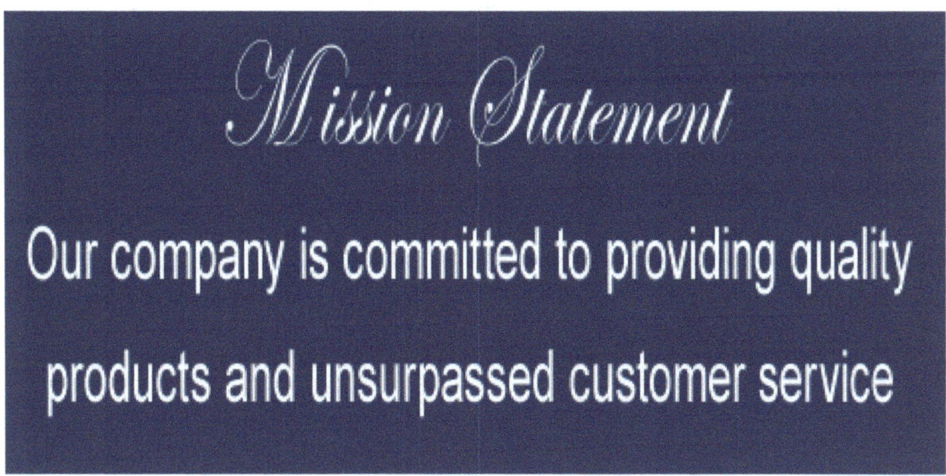

FIGURE 4.1 Mission Statement

Organizational culture refers to the implicit values and beliefs that reflect the norms and traditions of an organization. An organization's vision, mission, and values statements are the foundation of organizational culture. Because individual organizations have their own vision, mission, and values statements, each organization has a different culture.[6] Organizational culture helps reflect the expected norms and behaviors that are inherent to an organization. Expected conduct is comprised of the unwritten rules and standards that reflect how employees should behave in different situations. The culture also informs the common communication styles that are inherent to an organization, including both formal and informal channels. The culture may also be manifested outwardly through various symbols and artifacts that are embedded within the organization. These may include specific logos, objects, or other physical manifestations of elements that represent the organization's culture. Some organizations may also reflect their cultural values through activities or ceremonies held within the community.

As health care continues to evolve and new models of care are introduced, nursing managers must develop innovative approaches that address change while aligning with that organization's vision, mission, and values. Leaders embrace the organization's mission, identify how individuals' work contributes to it, and ensure that outcomes advance the organization's mission and purpose. Leaders use vision, mission, and values

4. "Mission_statement.jpg" by RadioFan (talk) is licensed under CC BY-SA 3.0
5. Wagner, J. (2018). *Leadership and Influencing Change in Nursing.* University of Regina Press. https://leadershipandinfluencingchangeinnursing.pressbooks.com/chapter/chapter-5-providing-nursing-leadership-within-the-health-care-system/
6. Wagner, J. (2018). *Leadership and Influencing Change in Nursing.* University of Regina Press. https://leadershipandinfluencingchangeinnursing.pressbooks.com/chapter/chapter-5-providing-nursing-leadership-within-the-health-care-system/

statements for guidance when determining appropriate responses to critical events and unforeseen challenges that are common in a complex health care system. Successful organizations require employees to be committed to following these strategic guidelines during the course of their work activities. Employees who understand the relationship between their own work and the mission and purpose of the organization will contribute to a stronger health care system that excels in providing quality client care. The vision, mission, and values provide a common organization-wide frame of reference for decision-making for both leaders and staff.[7]

It is important for employees in health care organizations to have an understanding of how their roles and responsibilities connect to the broader mission and vision of the organization. This alignment fosters a cohesive work environment where each staff member is motivated by a shared purpose, leading to more effective and high-quality client care. It is important that both the leader and employee have clarity in the underlying vision, mission, and values of an organization. This involves responsibility for both the leader and employee. Leaders must articulate the organization's vision, mission, and values clearly and consistently. This involves regular communication through meetings, written materials, etc. Employees share in the responsibility by being empowered to ask questions and seek clarification on how their daily tasks contribute to the organization's overarching goals.

Learning Activity

Investigate the mission, vision, and values of a potential employer, as you would do prior to an interview for a job position.

Reflective Questions

1. How well do the organization's vision and values align with your personal values regarding health care?
2. How well does the organization's mission align with your professional objective in your resume?

Followership

Followership is described as the upward influence of individuals on their leaders and their teams. The actions of followers have an important influence on staff performance and client outcomes. Being an effective follower requires individuals to contribute to the team not only by doing as they are told, but also by being aware and raising relevant concerns. Effective followers realize that they can initiate change and disagree or challenge their leaders if they feel their organization or unit is failing to promote wellness and deliver safe, value-driven, and compassionate care. Leaders who gain the trust and dedication of followers are more effective in their leadership role. Everybody has a voice and a responsibility to take ownership of the workplace culture, and good followership contributes to the establishment of high-functioning and safety-conscious teams.[8] Key elements of effective followership include proactive engagement, constructive communication, collaboration, advocacy, continuous improvement, and a supportive leadership environment.

---

7. Wagner, J. (2018). *Leadership and Influencing Change in Nursing.* University of Regina Press. https://leadershipandinfluencingchangeinnursing.pressbooks.com/chapter/chapter-5-providing-nursing-leadership-within-the-health-care-system/
8. Wagner, J. (2018). *Leadership and Influencing Change in Nursing.* University of Regina Press. https://leadershipandinfluencingchangeinnursing.pressbooks.com/chapter/chapter-5-providing-nursing-leadership-within-the-health-care-system/

In order to demonstrate proactive engagement, followers must also be initiators. Effective followers do not passively wait for instruction but rather take initiative to address issues, propose solutions, and contribute to ideas. They recognize the importance of their voice in engaging in problem-solving and understand that being an effective follower does not mean being passive in their role. Effective followers also employ a keen situational awareness where they maintain vigilant assessment of the environment and potential risks, ensuring that they act in the best interests of clients. They must be confident that they can raise concerns if they identify potential problems or unsafe practices. This reflects a culture where followers feel that their feedback is welcomed and valued. Effective followership also involves communication practices in which the message is clearly conveyed, measures to confirm the message are employed, and the confirmation is received. To be an effective follower, support of the team's goals must be a central tenet of one's work. Collaboration with others involves supporting colleagues and working together toward the common goal even when viewpoints may differ. Identifying strategies that create a respectful opportunity to debate and exploring different opinions are important to effective followership. Additionally, followers must take accountability for their own actions while understanding how their role and performance impact the function of the team, as well as client outcomes. Effective followers also practice ethical advocacy, ensuring that the needs of clients are prioritized and respected. This advocacy also involves the ability to courageously challenge any decisions or actions that may jeopardize care or organizational values. Finally, effective followers engage in continuous learning to enhance their skills and knowledge. They seek feedback and use the feedback to contribute to their own performance and also the growth of the team. Effective followership is further cultivated when leaders and followers come together with mutual respect, trust, and work with a purposeful drive toward shared goals that reflect the organization's mission.

Team members impact client safety by following teamwork guidelines for good followership. For example, strategies such as closed-loop communication are important tools to promote client safety.

Read more about communication and teamwork strategies in the "Collaboration Within the Interprofessional Team" chapter.

Leadership and Management Characteristics

Leadership and management are terms often used interchangeably, but they are two different concepts with many overlapping characteristics. **Leadership** is the art of establishing direction and influencing and motivating others to achieve their maximum potential to accomplish tasks, objectives, or projects.[9,10] See Figure 4.2[11] for an illustration of team leadership. There is no universally accepted definition or theory of nursing leadership, but there is increasing clarity about how it differs from management.[12] **Management** refers to

9. Northhouse, P. (2004). *Leadership: Theory and practice* (9th ed.). Sage Publications.

10. Specchia, M. L., Cozzolino, M. R., Carini, E., Di Pilla, A., Galletti, C., Ricciardi, W., & Damiani, G. (2021). Leadership styles and nurses' job satisfaction. Results of a systematic review. *International Journal of Environmental Research and Public Health, 18*(4), 1552. https://doi.org/10.3390/ijerph18041552

11. "3D_Team_Leadership_Arrow_Concept.jpg" by lumaxart is licensed under CC BY-SA 2.0

12. Scully, N. J. (2015). Leadership in nursing: The importance of recognising inherent values and attributes to secure a positive future for the profession. *Collegian, 22*(4), 439-444. https://doi.org/10.1016/j.colegn.2014.09.004

roles that focus on tasks such as planning, organizing, prioritizing, budgeting, staffing, coordinating, and reporting.[13] The overriding function of management has been described as providing order and consistency to organizations, whereas the primary function of leadership is to produce change and movement.[14] View a comparison of the characteristics of management and leadership in Table 4.2a.

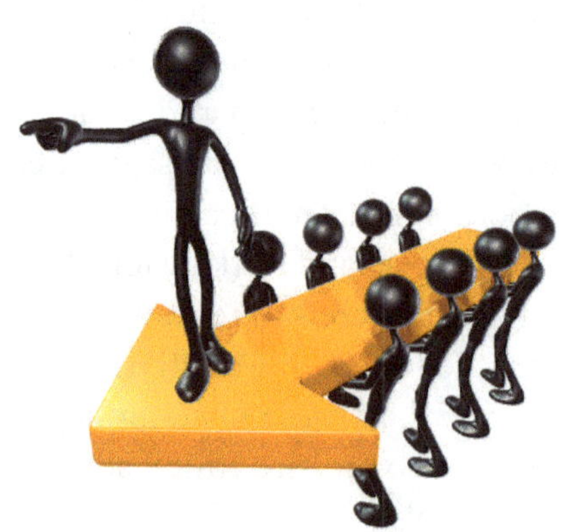

FIGURE 4.2 Leadership

TABLE 4.2A. Management and Leadership Characteristics[15]

MANAGEMENT	LEADERSHIP
Planning, Organizing, and Prioritizing • Establish agenda • Set goals and time frames • Prioritize tasks • Establish policies and procedures	**Establishing Direction** • Create a shared vision • Identify issues requiring change • Set strategies • Implement evidence-based practices
Budgeting and Staffing • Allocate resources • Hire and terminate employees • Make assignments	**Influencing Others** • Listen to team members' concerns • Communicate effectively • Advocate for clients, family members, communities, and the nursing profession • Build effective teamwork
Coordinating and Problem-Solving • Generate solutions • Develop incentives • Take corrective actions • Participate in quality improvement initiatives	**Motivating** • Inspire, energize, and empower team members • Promote professional growth

13. Hannaway, J. (1989). *Managers managing: The workings of an administrative system.* Oxford University Press, p. 39.
14. Northouse, P. (2004). *Leadership: Theory and practice* (9th ed.). Sage Publications.
15. Northouse, P. (2004). *Leadership: Theory and practice* (9th ed.). Sage Publications.

Leader Vs. Manager Case Activity

Utilizing the information from the table above, review the following cases and identify whether the individual is serving as a leader or manager based upon the actions taken within the case scenario. Include supportive rationale for your decision regarding the role.

Case 1: Sima, the head nurse, reviews the upcoming schedule and allocates resources to ensure each shift is adequately staffed. She also makes assignments for the nursing staff based on their skills and client needs. Additionally, she is responsible for hiring new staff and, when necessary, terminating employees who do not meet performance standards.

Case 2: Juan, a senior nurse, is passionate about improving client care. He identifies an issue with the current handoff process between shifts and proposes a new strategy that incorporates evidence-based practices to enhance communication and reduce errors. He reaches out to his team at their monthly department meetings in order to develop a shared vision for this change and encourages them to partner with him on the new process.

Case 3: Maria, a unit supervisor, holds a meeting to set specific goals and time frames for the department's upcoming projects. She prioritizes tasks for the team and establishes policies and procedures to ensure these tasks are completed efficiently and within the given deadlines.

Case 4: Emily, the nurse director, is tasked with preparing the budget for the upcoming fiscal year. She allocates resources effectively to ensure all departments are adequately funded. Emily also manages the staffing needs, ensuring that the hiring and termination processes are handled efficiently.

Case 5: Rachel, an experienced nurse, takes the time to build effective teamwork within her unit. She advocates for her clients, their families, and the nursing profession as a whole. Rachel communicates openly and listens to her team's concerns, ensuring everyone feels valued and heard.

Not all nurses are managers, but all nurses are leaders because they encourage individuals to achieve their goals. The American Nurses Association (ANA) established *Leadership* as a Standard of Professional Performance for all registered nurses. Standards of Professional Performance are "authoritative statements of action and behaviors that all registered nurses, regardless of role, population, specialty, and setting, are expected to perform competently."[16] See the competencies of the ANA *Leadership* standard in the following box and additional content in other chapters of this book.

16. American Nurses Association. (2021). *Nursing: Scope and standards of practice* (4th ed.). American Nurses Association.

Competencies of ANA's Leadership Standard of Professional Performance

- Promotes effective relationships to achieve quality outcomes and a culture of safety
- Leads decision-making groups
- Engages in creating an interprofessional environment that promotes respect, trust, and integrity
- Embraces practice innovations and role performance to achieve lifelong personal and professional goals
- Communicates to lead change, influence others, and resolve conflict
- Implements evidence-based practices for safe, quality health care and health care consumer satisfaction
- Demonstrates authority, ownership, accountability, and responsibility for appropriate delegation of nursing care
- Mentors colleagues and others to embrace their knowledge, skills, and abilities
- Participates in professional activities and organizations for professional growth and influence
- Advocates for all aspects of human and environmental health in practice and policy

Read additional content related to leadership and management activities in corresponding chapters of this book:

- Read about the culture of safety in the "Legal Implications" chapter.
- Read about effective interprofessional teamwork and resolving conflict in the "Collaboration Within the Interprofessional Team" chapter.
- Read about quality improvement and implementing evidence-based practices in the "Quality and Evidence-Based Practice" chapter.
- Read more about delegation, supervision, and accountability in the "Delegation and Supervision" chapter.
- Read about professional organizations and advocating for clients, communities, and their environments in the "Advocacy" chapter.
- Read about budgets and staffing in the "Health Care Economics" chapter.
- Read about prioritization in the "Prioritization" chapter.

Leadership Theories and Styles

In the 1930s Kurt Lewin, the father of social psychology, originally identified three leadership styles: authoritarian, democratic, and laissez-faire.[17,18]

17. Carlin, D. (2019). Democratic, authoritarian, laissez-faire: What type of leader are you? *Forbes*. https://www.forbes.com/sites/davidcarlin/2019/10/18/democratic-authoritarian-laissez-faire-what-type-of-leader-are-you/?sh=618359422a6b

18. Lewin, K., Lippitt, R., & White, R. K. (1939). Patterns of aggressive behavior in experimentally created "social climates." *Journal of Social Psychology, 10*(2), 271-301. https://doi.org/10.1080/00224545.1939.9713366

Authoritarian leadership means the leader has full power. Authoritarian leaders tell team members what to do and expect team members to execute their plans. When fast decisions must be made in emergency situations, such as when a client "codes," the authoritarian leader makes quick decisions and provides the group with direct instructions. However, there are disadvantages to authoritarian leadership. Authoritarian leaders are more likely to disregard creative ideas of other team members, causing resentment and stress.[19]

Democratic leadership balances decision-making responsibility between team members and the leader. Democratic leaders actively participate in discussions, but also make sure to listen to the views of others. For example, a nurse supervisor may hold a meeting regarding an increased incidence of client falls on the unit and ask team members to share their observations regarding causes and potential solutions. The democratic leadership style often leads to positive, inclusive, and collaborative work environments that encourage team members' creativity. Under this style, the leader still retains responsibility for the final decision.[20]

Laissez-faire is a French word that translates to English as, "leave alone." Laissez-faire leadership gives team members total freedom to perform as they please. Laissez-faire leaders do not participate in decision-making processes and rarely offer opinions. The laissez-faire leadership style can work well if team members are highly skilled and highly motivated to perform quality work. However, without the leader's input, conflict and a culture of blame may occur as team members disagree on roles, responsibilities, and policies. By not contributing to the decision-making process, the leader forfeits control of team performance.[21]

Over the decades, Lewin's original leadership styles have evolved into many styles of leadership in health care, such as passive-avoidant, transactional, transformational, servant, resonant, and authentic.[22,23] Many of these leadership styles have overlapping characteristics. See Figure 4.3[24] for a comparison of various leadership styles in terms of engagement.

Effort
Energy needed from leader
Transformational leadership
Motivate and empower others
Transactional leadership
Command and incentivize
Laissez faire leadership
Free agent/ market behavior
Engagement
Extent to which leader changes attitudes and behaviours of others

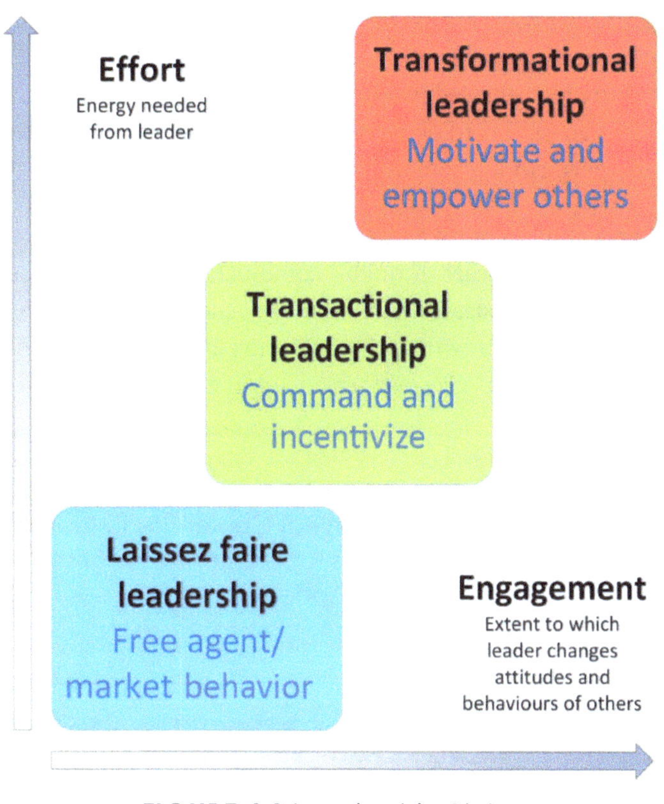

FIGURE 4.3 Leadership Styles

19. Carlin, D. (2019). Democratic, authoritarian, laissez-faire: What type of leader are you? *Forbes*. https://www.forbes.com/sites/davidcarlin/2019/10/18/democratic-authoritarian-laissez-faire-what-type-of-leader-are-you/?sh=618359422a6b

20. Carlin, D. (2019). Democratic, authoritarian, laissez-faire: What type of leader are you? *Forbes*. https://www.forbes.com/sites/davidcarlin/2019/10/18/democratic-authoritarian-laissez-faire-what-type-of-leader-are-you/?sh=618359422a6b

21. Carlin, D. (2019). Democratic, authoritarian, laissez-faire: What type of leader are you? *Forbes*. https://www.forbes.com/sites/davidcarlin/2019/10/18/democratic-authoritarian-laissez-faire-what-type-of-leader-are-you/?sh=618359422a6b

22. Northouse, P. (2004). *Leadership: Theory and practice* (9th ed.). Sage Publications.

23. Specchia, M. L., Cozzolino, M. R., Carini, E., Di Pilla, A., Galletti, C., Ricciardi, W., & Damiani, G. (2021). Leadership styles and nurses' job satisfaction. Results of a systematic review. *International Journal of Environmental Research and Public Health, 18*(4), 1552. https://doi.org/10.3390/ijerph18041552

24. "Full_Range_Leadership_model.jpg" by John Pons is licensed under Public Domain, CC0

Passive-avoidant leadership is similar to laissez-faire leadership and is characterized by a leader who avoids taking responsibility and confronting others. Employees perceive the lack of control over the environment resulting from the absence of clear directives. Organizations with this type of leader have high staff turnover and low retention of employees. These types of leaders tend to react and take corrective action only after problems have become serious and often avoid making any decisions at all.[25]

Transactional leadership involves both the leader and the follower receiving something for their efforts; the leader gets the job done and the follower receives pay, recognition, rewards, or punishment based on how well they perform the tasks assigned to them.[26] Staff generally work independently with no focus on cooperation among employees or commitment to the organization.[27]

Transformational leadership involves leaders motivating followers to perform beyond expectations by creating a sense of ownership in reaching a shared vision.[28] It is characterized by a leader's charismatic influence over team members and includes effective communication, valued relationships, and consideration of team member input. Transformational leaders know how to convey a sense of loyalty through shared goals, resulting in increased productivity, improved morale, and increased employees' job satisfaction.[29] They often motivate others to do more than originally intended by inspiring them to look past individual self-interest and perform to promote team and organizational interests.[30]

Servant leadership focuses on the professional growth of employees while simultaneously promoting improved quality care through a combination of interprofessional teamwork and shared decision-making. Servant leaders assist team members to achieve their personal goals by listening with empathy and committing to individual growth and community-building. They share power, put the needs of others first, and help individuals optimize performance while forsaking their own personal advancement and rewards.[31]

Visit the Greenleaf Center site to learn more about servant leadership. Access supplementary digital content in the online book using this QR code.

25. Specchia, M. L., Cozzolino, M. R., Carini, E., Di Pilla, A., Galletti, C., Ricciardi, W., & Damiani, G. (2021). Leadership styles and nurses' job satisfaction. Results of a systematic review. *International Journal of Environmental Research and Public Health, 18*(4), 1552. https://doi.org/10.3390/ijerph18041552
26. Northouse, P. (2004). *Leadership: Theory and practice* (9th ed.). Sage Publications.
27. Specchia, M. L., Cozzolino, M. R., Carini, E., Di Pilla, A., Galletti, C., Ricciardi, W., & Damiani, G. (2021). Leadership styles and nurses' job satisfaction. Results of a systematic review. *International Journal of Environmental Research and Public Health, 18*(4), 1552. https://doi.org/10.3390/ijerph18041552
28. Northouse, P. (2004). *Leadership: Theory and practice* (9th ed.). Sage Publications.
29. Specchia, M. L., Cozzolino, M. R., Carini, E., Di Pilla, A., Galletti, C., Ricciardi, W., & Damiani, G. (2021). Leadership styles and nurses' job satisfaction. Results of a systematic review. *International Journal of Environmental Research and Public Health, 18*(4), 1552. https://doi.org/10.3390/ijerph18041552
30. Specchia, M. L., Cozzolino, M. R., Carini, E., Di Pilla, A., Galletti, C., Ricciardi, W., & Damiani, G. (2021). Leadership styles and nurses' job satisfaction. Results of a systematic review. *International Journal of Environmental Research and Public Health, 18*(4), 1552. https://doi.org/10.3390/ijerph18041552
31. Specchia, M. L., Cozzolino, M. R., Carini, E., Di Pilla, A., Galletti, C., Ricciardi, W., & Damiani, G. (2021). Leadership styles and nurses' job satisfaction. Results of a systematic review. *International Journal of Environmental Research and Public Health, 18*(4), 1552. https://doi.org/10.3390/ijerph18041552

Resonant leaders are in tune with the emotions of those around them, use empathy, and manage their own emotions effectively. Resonant leaders build strong, trusting relationships and create a climate of optimism that inspires commitment even in the face of adversity. They create an environment where employees are highly engaged, making them willing and able to contribute with their full potential.[32]

Authentic leaders have an honest and direct approach with employees, demonstrating self-awareness, internalized moral perspective, and relationship transparency. They strive for trusting, symmetrical, and close leader–follower relationships; promote the open sharing of information; and consider others' viewpoints.[33]

TABLE 4.2B. Characteristics of Leadership Styles

Authoritarian	Democratic	Laissez-Faire or Passive-Avoidant
• Demonstrate centralized decision-making • Use power to control others • Motivate through fear or reward • Disregard needs of group members	• Demonstrate participatory decision-making • Display multidirectional communication • Build close, personal relationships • Encourage goal attainment	• Demonstrate passive, permissive, or absent decision-making

Transactional	Transformational	Servant
• Promote both parties receiving something for efforts • Motivate with external rewards • Reward good performance and penalize low performance • Do not focus on team cooperation or commitment to the organization	• Create ownership with shared, inspiring vision • Demonstrate effective communication • Value relationships • Consider individuals' needs and abilities	• Focus on growth and well-being of team members • Share in decision-making • Develop team members to their highest potential

32. Specchia, M. L., Cozzolino, M. R., Carini, E., Di Pilla, A., Galletti, C., Ricciardi, W., & Damiani, G. (2021). Leadership styles and nurses' job satisfaction. Results of a systematic review. *International Journal of Environmental Research and Public Health, 18*(4), 1552. https://doi.org/10.3390/ijerph18041552

33. Specchia, M. L., Cozzolino, M. R., Carini, E., Di Pilla, A., Galletti, C., Ricciardi, W., & Damiani, G. (2021). Leadership styles and nurses' job satisfaction. Results of a systematic review. *International Journal of Environmental Research and Public Health, 18*(4), 1552. https://doi.org/10.3390/ijerph18041552

TABLE 4.2B. Continued...

Resonant Leaders	Authentic Leaders
• Build strong, trusting relationships • Tune into the emotions of those around them, use empathy, and manage their own emotions effectively • Create a climate of optimism	• Use an honest and direct approach • Develop close leader–follower relationships • Promote the open sharing of information • Consider others' viewpoints

Outcomes of Various Leadership Styles

Leadership styles affect team members, client outcomes, and the organization. A systematic review of the literature published in 2021 showed significant correlations between leadership styles and nurses' job satisfaction. Transformational leadership style had the greatest positive correlation with nurses' job satisfaction, followed by authentic, resonant, and servant leadership styles. Passive-avoidant and laissez-faire leadership styles showed a negative correlation with nurses' job satisfaction.[34] In this challenging health care environment, managers and nurse leaders must promote technical and professional competencies of their staff, but they must also act to improve staff satisfaction and morale by using appropriate leadership styles with their team.[35]

Systems Theory

Systems theory is based on the concept that systems do not function in isolation but rather there is an interdependence that exists between their parts. Systems theory assumes that most individuals strive to do good work but are affected by diverse influences within the system. Efficient and functional systems account for these diverse influences and improve outcomes by studying patterns and behaviors across the system.[36]

Many health care agencies have adopted a culture of safety based on systems theory. A **culture of safety** is an organizational culture that embraces error reporting by employees with the goal of identifying systemic causes of problems that can be addressed to improve client safety. According to The Joint Commission, a culture of safety includes the following components[37]:

- **Just Culture:** A culture where people feel safe raising questions and concerns and report safety events in an environment that emphasizes a nonpunitive response to errors and near misses. Clear lines are drawn by managers between human error, at-risk, and reckless employee behaviors. See Figure 4.4[38] for an illustration of Just Culture.

34. Specchia, M. L., Cozzolino, M. R., Carini, E., Di Pilla, A., Galletti, C., Ricciardi, W., & Damiani, G. (2021). Leadership styles and nurses' job satisfaction. Results of a systematic review. *International Journal of Environmental Research and Public Health, 18*(4), 1552. https://doi.org/10.3390/ijerph18041552
35. Specchia, M. L., Cozzolino, M. R., Carini, E., Di Pilla, A., Galletti, C., Ricciardi, W., & Damiani, G. (2021). Leadership styles and nurses' job satisfaction. Results of a systematic review. *International Journal of Environmental Research and Public Health, 18*(4), 1552. https://doi.org/10.3390/ijerph18041552
36. Anderson, B. R. (2016). Improving health care by embracing systems theory. *The Journal of Thoracic and Cardiovascular Surgery, 152*(2), 593-594. https://www.jtcvs.org/article/S0022-5223(16)30001-0/pdf
37. The Joint Commission. (2017). The essential role of leadership in developing a safety culture. *Sentinel Event Alert,* Issue 57. https://www.jointcommission.org/-/media/tjc/documents/resources/patient-safety-topics/sentinel-event/sea_57_safety_culture_leadership_0317pdf.pdf
38. "Just Culture Infographic.png" by Valeria Palarski 2020. Used with permission.

- **Reporting Culture:** People realize errors are inevitable and are encouraged to speak up for client safety by reporting errors and near misses. For example, nurses complete an "incident report" according to agency policy when a medication error occurs, or a client falls. Error reporting helps the agency manage risk and reduce potential liability.
- **Learning Culture:** People regularly collect information and learn from errors and successes while openly sharing data and information and applying best evidence to improve work processes and client outcomes.

Just Culture

The American Nurses Association (ANA) officially endorses the Just Culture model. In 2019 the ANA published a position statement on Just Culture, stating, "Traditionally, healthcare's culture has held individuals accountable for all errors or mishaps that befall clients under their care. By contrast, a Just Culture recognizes that individual practitioners should not be held accountable for system failings over which they have no control. A Just Culture also recognizes many individual or 'active' errors represent predictable interactions between human operators and the systems in which they work. However, in contrast to a culture that touts 'no blame' as its governing principle, a Just Culture does not tolerate conscious disregard of clear risks to clients or gross misconduct (e.g., falsifying a record or performing professional duties while intoxicated)."

The Just Culture model categorizes human behavior into three causes of errors. Consequences of errors are based on whether the error is a simple human error or caused by at-risk or reckless behavior.

- **Simple human error:** A simple human error occurs when an individual inadvertently does something other than what should have been done. Most medical errors are the result of human error due to poor processes, programs, education, environmental issues, or situations. These errors are managed by correcting the cause, looking at the process, and fixing the deviation. For example, a nurse appropriately checks the rights of medication administration three times, but due to the similar appearance and names of two different medications stored next to each other in the medication dispensing system, administers the incorrect medication to a client. In this example, a root cause analysis reveals a system issue that must be modified to prevent future client errors (e.g., change the labelling and storage of look alike-sound alike medication).
- **At-risk behavior:** An error due to at-risk behavior occurs when a behavioral choice is made that increases risk where the risk is not recognized or is mistakenly believed to be justified. For example, a nurse scans a client's medication with a barcode scanner prior to administration, but an error message appears on the scanner. The nurse mistakenly interprets the error to be a technology problem and proceeds to administer the medication instead of stopping the process and further investigating the error message, resulting in the wrong dosage of a medication being administered to the client. In this case, ignoring the error message on the scanner can be considered "at-risk behavior" because the behavioral choice was considered justified by the nurse at the time.
- **Reckless behavior:** Reckless behavior is an error that occurs when an action is taken with conscious disregard for a substantial and unjustifiable risk.[39] For example, a nurse arrives at work intoxicated and administers the wrong medication to the wrong client. This error is considered due to reckless behavior because the decision to arrive intoxicated was made with conscious disregard for substantial risk.

39. American Nursing Association. (2010). *Position statement: Just culture.* https://www.nursingworld.org/~4afe07/globalassets/practiceandpolicy/health-and-safety/just_culture.pdf

These examples show three different causes of medication errors that would result in different consequences to the employee based on the Just Culture model. Under the Just Culture model, after root cause analysis is completed, system-wide changes are made to decrease factors that contributed to the error. Managers appropriately hold individuals accountable for errors if they were due to simple human error, at-risk behavior, or reckless behaviors.

If an individual commits a simple human error, managers console the individual and consider changes in training, procedures, and processes. In the "simple human error" above, system-wide changes would be made to change the label and location of the medication to prevent future errors from occurring with the same medication.

Individuals committing at-risk behavior are held accountable for their behavioral choice and often require coaching with incentives for less risky behaviors and situational awareness. In the "at-risk behavior" example above where the nurse ignored an error message on the barcode scanner, mandatory training on using a barcode scanner and responding to errors would be implemented, and the manager would track the employee's correct usage of the barcode scanner for several months following training.

If an individual demonstrates reckless behavior, remedial action and/or punitive action is taken.[40] In the "reckless behavior" example above, the manager would report the nurse's behavior to the state's Board of Nursing with mandatory substance abuse counseling to maintain their nursing license. Employment may be terminated with consideration of patterns of behavior.

A Just Culture in which employees aren't afraid to report errors is a highly successful way to enhance client safety, increase staff and client satisfaction, and improve outcomes. Success is achieved through good communication, effective management of resources, and an openness to changing processes to ensure the safety of clients and employees. The infographic in Figure 4.4[41] illustrates the components of a culture of safety and Just Culture.

The principles of culture of safety, including Just Culture, Reporting Culture, and Learning Culture are also being adopted in nursing education. It's understood that mistakes are part of learning and that a shared accountability model promotes individual- and system-level learning for improved client safety. Under a shared accountability model, students are responsible for the following[42]:

- Being fully prepared for clinical experiences, including laboratory and simulation assignments
- Being rested and mentally ready for a challenging learning environment
- Accepting accountability for their part in contributing to a safe learning environment
- Behaving professionally
- Reporting their own errors and near mistakes
- Keeping up-to-date with current evidence-based practice
- Adhering to ethical and legal standards

40. American Nursing Association. (2010). *Position statement: Just culture.* https://www.nursingworld.org/~4afe07/globalassets/practiceandpolicy/health-and-safety/just_culture.pdf
41. "Just Culture Infographic.png" by Valeria Palarski 2020. Used with permission.
42. Barnsteiner, J., & Disch, J. (2017). Creating a fair and just culture in schools of nursing. *American Journal of Nursing, 117*(11), 42-48. https://doi.org/10.1097/01.NAJ.0000526747.84173.97.

Just Culture
investigate for safety
respect others
flatten hierarchies
embrace different perspectives
champion innovation
be fair
be consistent
seek improvement
welcome challenge
E=MC²
strive for learning
be kind
trust
encourage curiosity
be transparent
embrace different perspectives

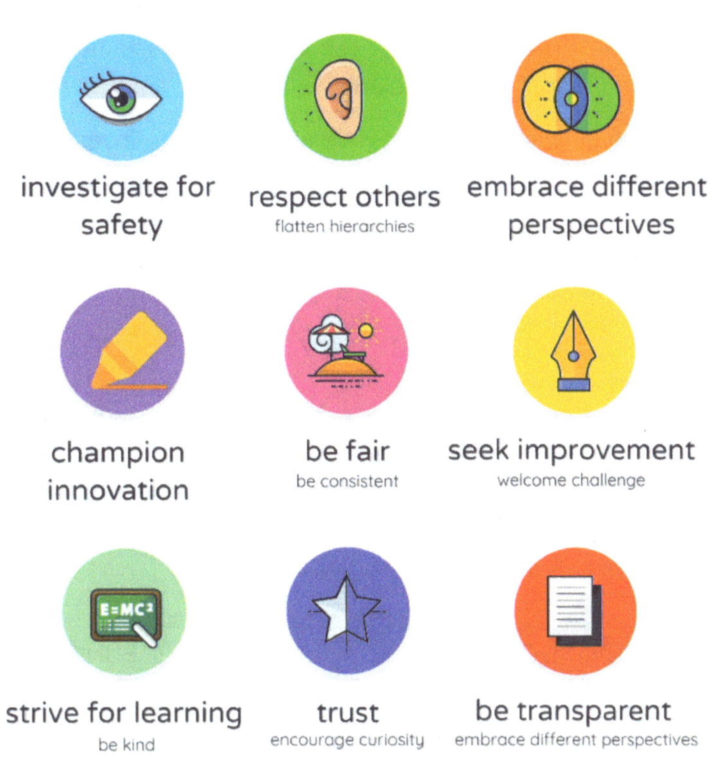

FIGURE 4.4 Just Culture. Used with permission.

Students know they will be held accountable for their actions but will not be blamed for system faults that lie beyond their control. They can trust that a fair process will be used to determine what went wrong if a client care error or near miss occurs. Student errors and near misses are addressed based on an investigation determining if it was simple human error, an at-risk behavior, or reckless behavior. For example, a simple human error by a student can be addressed with coaching and additional learning opportunities to remedy the knowledge deficit. However, if a student acts with recklessness (for example, repeatedly arrives to clinical unprepared despite previous faculty feedback or falsely documents an assessment or procedure), they are appropriately and fairly disciplined, which may include dismissal from the program.[43]

See Table 4.2c describing classifications of errors using the Just Culture model.

43. Barnsteiner, J., & Disch, J. (2017). Creating a fair and just culture in schools of nursing. *American Journal of Nursing, 117*(11), 42-48. https://doi.org/10.1097/01.NAJ.0000526747.84173.97.

TABLE 4.2C. Classification of Errors Using the Just Culture Model

Human Error	At-Risk Behavior	Reckless Behavior
The caregiver made an error while working appropriately and focusing on the client's best interests.	The caregiver made a potentially unsafe choice resulting from faulty or self-serving decision-making.	The caregiver knowingly violated a rule and/or made a dangerous or unsafe choice.
Investigation reveals system factors contributing to similar errors by others with similar knowledge and skills.	Investigation reveals the system supports risky action and the caregiver requires coaching.	Investigation reveals the caregiver is accountable and needs retraining.
Manage by fixing system errors in processes, procedures, training, design, or environment.	Manage by coaching the caregiver and fixing any system issues: • Remove incentives for at-risk behaviors • Create incentives for safe behaviors • Increase situational awareness	Manage by disciplining the caregiver. If the system supports reckless behavior, it requires fixing.
CONSOLE	COACH	PUNISH

Systems leadership refers to a set of skills used to catalyze, enable, and support the process of systems-level change that is encouraged by the Just Culture model. Systems leadership is comprised of three interconnected elements:[44]

- **The Individual:** The skills of collaborative leadership to enable learning, trust-building, and empowered action among stakeholders who share a common goal
- **The Community:** The tactics of coalition building and advocacy to develop alignment and mobilize action among stakeholders in the system, both within and between organizations
- **The System:** An understanding of the complex systems shaping the challenge to be addressed

Just Culture Cases

Review the following case descriptions. Identify the classification of error that has occurred and the recommended actions that should occur.

A chief nursing officer receives a daily report of organization incident reports and reviews the following incident:

44. Dreier, L., Nabarro, D., & Nelson, J. (2019). *Systems leadership for sustainable development: Strategies for achieving system change.* CR Initiative at Harvard Kennedy School. https://www.hks.harvard.edu/sites/default/files/centers/mrcbg/files/Systems%20Leadership.pdf

Incident Description

Client Mr. Joe Doden, Room 13067, Medical-Surgical floor

On the afternoon of May 15, 2024, Nurse Sarah was responsible for administering Mr. Joe Doden's insulin dose. The insulin vials used by the hospital had recently been redesigned by the manufacturer, which led to changes in the labeling. The client was scheduled to receive ten units of regular insulin at 14:30. However, at 1450 the client turns on his call light, reports feeling unwell. He is shaky, confused, and sweating profusely. The client's glucose is checked, and he is found to be hypoglycemic. He is treated based upon the hypoglycemia protocol and recovers without further complication.

Case Investigation A

Action: Sarah RN who administered the insulin was following the protocol but mistakenly read the dosage due to a poorly designed label on the insulin vial. The nurse was focused on the client's best interests and followed all required steps.

Findings: The investigation revealed that the labeling on the insulin vials was confusing and had led to similar errors by other nurses in the past. The system's design flaw contributed significantly to the error.

Question A: How would you classify this error? What actions should be taken?

Case Investigation B

Action: Sarah RN, due to time pressure and a high client load, decided to skip the double-check protocol for administering the same insulin dose, believing it would save time without causing harm.

Findings: The investigation revealed that the hospital's workload and time pressures often led to shortcuts in following safety protocols.

Question B: How would you classify this error? What actions should be taken?

Case Investigation C

Action: Sarah RN is familiar with the protocol and knowingly bypassed the double-check system, dismissing its importance and administering a medication dose on her own.

Findings: The investigation found that the nurse had a history of disregarding safety protocols, showing a pattern of reckless behavior. This behavior was not supported by the hospital's policies or environment.

Question C: How would you classify this error? What actions should be taken?

4.3 IMPLEMENTING CHANGE

Change is constant in the health care environment. **Change** is defined as the process of altering or replacing existing knowledge, skills, attitudes, systems, policies, or procedures.[45] The outcomes of change must be consistent with an organization's mission, vision, and values. Although change is a dynamic process that requires alterations in behavior and can cause conflict and resistance, change can also stimulate positive behaviors and attitudes and improve organizational outcomes and employee performance. Change can result from identified problems or from the incorporation of new knowledge, technology, management, or leadership. Problems may be identified from many sources, such as quality improvement initiatives, employee performance evaluations, or accreditation survey results.[46]

Nurse managers must deal with the fears and concerns triggered by change. They should recognize that change may not be easy and may be met with enthusiasm by some and resistance by others. Leaders should identify individuals who will be enthusiastic about the change (referred to as "early adopters"), as well as those who will be resisters (referred to as "laggers"). Early adopters should be involved to build momentum, and the concerns of resisters should be considered to identify barriers. Data should be collected, analyzed, and communicated so the need for change (and its projected consequences) can be clearly articulated. Managers should articulate the reasons for change, the way(s) the change will affect employees, the way(s) the change will benefit the organization, and the desired outcomes of the change process.[47] See Figure 4.5[48] for an illustration of communicating upcoming change.

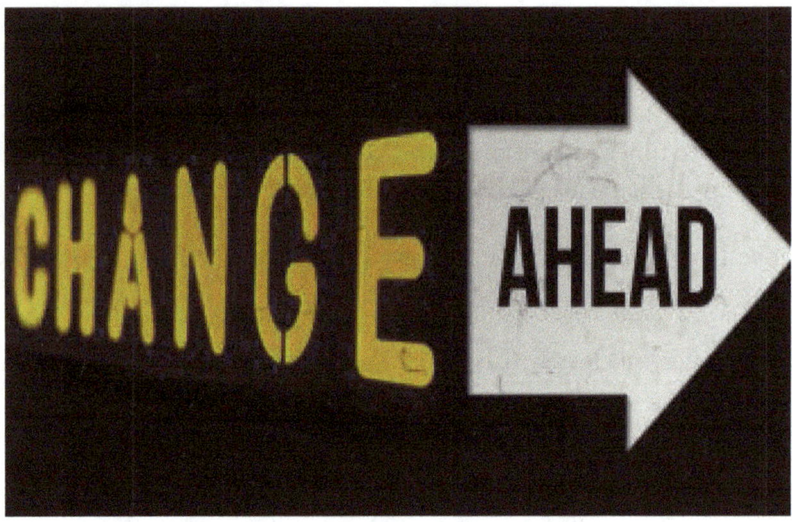

FIGURE 4.5 Identifying Upcoming Change

45. Ana, B. H., & Hendricks-Jackson, L. (2017). *Nursing professional development review and resource manual* (4th ed.). American Nurses Association, Nursing Knowledge Center. https://www.nursingworld.org/~49379b/globalassets/catalog/sample-chapters/npdsamplechapter.pdf
46. Ana, B. H., & Hendricks-Jackson, L. (2017). *Nursing professional development review and resource manual* (4th ed.). American Nurses Association, Nursing Knowledge Center. https://www.nursingworld.org/~49379b/globalassets/catalog/sample-chapters/npdsamplechapter.pdf
47. Ana, B. H., & Hendricks-Jackson, L. (2017). *Nursing professional development review and resource manual* (4th ed.). American Nurses Association, Nursing Knowledge Center. https://www.nursingworld.org/~49379b/globalassets/catalog/sample-chapters/npdsamplechapter.pdf
48. "Change-1080x675.jpg" by Amman Wahab Nizamani is licensed under CC BY-SA 4.0

Change Theories

There are several change theories that nurse leaders may adopt when implementing change. Two traditional change theories are known as Lewin's Unfreeze-Change-Refreeze Model and Lippitt's Seven-Step Change Theory.[49]

Lewin's Change Model

Kurt Lewin, the father of social psychology, introduced the classic three-step model of change known as Unfreeze-Change-Refreeze Model that requires prior learning to be rejected and replaced. Lewin's model has three major concepts: driving forces, restraining forces, and equilibrium. Driving forces are those that push in a direction and cause change to occur. They facilitate change because they push the person in a desired direction. They cause a shift in the equilibrium towards change. Restraining forces are those forces that counter the driving forces. They hinder change because they push the person in the opposite direction. They cause a shift in the equilibrium that opposes change. Equilibrium is a state of being where driving forces equal restraining forces, and no change occurs. It can be raised or lowered by changes that occur between the driving and restraining forces.[50,51]

- **Step 1: Unfreeze the status quo.** Unfreezing is the process of altering behavior to agitate the equilibrium of the current state. This step is necessary if resistance is to be overcome and conformity achieved. Unfreezing can be achieved by increasing the driving forces that direct behavior away from the existing situation or status quo while decreasing the restraining forces that negatively affect the movement from the existing equilibrium. Nurse leaders can initiate activities that can assist in the unfreezing step, such as motivating participants by preparing them for change, building trust and recognition for the need to change, and encouraging active participation in recognizing problems and brainstorming solutions within a group.[52]
- **Step 2: Change.** Change is the process of moving to a new equilibrium. Nurse leaders can implement actions that assist in movement to a new equilibrium by persuading employees to agree that the status quo is not beneficial to them; encouraging them to view the problem from a fresh perspective; working together to search for new, relevant information; and connecting the views of the group to well-respected, powerful leaders who also support the change.[53]
- **Step 3: Refreeze.** Refreezing refers to attaining equilibrium with the newly desired behaviors. This step must take place after the change has been implemented for it to be sustained over time. If this step does not occur, it is very likely the change will be short-lived and employees will revert to the old equilibrium. Refreezing integrates new values into community values and traditions. Nursing leaders can reinforce new patterns of behavior and institutionalize them by adopting new policies and procedures.[54]

---

49. Ana, B. H., & Hendricks-Jackson, L. (2017). *Nursing professional development review and resource manual* (4th ed.). American Nurses Association, Nursing Knowledge Center. https://www.nursingworld.org/~49379b/globalassets/catalog/sample-chapters/npdsamplechapter.pdf
50. Ana, B. H., & Hendricks-Jackson, L. (2017). *Nursing professional development review and resource manual* (4th ed.). American Nurses Association, Nursing Knowledge Center. https://www.nursingworld.org/~49379b/globalassets/catalog/sample-chapters/npdsamplechapter.pdf
51. Nursing Theory. (2023). *Lewin's change theory.* https://nursing-theory.org/theories-and-models/lewin-change-theory.php
52. Kritsonis, A. (2005). Comparison of change theories. *International Journal of Scholarly Academic Intellectual Diversity, 8*(1). https://globalioc.com/wp-content/uploads/2018/09/Kritsonis-Alicia-Comparison-of-Change-Theories.pdf
53. Kritsonis, A. (2005). Comparison of change theories. *International Journal of Scholarly Academic Intellectual Diversity, 8*(1). https://globalioc.com/wp-content/uploads/2018/09/Kritsonis-Alicia-Comparison-of-Change-Theories.pdf
54. Kritsonis, A. (2005). Comparison of change theories. *International Journal of Scholarly Academic Intellectual Diversity, 8*(1). https://globalioc.com/wp-content/uploads/2018/09/Kritsonis-Alicia-Comparison-of-Change-Theories.pdf

EXAMPLE USING LEWIN'S CHANGE THEORY

A new nurse working in a rural medical-surgical unit identifies that bedside handoff reports are not currently being used during shift reports.

Step 1: Unfreeze: The new nurse recognizes a change is needed for improved client safety and discusses the concern with the nurse manager. Current evidence-based practice is shared regarding bedside handoff reports between shifts for client safety.[55] The nurse manager initiates activities such as scheduling unit meetings to discuss evidence-based practice and the need to incorporate bedside handoff reports.

Step 2: Change: The nurse manager gains support from the director of nursing to implement organizational change and plans staff education about bedside report checklists and the manner in which they are performed.

Step 3: Refreeze: The nurse manager adopts bedside handoff reports in a new unit policy and monitors staff for effectiveness.

LIPPITT'S SEVEN-STEP CHANGE THEORY

Lippitt's Seven-Step Change Theory expands on Lewin's change theory by focusing on the role of the change agent. A **change agent** is anyone who has the skill and power to stimulate, facilitate, and coordinate the change effort. Change agents can be internal, such as nurse managers or employees appointed to oversee the change process, or external, such as an outside consulting firm. External change agents are not bound by organizational culture, politics, or traditions, so they bring a different perspective to the situation and challenge the status quo. However, this can also be a disadvantage because external change agents lack an understanding of the agency's history, operating procedures, and personnel.[56] The seven-step model includes the following steps[57]:

- **Step 1: Diagnose the problem.** Examine possible consequences, determine who will be affected by the change, identify essential management personnel who will be responsible for fixing the problem, collect data from those who will be affected by the change, and ensure those affected by the change will be committed to its success.
- **Step 2: Evaluate motivation and capability for change.** Identify financial and human resources capacity and organizational structure.
- **Step 3: Assess the change agent's motivation and resources, experience, stamina, and dedication.**

55. Agency for Healthcare Research and Quality. (2010). *Bedside shift report checklist.* https://www.ahrq.gov/sites/default/files/wysiwyg/professionals/systems/hospital/engagingfamilies/strategy3/Strat3_Tool_2_Nurse_Chklst_508.pdf
56. Lunenburg, F. C. (2010). Managing change: The role of the change agent. *International Journal of Management, Business, and Administration, 13*(1). https://naaee.org/sites/default/files/lunenburg_fred_c._managing_change_the_role_of_change_agent_ijmba_v13_n1_2010.pdf
57. Ana, B. H., & Hendricks-Jackson, L. (2017). *Nursing professional development review and resource manual* (4th ed.). American Nurses Association, Nursing Knowledge Center. https://www.nursingworld.org/~49379b/globalassets/catalog/sample-chapters/npdsamplechapter.pdf

- **Step 4: Select progressive change objectives.** Define the change process and develop action plans and accompanying strategies.
- **Step 5: Explain the role of the change agent to all employees and ensure the expectations are clear.**
- **Step 6: Maintain change.** Facilitate feedback, enhance communication, and coordinate the effects of change.
- **Step 7: Gradually terminate the helping relationship of the change agent.**

Example Using Lippitt's Seven-Step Change Theory

Refer to the previous example of using Lewin's change theory on a medical-surgical unit to implement bedside handoff reporting. The nurse manager expands on the Unfreeze-Change-Refreeze Model by implementing additional steps based on Lippitt's Seven-Step Change Theory:

- The nurse manager collects data from team members affected by the changes and ensures their commitment to success.
- Early adopters are identified as change agents on the unit who are committed to improving client safety by implementing evidence-based practices such as bedside handoff reporting.
- Action plans (including staff education and mentoring), timelines, and expectations are clearly communicated to team members as progressive change objectives. Early adopters are trained as "super-users" to provide staff education and mentor other nurses in using bedside handoff checklists across all shifts.
- The nurse manager facilitates feedback and encourages two-way communication about challenges as change is implemented on the unit. Positive reinforcement is provided as team members effectively incorporate change.
- Bedside handoff reporting is implemented as a unit policy, and all team members are held accountable for performing accurate bedside handoff reporting.

Read more about additional change theories in the Current Theories of Change Management pdf. Access supplementary digital content in the online book using this QR code.

Change Management

Change management is the process of making changes in a deliberate, planned, and systematic manner.[58] It is important for nurse leaders and nurse managers to remember a few key points about change management[59]:

58. Ana, B. H., & Hendricks-Jackson, L. (2017). *Nursing professional development review and resource manual* (4th ed.). American Nurses Association, Nursing Knowledge Center. https://www.nursingworld.org/~49379b/globalassets/catalog/sample-chapters/npdsamplechapter.pdf
59. Ana, B. H., & Hendricks-Jackson, L. (2017). *Nursing professional development review and resource manual* (4th ed.). American Nurses Association, Nursing Knowledge Center. https://www.nursingworld.org/~49379b/globalassets/catalog/sample-chapters/npdsamplechapter.pdf

- Employees will react differently to change, no matter how important or advantageous the change is purported to be. Recognizing this variability is crucial for effectively managing the transition process.
- Basic needs will influence reaction to change, such as the need to be part of the change process, the need to be able to express oneself openly and honestly, and the need to feel that one has some control over the impact of change. Ensuring these needs are met can significantly reduce resistance.
- Change often results in a feeling of loss due to changes in established routines. Employees may react with shock, anger, and resistance, but ideally will eventually accept and adopt change. Acknowledging these feelings and providing support can facilitate smoother transitions.
- Change must be managed realistically, without false hopes and expectations, yet with enthusiasm for the future. Employees should be provided information honestly and allowed to ask questions and express concerns. This transparency builds trust and helps in aligning everyone towards common goals.

Strategies for Effective Change Management

- **Engage Stakeholders Early:** Involve key stakeholders in the planning stages of the change process. Their input can provide valuable insights and help in identifying potential challenges early on.
- **Communicate Clearly and Frequently:** Clear and frequent communication is essential. Use multiple channels to disseminate information and ensure that the message is consistent and comprehensible to all staff members.
- **Provide Training and Resources:** Equip employees with the necessary skills and resources to adapt to the change. This might include training sessions, informational materials, or access to support personnel.
- **Build a Supportive Culture:** Create an environment where change is viewed positively. Encourage collaboration and create opportunities for employees to share their experiences and strategies for adapting to change.
- **Monitor and Adjust:** Continuously monitor the progress of the change initiative and be prepared to make adjustments as needed. Solicit feedback from employees and be responsive to their concerns.

There are multiple strategies that can employed to overcome resistance to change. First, it is important to understand the underlying reasons for resistance. Resistance is commonly aligned to feelings of fear, lack of trust in leadership, or logistical concerns regarding workload, seniority, etc. To implement change effectively, a leader should empower staff by making sure they feel that their voice is respected and valued. When individuals feel valued and hear, they are more likely to support change, even if they do not personally agree with all elements associated with the change. Leaders also must understand that change is stressful for individuals. Depending on the significance of change, a leader may take actions to ensure that employee assistance programs, support groups, or additional counseling services or resources are available. These additional resources can be beneficial for individuals as they work through the emotions associated with the proposed change. Additionally, the benefits for any change should be clearly described. It is important to highlight how the proposed change will help improve work processes and client care quality. It is also helpful to acknowledge and demonstrate appreciation for early adopters of the change. This can provide motivation and encouragement for others to follow suit and fosters a positive attitude toward future changes.

4.4 SPOTLIGHT APPLICATION

Jamie has recently completed his orientation to the emergency department at a busy Level 1 trauma center. The environment is fast-paced, and there are typically a multitude of clients who require care. Jamie appreciates his colleagues and the collaboration that is reflected among members of the health care team, especially in times of stress. Jamie is providing care for an 8-year-old client who has broken her arm when there is a call that there are three Level 1 trauma clients approximately five minutes from the ER. The trauma surgeon reports to the ER, and multiple members of the trauma team report to the ER intake bays. If you were Jamie, what leadership style would you hope the trauma surgeon uses with the team?

In a stressful clinical care situation, where rapid action and direction are needed, an autocratic leadership style is most effective. There is no time for debating different approaches to care in a situation where immediate intervention may be required. Concise commands, direction, and responsive action from the team are needed to ensure that client care interventions are delivered quickly to enhance chance of survival and recovery.

4.5 LEARNING ACTIVITIES

Learning Activities

(Answers to "Learning Activities" can be found in the "Answer Key" at the end of the book. Answers to interactive activities are provided as immediate feedback.)

Sample Scenario

An 89-year-old female resident with Alzheimer's disease has been living at the nursing home for many years. The family decides they no longer want aggressive measures taken and request to the RN on duty that the resident's code status be changed to Do Not Resuscitate (DNR). The evening shift RN documents a progress note that the family (and designated health care agent) requested that the resident's status be made DNR. Due to numerous other responsibilities and needs during the evening shift, the RN does not notify the attending physician or relay the information during shift change or on the 24-hour report. The day shift RN does not read the night shift's notes because of several immediate urgent situations. The family, who had been keeping vigil at the resident's bedside throughout the night, leaves to go home to shower and eat. Upon return the next morning, they find the room full of staff and discover the staff performed CPR after their loved one coded. The resident was successfully resuscitated but now lies in a vegetative state. The family is unhappy and is considering legal action. They approach you, the current nurse assigned to the resident's care, and state, "We followed your procedures to make sure this would not happen! Why was this not managed as we discussed?"[60]

60. Agency for Healthcare Research and Quality. (2023). *TeamSTEPPS long term care specialty scenarios.* https://www.ahrq.gov/sites/default/files/wysiwyg/professionals/education/curriculum-tools/teamstepps/longtermcare/scenarios/scenarios.pdf

Reflective Questions

1. As the current nurse providing client care, explain how you would therapeutically address this family's concerns and use one or more leadership styles.
2. As the charge nurse, explain how you would address the staff involved using one or more leadership styles.
3. Explain how change theory can be implemented to ensure this type of situation does not recur.

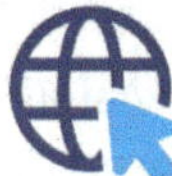

Interactive learning activities have been excluded from the print version of the text. Access free online learning activities in the online book using this QR code.

4.6 GLOSSARY

Change: The process of altering or replacing existing knowledge, skills, attitudes, systems, policies, or procedures.[61]

Change agent: Anyone who has the skill and power to stimulate, facilitate, and coordinate the change effort.

Change management: Process of making changes in a deliberate, planned, and systematic manner.

Core values: The foundational ideals that guide the organization's actions and decision-making processes.

Culture of safety: Organizational culture that embraces error reporting by employees with the goal of identifying systemic causes of problems that can be addressed to improve client safety. Just Culture is a component of a culture of safety.

Followership: The upward influence of individuals on their leaders and their teams.

Just Culture: A culture where people feel safe raising questions and concerns and report safety events in an environment that emphasizes a nonpunitive response to errors and near misses. Clear lines are drawn between human error, at-risk, and reckless employee behaviors.

Leadership: The art of establishing direction and influencing and motivating others to achieve their maximum potential to accomplish tasks, objectives, or projects.[62,63]

Management: Roles that focus on tasks such as planning, organizing, prioritizing, budgeting, staffing, coordinating, and reporting.[64]

Mission statement: An organization's statement that describes how the organization will fulfill its vision and establishes a common course of action for future endeavors.

Organizational culture: The implicit values and beliefs that reflect the norms and traditions of an organization. An organization's vision, mission, and values statements are the foundation of organizational culture.

Systems leadership: A set of skills used to catalyze, enable, and support the process of systems-level change that focuses on the individual, the community, and the system.

Systems theory: The concept that systems do not function in isolation but rather there is an interdependence that exists between their parts. Systems theory assumes that most individuals strive to do good work, but are affected by diverse influences within the system.

Values statement: The organization's established values that support its vision and mission and provide strategic guidelines for decision-making, both internally and externally, by members of the organization.

Vision statement: An organization's statement that defines why the organization exists, describes how the organization is unique and different from similar organizations, and specifies what the organization is striving to be.

---

61. Ana, B. H., & Hendricks-Jackson, L. (2017). *Nursing professional development review and resource manual* (4th ed.). American Nurses Association, Nursing Knowledge Center. https://www.nursingworld.org/~49379b/globalassets/catalog/sample-chapters/npdsamplechapter.pdf

62. Northouse, P. (2004). *Leadership: Theory and practice* (9th ed.). Sage Publications.

63. Specchia, M. L., Cozzolino, M. R., Carini, E., Di Pilla, A., Galletti, C., Ricciardi, W., & Damiani, G. (2021). Leadership styles and nurses' job satisfaction. Results of a systematic review. *International Journal of Environmental Research and Public Health, 18*(4), 1552. https://doi.org/10.3390/ijerph18041552

64. Hannaway, J. (1989). *Managers managing: The workings of an administrative system.* Oxford University Press, p. 39.

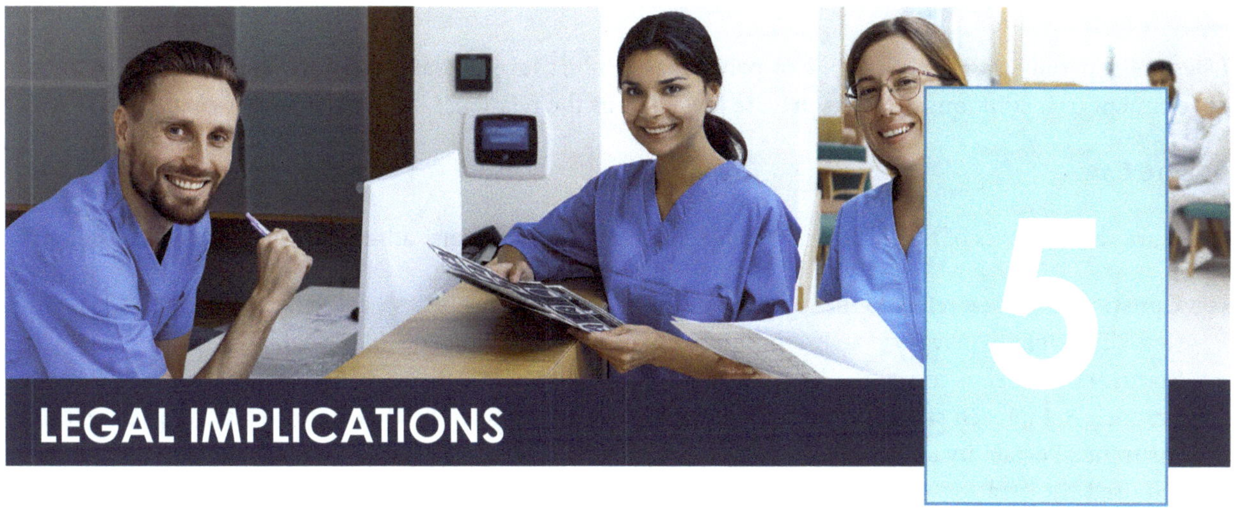

5.1 LEGAL IMPLICATIONS INTRODUCTION

LEARNING OBJECTIVES

- Examine competent practice within the legal framework of health care
- Analyze legal dilemmas of nursing practice utilizing professional and industry standards
- Examine how negligence and malpractice apply to nursing practice
- Practice within the legal framework of the Nurse Practice Act
- Examine the role of the nurse when observing illegal and/or unsafe practices

Nurses are responsible for being aware of the laws and regulations affecting their nursing care in the state(s) in which they are practicing. If allegations are made regarding a nurse's professional conduct or provision of client care, the excuse "I did not know" does not hold up in a court of law or with a state's Board of Nursing. This chapter will provide foundational legal knowledge for nursing practice in complex health care environments.

5.2 UNDERSTANDING THE LEGAL SYSTEM

Understanding the Legal System

There are several types of laws and regulations that affect nursing practice. **Laws** are rules and regulations created by a society and enforced by courts and professional licensure boards. Nurses are responsible for being aware of public and private laws that affect client care, as well as legal actions that can result when these laws are broken.

Laws are generally classified as public or private law. **Public law** regulates relations of individuals with the government or institutions, whereas **private law** governs the relationships between private parties.

Public Law

There are several types of public law, including constitutional, statutory, administrative, and criminal law.

- **Constitutional law** refers to the rights, privileges, and responsibilities established by the U.S. Constitution.[1] The right to privacy is an example of a client right based on constitutional law.
- **Statutory law** refers to written laws enacted by the federal or state legislature. For example, the Nurse Practice Act in each state is an example of statutory law enacted by that state's legislature. The Health Insurance Portability and Accountability Act (HIPAA) is an example of a federal statutory law. HIPAA required the creation of national standards to protect sensitive client health information from being disclosed without the client's consent or knowledge.
- **Administrative law** is law created by government agencies that have been granted the authority to establish rules and regulations to protect the public.[2] An example of federal administrative law is the regulations set by the Occupational Safety and Health Administration (OSHA). OSHA was established by Congress to ensure safe and healthy working conditions for employees by setting and enforcing federal standards. An example of administrative law at the state level is the State Board of Nursing (SBON). The SBON is a group of individuals in each state, established by that state's legislature, to develop, review, and enforce the Nurse Practice Act. The SBON also issues nursing licenses to qualified candidates, investigates reports of nursing misconduct, and implements consequences for nurses who have violated the Nurse Practice Act.
- **Criminal law** is a system of laws concerned with punishment of individuals who commit crimes.[3] A **crime** is a behavior defined by Congress or state legislature as deserving of punishment. Crimes are classified as felonies, misdemeanors, and infractions. Conviction for a crime requires evidence to show the defendant is guilty beyond a shadow of doubt. This means the prosecution must convince a jury there is no reasonable explanation other than guilty that can come from the evidence presented at trial. In the United States, an individual is considered innocent until proven guilty. See Figure 5.1[4] for an illustration of a trial with a jury.

Serious crimes that can result in imprisonment for longer than one year are called **felonies**. Felony convictions can also result in the loss of voting rights, the ability to own or use guns, and the loss of one's nursing license. An example of a felony committed by some nurses is drug diversion of controlled substances.

Misdemeanors are less serious crimes resulting in penalties of fines and/or imprisonment for less than one year. For example, in Wisconsin, misdemeanors are categorized as Class A, B, or C based on their sentencing. Class A misdemeanors are sentenced to a fine not to exceed $10,000 or imprisonment not to exceed nine months, or both. Class B misdemeanors are sentenced to a fine not to exceed $1,000 or imprisonment not to exceed 90 days, or both. Class C misdemeanors are sentenced to a fine not to exceed $500 or imprisonment not to exceed 30 days, or both.[5] Examples of misdemeanors include battery, possession of controlled substances, petty theft, disorderly conduct, and driving under the influence (DUI) charges.

1. Legal Information Institute. (n.d.) Cornell Law School. https://www.law.cornell.edu
2. Legal Information Institute. (n.d.) Cornell Law School. https://www.law.cornell.edu
3. Legal Information Institute. (n.d.) Cornell Law School. https://www.law.cornell.edu
4. "Courtroom Trial with Judge, Jury - Vector Image" designed by WannaPik is licensed under CC0
5. Wisconsin State Legislature. (2021). 939.51 *Classification of misdemeanors.* https://docs.legis.wisconsin.gov/statutes/statutes/939/iv/51

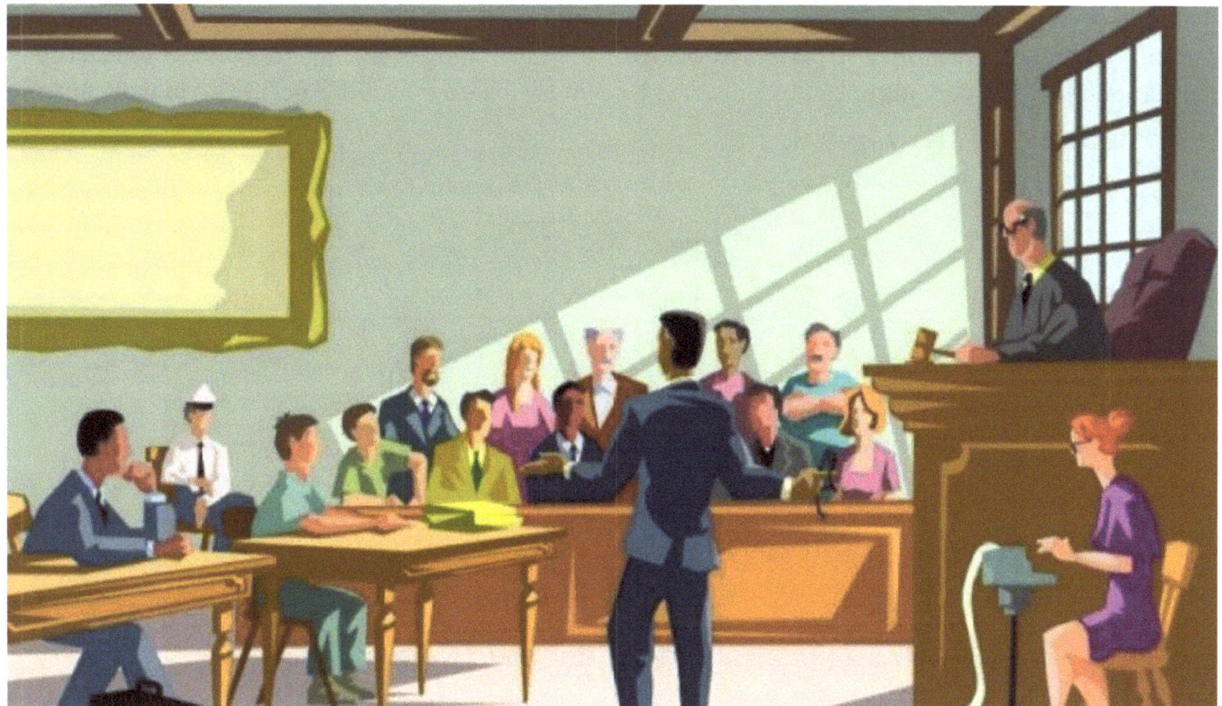

FIGURE 5.1 Trial by Jury

Although considered less serious crimes, misdemeanors can impact an individual's ability to obtain or maintain a nursing license.

Nurses who are found guilty of misdemeanors or felonies, regardless if the violation is related to the practice of nursing, must typically report these violations to their state's Board of Nursing.

Infractions are minor offenses, such as speeding tickets, that result in fines but not jail time. Infractions do not generally impact nursing licensure unless there is a significant quantity of them over a short period of time.

Sample Case

An LPN working for a hospice agency was accused of stealing a client's pain medications and substituting them with anti-seizure medication. The family asserted the actions of the LPN prolonged the client's suffering. The LPN served time in prison for diverting the client's medications.[6]

Private Law

Private law, also referred to as **civil law**, focuses on the rights, responsibilities, and legal relationships between private citizens. Civil law typically involves compensation to the injured party. Unlike criminal law

6. Nurses Service Organization (NSO) and CNA Financial Corporation. (2020). *Nurse professional liability exposure claim report: 4th edition: Minimizing risk, achieving excellence.* https://www.nso.com/Learning/Artifacts/Claim-Reports/Minimizing-Risk-Achieving-Excellence

that requires a jury to determine a defendant is guilty beyond reasonable doubt, civil law only requires a certainty of guilt of greater than 50 percent.[7] See Figure 5.2[8] illustrating balancing the evidence to determine the certainty of guilt. Any nurse can be impacted by civil law based on actions occurring in daily nursing practice.

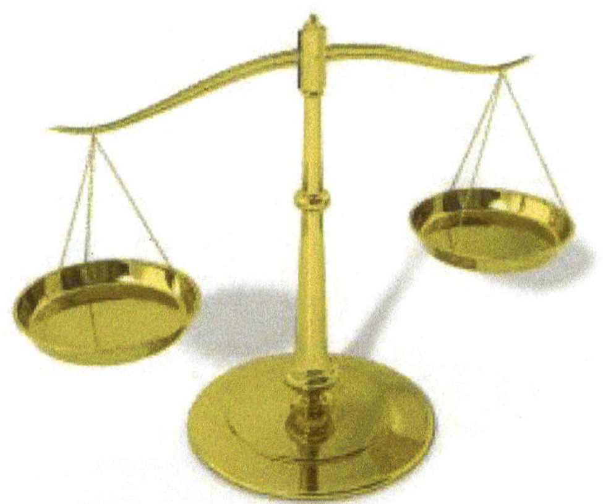

FIGURE 5.2 Balancing the Evidence to Determine Guilt

Civil law includes contract law and tort law. **Contracts** are binding written, verbal, or implied agreements. A **tort** is an act of commission or omission that gives rise to injury or harm to another and amounts to a civil wrong for which courts impose liability. In the context of torts, "injury" describes the invasion of any legal right, whereas "harm" describes a loss or detriment that an individual suffers.[9]

Two categories of torts affect nursing practice: intentional torts, such as intentionally hitting a person, and unintentional torts (also referred to as negligent torts), such as making an error by failing to follow agency policy.

INTENTIONAL TORTS

Intentional torts are wrongs that the defendant knew (or should have known) would be caused by their actions. Examples of intentional torts include assault, battery, false imprisonment, slander, libel, and breach of privacy or client confidentiality.

UNINTENTIONAL TORTS

Unintentional torts occur when the defendant's actions or inactions were unreasonably unsafe. Unintentional torts can result from acts of **commission** (i.e., doing something a reasonable nurse would not have done) or **omission** (i.e., failing to do something a reasonable nurse would do).[10]

---

7. Legal Information Institute. (n.d.) Cornell Law School. https://www.law.cornell.edu
8. "Balance Scales (Ethics)" by The Open University (OU) is licensed under CC BY-NC-ND 2.0
9. Legal Information Institute. (n.d.). Cornell Law School. https://www.law.cornell.edu
10. Brous, E. (2019). The elements of a nursing malpractice case, Part 2: Breach. *American Journal of Nursing, 119*(9), 42–46. https://doi.org/10.1097/01.NAJ.0000580256.10914.2e

Negligence and malpractice are examples of unintentional torts. Tort law exists to compensate clients injured by negligent practice, provide corrective judgement, and deter negligence with visible consequences of action or inaction.[11,12] Examples of common torts affecting nursing practice are discussed in further detail in the following subsections. See Table 5.2 for a comparison of public and private law.

TABLE 5.2. Comparison of Public and Private Law

Type of Law	Subtypes of Law and Examples
Public Law	• Statutory law (Nurse Practice Act and HIPAA) • Constitutional law (Right to Privacy) • Administrative law (State Board of Nursing and OSHA) • Criminal law (felonies and misdemeanors)
Private Law (Civil Law)	• Contract law – Written – Verbal – Implied • Tort law – Assault – Battery – Confidentiality – Consent – False imprisonment – Fraud – Negligence – Malpractice

Examples of Intentional and Unintentional Torts

ASSAULT AND BATTERY

Assault and battery are intentional torts. **Assault** is defined as intentionally putting another person in reasonable apprehension of an imminent harmful or offensive contact.[13] **Battery** is defined as intentional causation of harmful or offensive contact with another person without that person's consent.[14] Physical harm does not need to occur to be charged with assault or battery.

Battery convictions are often misdemeanors but can be felonies if serious bodily harm occurs. To avoid the risk of being charged with assault or battery, nurses must obtain consent from clients to provide hands-on care.

11. Legal Information Institute. (n.d.). Cornell Law School. https://www.law.cornell.edu
12. Mello, M. M., Frakes, M. D., Blumenkranz, E., & Studdert, D. M. (2020). Malpractice liability and health care quality: A review. *JAMA, 323*(4), 352–366. https://doi.org/10.1001/jama.2019.21411
13. Legal Information Institute. (n.d.). Cornell Law School. https://www.law.cornell.edu
14. Legal Information Institute. (n.d.). Cornell Law School. https://www.law.cornell.edu

FALSE IMPRISONMENT

False imprisonment is an intentional tort. False imprisonment is defined as an act of restraining another person and causing that person to be confined in a bounded area.[15] In nursing practice, restraints can be physical, chemical, or verbal. Nurses must strictly follow agency policies related to the use of restraints. Physical restraints typically require a provider order and documentation according to strict guidelines within specific time frames. See Figure 5.3[16] for an image of a simulated client in full physical medical restraints.

Chemical restraints include administering medications such as benzodiazepines and require clear documentation supporting their use. Verbal threats to keep an individual in an inpatient environment can also qualify as false imprisonment and should be avoided.

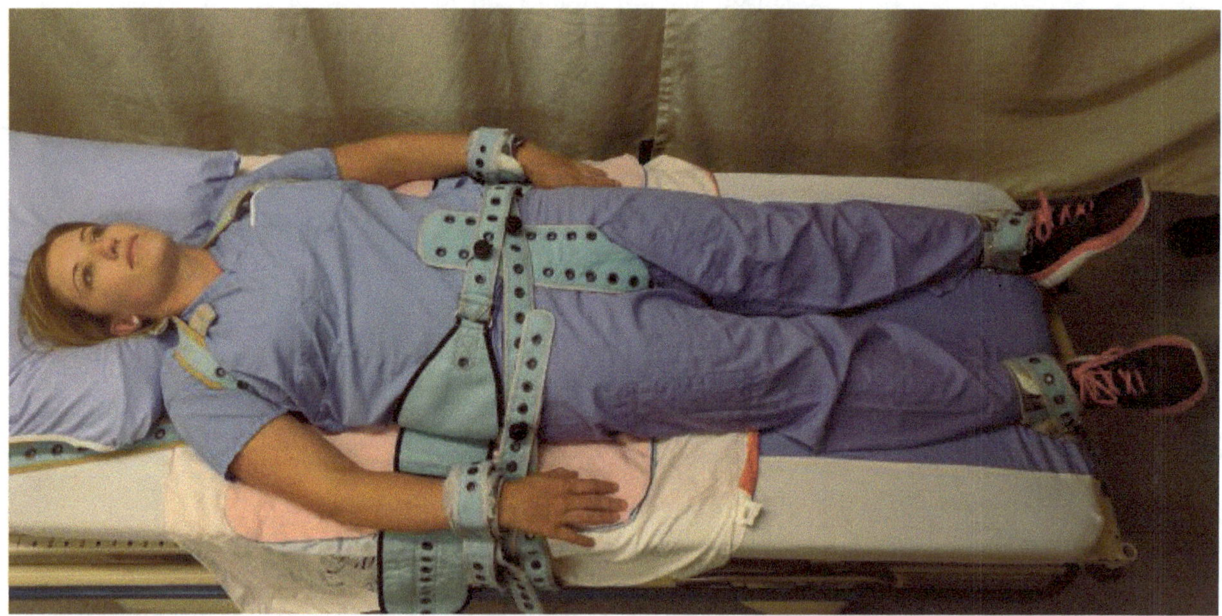

FIGURE 5.3 Full Physical Medical Restraints

BREACH OF PRIVACY AND CONFIDENTIALITY

Breaching privacy and confidentiality are intentional torts. **Confidentiality** is the right of an individual to have personal, identifiable medical information, referred to as protected health information (PHI), kept private. Protected Health Information (PHI) is defined as individually identifiable health information, including demographic data, that relates to the individual's past, present, or future physical or mental health or condition[17]; the provision of health care to the individual; and the past, present, or future payment for the provision of health care to the individual.

15. Legal Information Institute. (n.d.). Cornell Law School. https://www.law.cornell.edu
16. "PinelRestaint.jpg" by James Heilman, MD is licensed under CC BY-SA 4.0
17. U.S. Department of Health & Human Services. (2022). *Summary of the HIPAA Privacy Rule.* https://www.hhs.gov/hipaa/for-professionals/privacy/laws-regulations/index.html

This right is protected by federal regulations called the Health Insurance Portability and Accountability Act (HIPAA). HIPAA was enacted in 1996 and was prompted by the need to ensure privacy and protection of personal health records and data in an environment of electronic medical records and third-party insurance payers. There are two main sections of HIPAA law: the Privacy Rule and the Security Rule. The Privacy Rule addresses the use and disclosure of individuals' health information. The Security Rule sets national standards for protecting the confidentiality, integrity, and availability of electronically protected health information. HIPAA regulations extend beyond medical records and apply to client information shared with others. Therefore, all types of client information should be shared only with health care team members who are actively providing care to them.[18,19]

HIPAA violations may result in fines from $100 for an individual violation to $1.5 million for organizational violations. Criminal penalties, including jail time of up to ten years, may be imposed for violations involving the use of PHI for personal gain or malicious intent. Nursing students are also required to adhere to HIPAA guidelines from the moment they enter the clinical setting or risk being disciplined or expelled by their nursing program.

Sample Case

An RN accessed a client's medical records, as well as the records of the newborn son, although she was not assigned to their care because she believed the newborn was her biological grandchild. Although the chart was accessed for less than five seconds, it was unauthorized. The nurse was publicly reprimanded by the state's Board of Nursing, and her multistate licensure privileges were revoked. Expenses to defend the nurse exceeded $2,800.[20]

Read more about the HIPAA Privacy Rule. Access supplementary digital content in the online book using this QR code.

SLANDER AND LIBEL

Slander and libel are intentional torts. **Defamation of character** occurs when an individual makes negative, malicious, and false remarks about another person to damage their reputation. **Slander** is spoken defamation and **libel** is written defamation. Nurses must take care to communicate and document facts regarding client care without defamation in their oral and written communications with clients and coworkers.

18. Ernstmeyer, K., & Christman, E. (Eds.). (2024). *Nursing fundamentals 2E.* Open RN | WisTech Open. https://wtcs.pressbooks.pub/nursingfundamentals/
19. U.S. Department of Health & Human Services. (2022). *Summary of the HIPAA Privacy Rule.* https://www.hhs.gov/hipaa/for-professionals/privacy/laws-regulations/index.html
20. Nurses Service Organization (NSO) and CNA Financial Corporation. (2020). *Nurse professional liability exposure claim report: 4th edition:* Minimizing risk, achieving excellence.

FRAUD

Fraud is an intentional tort occurring when an individual is deceived for personal gain. An example of fraud is financial exploitation perpetrated by individuals who are in positions of trust.[21,22] A nurse may be charged with fraud for documenting interventions not performed or altering documentation to cover up an error. Fraud can result in civil and criminal charges and also suspension or revocation of a nurse's license.

NEGLIGENCE AND MALPRACTICE

Negligence and malpractice are types of unintentional torts. **Negligence** is the failure to exercise the ordinary care a reasonable person would use in similar circumstances. Wisconsin civil jury instruction states, "A person is not using ordinary care and is negligent, if the person, without intending to do harm, does something (or fails to do something) that a reasonable person would recognize as creating an unreasonable risk of injury or damage to a person or property."[23] **Malpractice** is a specific term used for negligence committed by a professional with a license. See Figure 5.4[24] for an illustration related to malpractice.

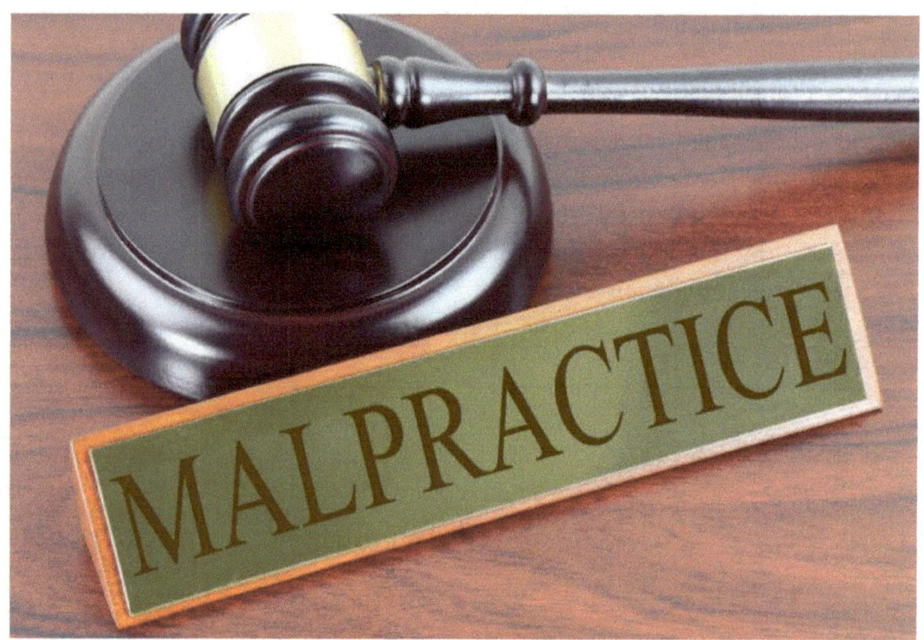

FIGURE 5.4 Malpractice

21. DeLiema, M. (2018). Elder fraud and financial exploitation: Application of routine activity theory. *The Gerontologist, 58*(4), 706–718. https://doi.org/10.1093/geront/gnw258
22. DeLiema, M., Deevy, M., Lusardi, A., & Mitchell, O. S. (2020). Financial fraud among older Americans: Evidence and implications. *The Journals of Gerontology. Series B, Psychological Sciences and Social Sciences, 75*(4), 861–868. https://doi.org/10.1093/geronb/gby151
23. Wis. JI—Civil 1005. (2016). https://wilawlibrary.gov/jury/civil/instruction.php?n=1005
24. "malpractice.jpg" by Nick Youngson hosted by Pix4free is licensed under CC BY-SA 3.0

ELEMENTS OF NURSING MALPRACTICE

Nurses and nursing students don't often get sued for malpractice, but when they do, it is important to understand the elements required to prove malpractice. All the following elements must be established in a court of law to prove malpractice[25]:

- **Duty:** A nurse-client relationship exists.
- **Breach:** The standard of care was not met and harm was a foreseeable consequence of the action or inaction.
- **Cause:** Injury was caused by the nurse's breach.
- **Harm:** Injury resulted in damages.

Parties bringing a lawsuit must be able to demonstrate their interests were harmed, providing a reason to stand before the court. The person bringing the lawsuit is called the **plaintiff**. The parties named in the lawsuit are called **defendants**. Most malpractice lawsuits name physicians or hospitals, although nurses can be individually named. Employers can be held liable for the actions of their employees.[26]

Malpractice lawsuits are concerned with the legal obligations nurses have to their clients to adhere to current standards of practice. These legal obligations are referred to as the **duty of reasonable care**. Nurses are required to adhere to standards of practice when providing care to clients they have been assigned. This includes following organizational policies and procedures, maintaining clinical competency, and confining their activities to the authorized scope of practice as defined by their state's Nurse Practice Act. Nurses also have a legal duty to be physically, mentally, and morally fit for practice. When nurses do not meet these professional obligations, they are said to have breached their duties to clients.[27]

Duty

In the work environment, a duty is created when the nurse accepts responsibility for a client and establishes a nurse-client relationship. This generally occurs during inpatient care upon acceptance of a handoff report from another nurse. Outside the work environment, a nurse-client relationship is created when the nurse volunteers services. Some states have statutes requiring notification of authorities (also referred to as mandatory reporting) or summoning assistance.[28]

GOOD SAMARITAN LAW

The **Good Samaritan Law** provides protections against negligence claims to individuals who render aid to people experiencing medical emergencies outside of clinical environments. All 50 states in the United States have a version of a Good Samaritan Law. See Figure 5.5[29] for historical artwork depicting a Good Samaritan. Differences exist in state laws regarding protection of bystanders who provide aid. For example, in

25. Brous, E. (2019). The elements of a nursing malpractice case, Part 1: Duty. *American Journal of Nursing, 119*(7), 64–67. https://doi.org/10.1097/01.NAJ.0000569476.17357.f5
26. Brous, E. (2019). The elements of a nursing malpractice case, Part 1: Duty. *American Journal of Nursing, 119*(7), 64–67. https://doi.org/10.1097/01.NAJ.0000569476.17357.f5
27. Brous, E. (2019). The elements of a nursing malpractice case, Part 1: Duty. *American Journal of Nursing, 119*(7), 64–67. https://doi.org/10.1097/01.NAJ.0000569476.17357.f5
28. Brous, E. (2019). The elements of a nursing malpractice case, Part 1: Duty. *American Journal of Nursing, 119*(7), 64–67. https://doi.org/10.1097/01.NAJ.0000569476.17357.f5
29. "The_good_samaritan_helping_a_stranger_who_has_been_ignored_b_Wellcome_V0015249.jpg" by S. Smith after C. L. Eastlake is licensed under CC BY 4.0

Wisconsin, the law states, "Any person who renders emergency care at the scene of any emergency or accident in good faith is immune from civil liability for the person's acts or omissions in rendering such emergency care."[30] There are a few states that require some emergency bystander action, so nurses should review the law in states they are visiting. It is also important to keep in mind that although anyone can file a lawsuit against someone who provides bystander aid, the Good Samaritan laws typically negate any penalty to the person rendering aid.

Although the majority of Good Samaritan laws are at the state level, the federal Aviation Medical Assistance Act (AMAA) provides liability protection for aid given on aircraft. The most common in-flight medical emergencies involve syncope, as well as gastrointestinal, respiratory, and cardiac events.[31] Note that consent for care by an unconscious person is implied, but consent must be obtained from alert individuals.

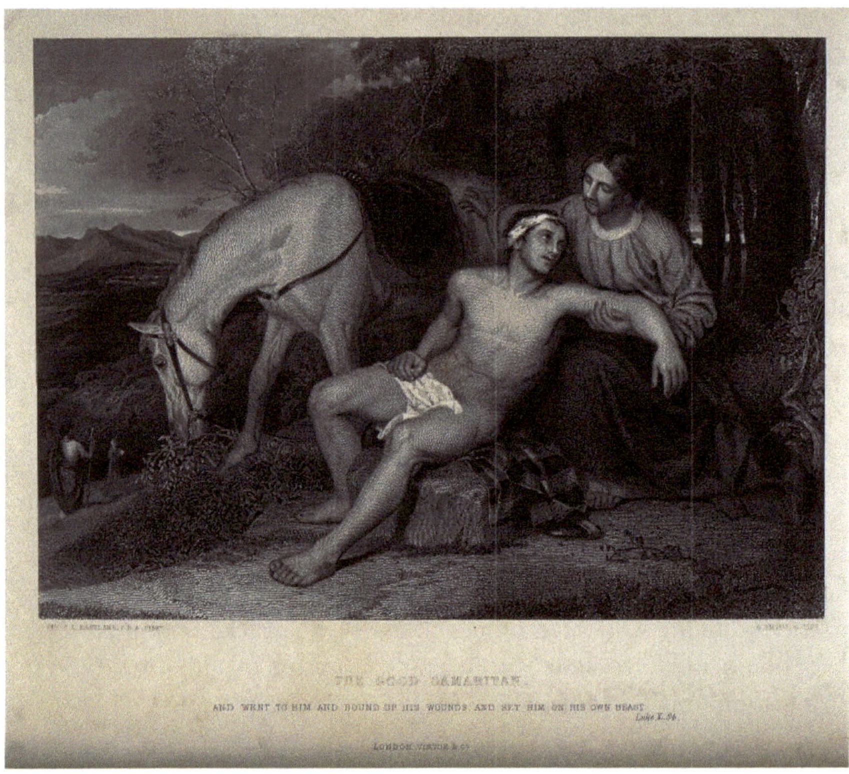

FIGURE 5.5 Good Samaritan

MANDATORY REPORTING

Nurses are legally responsible for reporting certain crimes. Mandatory reporting requirements vary based on the state of practice, but there are some commonalities. For example, nurses are mandated to report suspected abuse of children, the elderly, and the disabled (if they have been deemed as incompetent by a court of law or as incapacitated by qualified health care providers).

---

30. Otis, A. (2017). *Civil immunity under Wisconsin's Good Samaritan Law [Memo].* Wisconsin Legislative Council. https://docs.legis.wisconsin.gov/misc/lc/information_memos/2017/im_2017_03

31. West, B. & Varacallo, M. A. (2022). *Good Samaritan Laws.* StatPearls [Internet]. https://www.ncbi.nlm.nih.gov/books/NBK542176/

Nurses are also mandated to report gunshot wounds, dog bites, some communicable diseases, and unsafe or illegal practices of other health care team members. Reporting responsibility often begins at the organizational level. The nurse may also need to identify the appropriate local, state, or federal authorities to submit the report and pursue it to its resolution.

> **Sample Statute Regarding Duty to Assist**
>
> A Minnesota statute states that a person at the scene of an emergency who knows that another person is exposed to or has suffered grave physical harm shall, to the extent that the person can do so without danger or peril to self or others, give reasonable assistance to the exposed person. Reasonable assistance may include obtaining or attempting to obtain aid from law enforcement or medical personnel. A person who violates this is guilty of a petty misdemeanor.[32]

IMPLICATIONS FOR NURSES

Duty can be established in many ways. Nurses have a duty of reasonable care for a client they have been assigned. They may also have a duty in other circumstances. Therefore, nurses should understand the following[33]:

- Recognize that a nurse-client relationship is established upon acceptance of responsibility for a client, whether after a handoff report in the workplace or during volunteered services.
- Assume that on-call or supervisory responsibilities create a duty to clients, even in the absence of an expressed nurse-client relationship.
- Know if there is a duty to rescue statute in their state, and if so, what it demands.

Breach of Duty

The second element of malpractice is breach of duty. After a plaintiff has established the first element in a malpractice suit, that the nurse owed a duty to the plaintiff, the plaintiff must then demonstrate that the nurse breached that duty by failing to comply with the duty of reasonable care.[34]

To demonstrate that a nurse breached their duty to a client, the plaintiff must prove the nurse departed from acceptable standards of practice. The plaintiff must establish how a reasonably prudent nurse in the same or similar circumstances would act and then show that the defendant nurse departed from that standard of practice. The plaintiff must claim the nurse did something a reasonably prudent nurse would not have done (an act of commission) or failed to do something a reasonable nurse would have done (an act of omission).[35]

Experts are needed during court hearings to explain things outside the knowledge of non-nurse jurors. In reaching their opinions, experts review many materials, including the state's Nurse Practice Act and organizational policies, to determine whether the nurse adhered to them. To qualify as a nurse expert, the person

32. Brous, E. (2019). The elements of a nursing malpractice case, Part 1: Duty. *American Journal of Nursing, 119*(7), 64–67. https://doi.org/10.1097/01.NAJ.0000569476.17357.f5
33. Brous, E. (2019). The elements of a nursing malpractice case, Part 1: Duty. *American Journal of Nursing, 119*(7), 64–67. https://doi.org/10.1097/01.NAJ.0000569476.17357.f5
34. Brous, E. (2019). The elements of a nursing malpractice case, Part 2: Breach. *American Journal of Nursing, 119*(9), 42–46. https://doi.org/10.1097/01.NAJ.0000580256.10914.2e
35. Brous, E. (2019). The elements of a nursing malpractice case, Part 2: Breach. *American Journal of Nursing, 119*(9), 42–46. https://doi.org/10.1097/01.NAJ.0000580256.10914.2e

testifying must have relevant experience, education, skill, and knowledge. They typically have advanced degrees, are published in nursing literature, have spoken at professional conferences, and belong to professional organizations. Medical malpractice trials take place primarily in state courts, so experts are deemed qualified based on state requirements.

Sample Case Regarding Breach of Duty[36]

Mary Jones was an 87-year-old woman who presented to the hospital with dizziness, nausea, intermittent slurred speech, an unsteady gait, and a history of four falls at home that day. Significant medical history included heart disease and multiple medications. The admitting nurse assessed her as being at risk for falls and placed her on universal fall precautions. The fall precautions included keeping the bed in the lowest position, instructing her on the use of the call light and ensuring the call light was within her reach, providing a bedside commode, and placing her in a room close to the nurses' station where she could be observed. However, the nurse did not use a formal scoring system for fall risk assessment that was set forth in a nursing procedures textbook. Additionally, bed alarms had not been working at this agency for a year.

Five days later, a nurse responded to a sound coming from Mrs. Jones's room and found her lying on the bathroom floor. She was conscious and able to move all extremities but complained of left knee and elbow pain. The physician was notified, and Mrs. Jones was sent for X-rays and a CT scan. When Mrs. Jones returned to her room, the nurse observed she was diaphoretic and deteriorating. The nurse took Mrs. Jones to the emergency department, where she lost consciousness. She was evaluated by a neurosurgeon, intubated, and airlifted to a different hospital for a higher level of care. She never regained consciousness and died the next day from intracranial bleeding that was aggravated by anticoagulant therapy.

Mrs. Jones's estate brought a lawsuit alleging nursing malpractice. The estate's nursing expert stated the universal fall precautions had been inadequate for a high-risk client and additional measures should have been instituted. The expert testified that not only had the admitting nurse not adhered to the formal scoring system for fall risk assessment in the nursing procedures textbook, but also the standard of care required nurses to use bed alarms, institute 15-minute rounds, or place a sitter in the room.

A defense expert used The Joint Commission's National Patient Safety Goals to define the standard of care and testified it was her opinion the nurse had met that standard. The organizational policy did not require bed alarms as part of its fall prevention plan. Although the nurses did not use the formal scoring system in a textbook to assess the client's risk, they clearly identified her as being at risk for falling; assessed her frequently; maintained her bed in the lowest position; kept the wheels of her bed locked and her side rails up; and kept the call light within her reach. They instructed her on the use of the call light and placed her in a room where she could be readily observed.

The court entered the judgment for the defendant hospital, noting that "under the circumstances, it is a close call on whether the hospital, by not having functioning bed alarms and staff not checking on Mary more frequently, breached the standard of care."[37] In this case, the plaintiff's expert had not demonstrated the standard of care was breached.

36. Mello, M. M., Frakes, M. D., Blumenkranz, E., & Studdert, D. M. (2020). Malpractice liability and health care quality: A review. *JAMA, 323*(4), 352–366. https://doi.org/10.1001/jama.2019.21411

37. Brous, E. (2019). The elements of a nursing malpractice case, Part 2: Breach. *American Journal of Nursing, 119*(9), 42–46. https://doi.org/10.1097/01.NAJ.0000580256.10914.2e

IMPLICATIONS FOR NURSES

Nurses defending themselves against allegations of professional malpractice must demonstrate their actions conformed with accepted standards of practice. They must convince a jury they acted as a reasonably prudent nurse would have in the same or similar circumstances. Nurses should always follow these practices[38]:

- Adhere to organizational policies and procedures. Work-arounds can create liability. The standard of practice is to adhere to agency policy. Failing to do so creates an assumption of departure from standards.
- Document in a manner that permits accurate reconstruction of client assessments and the sequence of events, especially when notifying providers regarding clinical concerns.
- Maintain competence through continuing education, participation in professional conferences, membership in professional organizations, and subscriptions to professional journals.
- When using an interpreter, ensure that properly trained interpreters are used and document the name of the interpreter. The use of family, friends, or other untrained interpreters is unsafe practice and is not consistent with acceptable standards of practice.
- Maintain professional boundaries. Personal relationships with clients or their families can be red flags for juries and can be viewed as evidence of departure from professional standards.

Cause

The third element of malpractice is cause. After the plaintiff has established the nurse owed a duty to a client and then breached that duty, they must then demonstrate that damages or harm were caused by that breach. Plaintiffs cannot prevail by only demonstrating the nurse departed from acceptable standards of practice but must also prove that such departures were the cause of any injuries.[39] Additionally, nurses are held accountable for foreseeability, meaning a nurse of ordinary skill, care, and diligence could anticipate the risk of harm of departing from standards of practice in similar circumstances.[40]

Plaintiffs must be able to link the defendant's acts or omissions to the harm for which they are seeking compensation. This requires expert testimony from a physician because it requires a medical diagnosis. Unlike in criminal cases, in which the standard of proof is that elements of prosecution must be proven "beyond reasonable doubt," the elements of a malpractice lawsuit must be proven by a "preponderance of evidence." Expert testimony is required to demonstrate "medical certainty" that the nurse's breach was the cause of an actual injury.

---

38. Brous, E. (2019). The elements of a nursing malpractice case, Part 2: Breach. *American Journal of Nursing, 119*(9), 42–46. https://doi.org/10.1097/01.NAJ.0000580256.10914.2e
39. Brous, E. (2019). The elements of a nursing malpractice case, Part 3A: Causation: A plaintiff must prove not only that a provider departed from acceptable standards of practice--but that this departure caused an injury. *American Journal of Nursing, 119*(11), 54–59. https://doi.org/10.1097/01.naj.0000605380.52689.af
40. Brous, E. (2020). The elements of a nursing malpractice case, Part 3B: Causation. *American Journal of Nursing, 120*(1), 63–66. https://doi.org/10.1097/01.naj.0000652128.66135.55

Sample Cases Regarding Causation

Case 1

Janusz Osiecki was admitted to a subacute nursing facility to recover from Guillain-Barre syndrome. The standard of nursing care for this client included respiratory assessments and tracheostomy care. One morning, three weeks into his stay, he was found unresponsive, without pulse or respirations. His wife brought a wrongful death lawsuit, and expert witnesses testified the nurses breached the standard of care in not performing respiratory and tracheostomy assessments every two hours. Their rationale was that the purpose of the assessments was to detect and report pulmonary congestion, and if the nurses had done so in a timely manner, Mr. Osiecki could have received medical care that would have saved his life. A jury awarded the widow $577,005 for wrongful death and $250,000 for harm to family relationships.[41]

Case 2

A client identified as "C" was locked in a seclusion room after presenting to a hospital with psychosis and continuing bizarre behavior, hallucinations, irrationality, lack of contact with reality, and agitation. She was in the seclusion room undergoing treatment for over a week when she suffered a grand mal seizure. A psychiatrist ordered antipsychotic medication. The medication order was not noted by nursing staff until the next day, at which point it was discovered the medication was unavailable at the pharmacy. The psychiatrist was not made aware the medication was unavailable, and the client went without the prescribed medication for three days. The nurses also did not notify the psychiatrist during those three days that C was becoming increasingly more agitated and hallucinating. On the fourth day, C attempted to leave the unit and told staff she was hearing voices instructing her to harm herself. She was returned to seclusion and remained there without being assessed or treated. Four hours later, she was found unconscious with her head wedged between the side rail and the mattress. She suffered brain damage that left her in a permanent semicomatose state.

C's estate brought a lawsuit alleging it was negligent to leave C in a steel bed in a seclusion room without constant observation. The jury awarded $3.6 million. The hospital appealed, but the appellate court upheld the jury verdict and explained that particular injuries do not need to be foreseen, only the general harm that can occur. The court stated, "It is not extraordinary that a psychotic client who is delusional...might wedge herself between a mattress and side rail in an attempt to hurt herself."[42]

41. Brous, E. (2019). The elements of a nursing malpractice case, Part 3A: Causation: A plaintiff must prove not only that a provider departed from acceptable standards of practice--but that this departure caused an injury. *American Journal of Nursing, 119*(11), 54–59. https://doi.org/10.1097/01.naj.0000605380.52689.af

42. Brous, E. (2020). The elements of a nursing malpractice case, Part 3B: Causation. *American Journal of Nursing, 120*(1), 63–66. https://doi.org/10.1097/01.naj.0000652128.66135.55

IMPLICATIONS FOR NURSES

Nurses can reduce their liability by adhering to professional standards and documenting their observations and communications. Nurses should always follow these standards[43]:

- Follow the chain of command when there are concerns about unclear or potentially unsafe orders. Pursue concerns to resolution, documenting precisely who is notified and at what times.
- Document observations to justify clinical decisions. Variance charting (i.e., only charting things that vary from the norm) does not provide sufficient evidence of compliance with the standards of care.
- Adhere to organizational policies and procedures with an understanding that a failure to do so creates foreseeable harm to clients.

Harm

The fourth element of malpractice is harm. In a civil lawsuit, after a plaintiff has established the nurse owed a duty to the client and breached that duty and injury was caused by the nurse's breach, they must prove the injury resulted in damages. They request repayment for what they have lost.[44]

There are several types of injuries for which clients or their representatives seek compensation. Injuries can be physical, emotional, financial, professional, marital, or any combination of these. Physical injuries include loss of function, disfigurement, physical or mental impairment, exacerbation of prior medical problems, the need for additional medical care, and death. Economic injuries can include lost wages, additional medical expenses, rehabilitation, durable medical expenses, the need for architectural changes to one's home, the loss of earning capacity, the need to hire people to do things the plaintiff can no longer do, and the loss of financial support. Emotional injuries can include psychological damage, emotional distress, or other forms of mental suffering.[45]

Determining the specific amount a plaintiff needs can require expert witness testimony from a person known as a life care planner who is trained in analyzing and evaluating medical costs, as well as the subjective determination of a jury. Damages fall into several categories, including compensatory (economic) damages, noneconomic damages, and punitive damages.[46] See Figure 5.6[47] for an illustration of damages.

43. Brous, E. (2020). The elements of a nursing malpractice case, Part 3B: Causation. *American Journal of Nursing, 120*(1), 63–66. https://doi.org/10.1097/01.naj.0000652128.66135.55
44. Brous, E. (2020). The elements of a nursing malpractice case, Part 4: Harm. *American Journal of Nursing, 120*(3), 61–64. https://doi.org/10.1097/01.naj.0000656360.21284.50
45. Brous, E. (2020). The elements of a nursing malpractice case, Part 4: Harm. *American Journal of Nursing, 120*(3), 61–64. https://doi.org/10.1097/01.naj.0000656360.21284.50
46. Brous, E. (2020). The elements of a nursing malpractice case, Part 4: Harm. *American Journal of Nursing, 120*(3), 61–64. https://doi.org/10.1097/01.naj.0000656360.21284.50
47. "damages.jpg" by Nick Youngson hosted by Pix4free is licensed under CC BY-SA 3.0

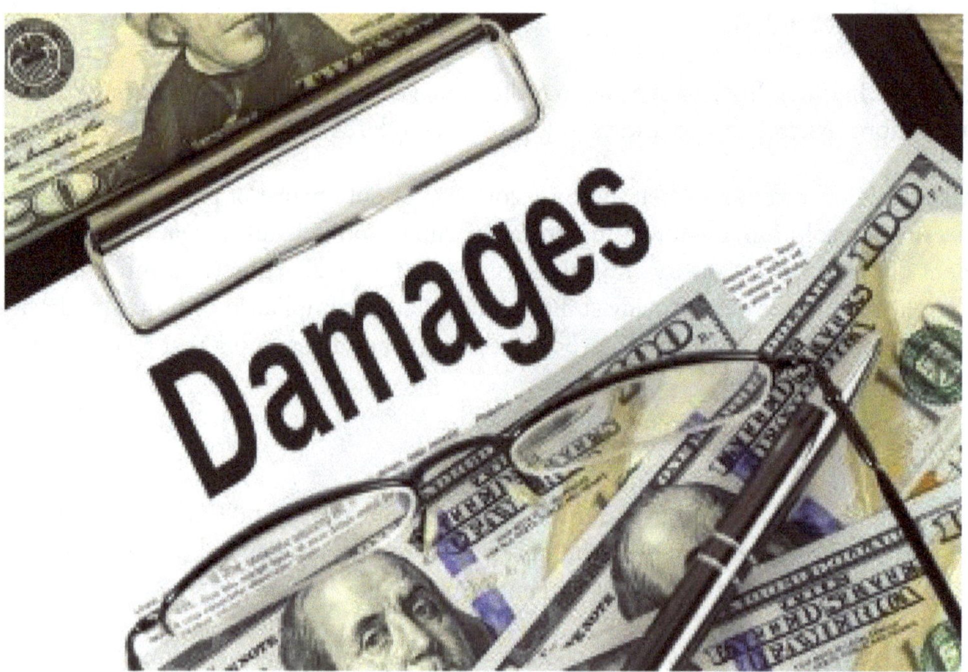

FIGURE 5.6 Damages

Economic damages (also referred to as actual damages) can be quantified. They are intended to restore the plaintiff to the position they were in before being injured. Compensatory damages are objectively calculated to provide the plaintiff with the amount of money necessary to replace what was lost.[48]

Noneconomic damages are subjective and can include things such as emotional distress, pain and suffering, loss of enjoyment of life, reputation damage, loss of companionship, or loss of parental guidance. They are more difficult to quantify than economic damages.[49]

Punitive damages are awards not related to the actual injury but are intended to punish the defendant(s) and deter others from engaging in similar conduct. In professional malpractice cases, punitive damages are difficult for plaintiffs to obtain because they must be related to outrageous conduct, such as gross negligence, recklessness, willful actions, or fraud.[50]

48. Brous, E. (2020). The elements of a nursing malpractice case, Part 4: Harm. *American Journal of Nursing, 120*(3), 61–64. https://doi.org/10.1097/01.naj.0000656360.21284.50
49. Brous, E. (2020). The elements of a nursing malpractice case, Part 4: Harm. *American Journal of Nursing, 120*(3), 61–64. https://doi.org/10.1097/01.naj.0000656360.21284.50
50. Brous, E. (2020). The elements of a nursing malpractice case, Part 4: Harm. *American Journal of Nursing, 120*(3), 61–64. https://doi.org/10.1097/01.naj.0000656360.21284.50

Sample Case Related to Damages[51]

Betty Shiflett fell out of bed in the recovery room after undergoing knee surgery. Three days later, she reported a clicking sound and pain in her knee to one of the nurses. Although the nurse documented these symptoms, she did not convey the information to the physician. A physical therapist reported these symptoms to the physician a week later. The physician then identified a previously undiagnosed nondisplaced left tibial fracture that was now avulsed. Two additional surgeries were unsuccessful, and Betty remained disabled, confined to a wheelchair, and in chronic pain.

Betty and her husband filed a lawsuit alleging negligence for the fall and the nurse's failure to report the symptoms to the physician. They also asserted a claim for a loss of consortium, meaning the spouse or family had also been harmed. The harm suffered is a loss of companionship, conjugal relations, support and services, or marital quality. The jury awarded total damages of $2,391,620 with the following breakdown:

- $791,620 for future medical expenses
- $800,000 for past noneconomic damages
- $500,000 for future noneconomic damages
- $300,000 for loss of consortium with spouse

Implications for Nurses

Nurses can reduce their liability exposure by following these principles[52]:

- Practicing according to current standards of practice.
- Maintaining professional liability insurance to provide coverage for events and licensure defense.
- Avoiding work-arounds or deviations from organizational policies and procedures.
- Maintaining clinical competency, including awareness of standard-of-practice changes.
- Engaging the chain of command with client concerns and pursuing concerns to resolution.
- Documenting in a manner that permits accurate reconstruction of client assessments, notification of others, and the sequence of events.

5.3 PROFESSIONAL LIABILITY AND YOUR NURSING LICENSE

As discussed in the previous sections, professional liability occurs when a civil lawsuit compensates clients who allege they have suffered injury or damage as a result of professional negligence. Many nurses elect to purchase malpractice insurance to protect themselves from professional liability, especially if working in specialty areas that experience a high number of claims, such as in obstetrics or post-anesthesia care units

51. Brous, E. (2020). The elements of a nursing malpractice case, Part 4: Harm. *American Journal of Nursing, 120*(3), 61–64. https://doi.org/10.1097/01.naj.0000656360.21284.50
52. Brous, E. (2020). The elements of a nursing malpractice case, Part 4: Harm. *American Journal of Nursing, 120*(3), 61–64. https://doi.org/10.1097/01.naj.0000656360.21284.50

(PACUs). The Nursing Service Organization (NSO) works in association with the American Nurses Association to provide malpractice insurance for nurses interested in purchasing it.

Read more about malpractice insurance available for nurses at https://www.nso.com/. Access supplementary digital content in the online book using this QR code.

The civil justice system cannot make rulings regarding your nursing license. It is the responsibility of the State Board of Nursing to suspend or revoke an individual's nursing license based on a disciplinary process.

The State Board of Nursing (SBON) governs nursing practice according to that state's Nurse Practice Act. The purpose of the SBON is to protect the public through licensure, education, legislation, and discipline. A nursing license is a contract between the state and licensee in which the licensee agrees to provide nursing care according to that state's Nurse Practice Act. Deviation from the Nurse Practice Act is a breach of contract that can lead to limited or revoked licensure. The SBON can suspend or revoke an individual's nursing license to protect the public from unsafe nursing practice. Nursing scope of practice and standards of nursing care are defined in the Nurse Practice Act that is enacted by the state legislature and enforced by the SBON. Nurses must practice according to the Nurse Practice Act of the state in which they are providing client care.

A nurse may be named in a board licensing complaint, also called an allegation. Allegations can be directly related to a nurse's clinical responsibilities, or they can be nonclinical (such as substance abuse, unprofessional behavior, or billing fraud). A complaint can be filed against a nurse by anyone, such as a client, a client's family member, a colleague, or an employer. It can be filed anonymously. After a complaint is filed, the SBON follows a disciplinary process that includes investigation, proceedings, board actions, and enforcement. The process can take months or years to resolve, and it can be costly to hire legal representation.[53]

During the investigation process, investigators use various methods to determine the facts, such as interviewing parties who were present, reviewing documentation and records, performing drug screens (if impairment is alleged), and compiling pertinent facts related to the events and circumstances surrounding the complaint. Nurses being investigated may receive a letter, email, or phone call from the SBON, or they may be required to appear at a certain date and time for an interview with an investigator. It is recommended that nurses consult with an attorney before responding to the SBON within the deadline provided. Nurses should be cooperative but should be aware that whatever is shared will be provided to a prosecuting attorney and/or the SBON.[54]

After completion of the investigation, the prosecuting attorney will determine how to proceed. A conference may be scheduled where the nurse will be interviewed by a member of the SBON and possibly the prosecut-

53. Nurses Service Organization (NSO) and CNA Financial Corporation. (2020). *Nurse professional liability exposure claim report: 4th edition: Minimizing risk, achieving excellence.* https://www.nso.com/Learning/Artifacts/Claim-Reports/Minimizing-Risk-Achieving-Excellence

54. Nurses Service Organization (NSO) and CNA Financial Corporation. (2020). *Nurse professional liability exposure claim report: 4th edition: Minimizing risk, achieving excellence.* https://www.nso.com/Learning/Artifacts/Claim-Reports/Minimizing-Risk-Achieving-Excellence

ing attorney. It is recommended for the nurse to have an attorney present during proceedings. The nurse has the opportunity to present evidence supporting their case. A resolution may be offered after the conference that ends the matter.[55]

However, if the SBON believes there is significant evidence, a formal hearing is held where a disciplinary action is proposed. This formal hearing is similar to a civil trial. The hearing panel may include some or all of the SBON members. A court reporter records the entire proceeding and a transcript is created. Witnesses may be called to testify and the nurse undergoes cross-examination. When both sides have presented their cases, the hearing is concluded. The outcome of the formal hearing is a ruling by the administrative law judge and the SBON. The nurse may face disciplinary action such as a reprimand, limitation, suspension, or revocation of their license. Nondisciplinary actions, such as a warning or a remedial education order, may be set. See a description of possible disciplinary actions enforced by the Wisconsin State Board of Nursing in Table 5.3a.

TABLE 5.3A. Potential Disciplinary and Nondisciplinary Actions of the Wisconsin State Board of Nursing[56]

Disciplinary Options	**Reprimand:** The licensee receives a public warning for a violation. **Limitation of License:** The licensee has conditions or requirements imposed upon their license, their scope of practice, or both. **Suspension:** The license is completely and absolutely withdrawn and withheld for a period of time, including all rights, privileges, and authority previously conferred by the credential. **Revocation:** The license is completely and absolutely terminated, as well as all rights, privileges, and authority previously conferred by the credential.
Nondisciplinary Options	**Administrative Warning:** A warning is issued if the violation is of a minor nature or a first occurrence, and the warning will adequately protect the public. The issuance of an administrative warning is public information; however, the reason for issuance is not. **Remedial Education Order:** A remedial education order is issued when there is reason to believe that the deficiency can be corrected with remedial education, while sufficiently protecting the public.

55. Nurses Service Organization (NSO) and CNA Financial Corporation. (2020). *Nurse professional liability exposure claim report: 4th edition: Minimizing risk, achieving excellence.* https://www.nso.com/Learning/Artifacts/Claim-Reports/Minimizing-Risk-Achieving-Excellence

56. Wisconsin Department of Safety and Professional Services. (2021). *Board of nursing newsletter.* https://content.govdelivery.com/accounts/WIDSPS/bulletins/2d71e3d

Find and review your state's Nurse Practice Act at https://www.ncsbn.org/policy/npa.page.

Read more about Wisconsin's Board of Nursing and Administrative Code.

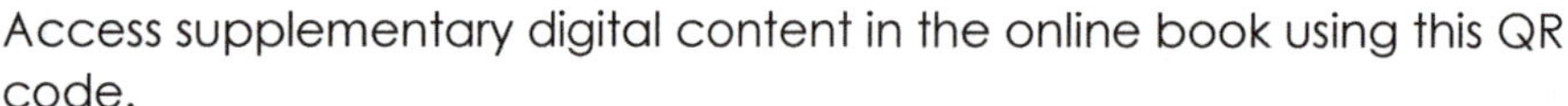

Access supplementary digital content in the online book using this QR code.

Liability considerations does not only apply when working in your professional nursing role, but also within your student nurse role. As you work as a student nurse, there are other role considerations that may impact the decision regarding professional liability. Please see Table 5.3b for a comparison of different types of liability.

TABLE 5.3B. Types of Liability

Type of Liability	Definition	Example
Supervisory Liability[57]	When a clinical supervisor or preceptor is held responsible for the actions of the student nurse or for failing to properly supervise them.	A clinical supervisor fails to provide proper guidance during a procedure, resulting in the student nurse administering the wrong medication to a client. The supervisor could be held liable for inadequate supervision.
Institutional Liability[58]	When the health care institution (e.g., hospital, clinic) is held responsible for the actions of its employees or for failing to implement adequate policies and procedures to prevent harm.	A hospital does not provide proper orientation or training programs for student nurses, leading to a student nurse making a critical error. The hospital could be held liable for not ensuring adequate training.
Student Liability[59]	When the student nurse is held responsible for their own actions that cause harm to clients or violate protocols.	A student nurse neglects to follow infection control protocols, resulting in a client's condition worsening. The student nurse could be held liable for their negligence.

57. Dyer, A. M. & Griffin, S. (2024). *Just culture, liability concerns, and ensuring a safe working environment.* AOCN, Association of periOperative Registered Nurses. https://www.aorn.org/article/just-culture#:~:text=This%20is%20called%20vicarious%20liability,the%20nurse's%20scope%20of%20practice

58. Oliva, A., Caputo, M., Grassi, S., Vetrugno, G., Marazza, M., Ponzanelli, G., Cauda, R., Scambia, G., Forti, G., Bellantone, R., & Pascali, V. (2020). Liability of health care professionals and institutions during COVID-19 pandemic in Italy: Symposium proceedings and position Statement. *Journal of Patient Safety 16*(4), e299-e302. https://doi.org/10.1097/PTS.0000000000000793

59. Nurses Service Organization (NSO) and CNA Financial Corporation. (2020). *Nurse professional liability exposure claim report: 4th edition: Minimizing risk, achieving excellence.* https://www.nso.com/Learning/Artifacts/Claim-Reports/Minimizing-Risk-Achieving-Excellence

5.4 FREQUENT ALLEGATIONS AND SBON INVESTIGATIONS

The Nurses Service Organization (NSO) reported the three most common allegations resulting in state board investigations in 2020 were related to the categories of professional conduct, scope of practice, and documentation errors or omissions.[60]

Professional Conduct

Common allegations related to professional conduct included drug diversion and substance abuse, professional misconduct, reciprocal actions, and wastage errors.

DRUG DIVERSION AND SUBSTANCE ABUSE

The most common allegations related to professional conduct for both RNs and LPN/VNs in 2020 were related to drug diversion and/or substance abuse. Examples include diverting medications for oneself or others and apparent intoxication from alcohol or drugs while on duty.

The National Council of State Boards of Nursing (NCSBN) created a brochure titled *Substance Abuse Disorder in Nursing* to address this common issue.[61] Many states have programs in place to assist nurses with substance abuse, such as Wisconsin Nursing Association's Nurses Caring for Nurses (Peer Assistance) program or New York State Nursing Association's Statewide Peer Assistance for Nurses (SPAN) program.[62,63]

PROFESSIONAL MISCONDUCT

Professional misconduct as defined by state regulations was the second most common allegation related to professional conduct. This category includes unprofessional conduct towards coworkers and clients, as well as allegations of falling asleep.

Sample Case

A home health RN was assigned to monitor an 11-month-old child from 1900 to 0700. The child was intubated and required constant monitoring to ensure the tubing remained secure while she was in her crib. However, the child's father found the RN sleeping and the child's tubing unsecured. The child did not suffer harm due to the incident, but the SBON publicly reprimanded the RN, and the costs to defend the nurse exceeded $2,400.[64]

---

60. Nurses Service Organization (NSO) and CNA Financial Corporation. (2020). *Nurse professional liability exposure claim report: 4th edition: Minimizing risk, achieving excellence.* https://www.nso.com/Learning/Artifacts/Claim-Reports/Minimizing-Risk-Achieving-Excellence
61. National Council State Board of Nursing. *Substance abuse disorder in nursing* [Brochure]. https://www.ncsbn.org/nursing-regulation/practice/substance-use-disorder.page
62. Wisconsin Nurses Association. (n.d.). *Nurses caring for nurses (peer assistance).* https://www.wisconsinnurses.org/about-wna/affiliates/nurses-caring-for-nurses-peer-assistance/
63. Statewide Peer Assistance For Nurses. https://www.statewidepeerassistance.org/
64. Nurses Service Organization (NSO) and CNA Financial Corporation. (2020). *Nurse professional liability exposure claim report: 4th edition: Minimizing risk, achieving excellence.* https://www.nso.com/Learning/Artifacts/Claim-Reports/Minimizing-Risk-Achieving-Excellence

RECIPROCAL ACTIONS

The third most common professional conduct allegation was reciprocal actions. Many cases involved nurses who were trying to contend with clients who were violent or aggressive and either retaliated against the client or responded to the client 's aggression in an inappropriate or unprofessional manner.

> **Sample Case**
>
> A client in an inpatient behavioral health unit became agitated, pulled a phone out of the wall, and threw it. The nurse entered the room and following a brief interaction, an altercation between the client and the nurse ensued. The nurse received a public reprimand and disciplinary actions from the SBON.[65]

WASTAGE ERRORS

Wastage errors were the fourth most common allegation. Wastage errors occurred when nurses neglected to perform accurate medication counts or did not appropriately document proper disposal of opioids and other drugs with a high potential for abuse.

> **Sample Case**
>
> An RN left two 15 milligram tablets of a benzodiazepine called Temazepam unattended in an area accessible to clients. The medication went missing and was apparently taken by a client. The nurse falsely documented the Temazepam as wastage, knowing the medication was actually missing. The SBON issued a $200 fine, and expenses to defend the nurse exceeded $7,200.[66]

Scope of Practice

Common allegations related to scope of practice include failure to maintain a minimum standard of practice and providing services beyond one's scope of practice.

FAILURE TO MAINTAIN MINIMUM STANDARD OF NURSING PRACTICE

The most common allegations related to scope of practice include failure to maintain a minimum standard of nursing practice. These cases include a breach of minimum professional standards, incompetence, and negligence.

65. Nurses Service Organization (NSO) and CNA Financial Corporation. (2020). *Nurse professional liability exposure claim report: 4th edition: Minimizing risk, achieving excellence.* https://www.nso.com/Learning/Artifacts/Claim-Reports/Minimizing-Risk-Achieving-Excellence

66. Nurses Service Organization (NSO) and CNA Financial Corporation. (2020). *Nurse professional liability exposure claim report: 4th edition: Minimizing risk, achieving excellence.* https://www.nso.com/Learning/Artifacts/Claim-Reports/Minimizing-Risk-Achieving-Excellence

Sample Case

A nurse working in home health failed to complete required client assessments and omitted pertinent client information in the health care record. This omission could have caused a disruption in the continuity of treatment resulting in client harm. The SBON determined the nurse failed to exercise the degree of learning, skill, care, and experience ordinarily possessed and exercised by a competent RN. The SBON placed the nurse on probation for three years, and the expenses associated with defending the nurse exceeded $5,400.[67]

Sample Case

An RN failed to follow agency policy and procedures by neglecting to properly verify identification of two clients and omitting the review of relevant laboratory results. As a result of bypassing standard safety procedures, the RN gave an extra unit of blood to one client that was intended for the other client, thereby depriving that client the extra unit of blood required based on her lab results. The SBON placed the nurse on probation for three years. However, the nurse did not comply with the terms of her probation by failing to report to the SBON when she applied for licensure in two other states. The nurse also failed to obtain approval prior to commencing employment. The nurse was ultimately ordered to surrender her license.[68]

Sample Case

A student nurse was instructed to discontinue an intravenous (IV) antibiotic for a client with a central venous catheter. When the student discontinued the IV, she unknowingly loosened the catheter connection from the lumen luer connector. The loosened line would likely have been discovered when the line was flushed per agency policy, but the student testified she did not know she was supposed to flush the catheter line or clamp it after the medication was discontinued. Shortly thereafter, the client became unresponsive, and a code was called. The disconnection was not discovered until the client was transferred to the intensive care unit three hours later. The client experienced an air embolism and died. A malpractice claim was awarded.[69]

67. Nurses Service Organization (NSO) and CNA Financial Corporation. (2020). *Nurse professional liability exposure claim report: 4th edition: Minimizing risk, achieving excellence.* https://www.nso.com/Learning/Artifacts/Claim-Reports/Minimizing-Risk-Achieving-Excellence

68. NNurses Service Organization (NSO) and CNA Financial Corporation. (2020). *Nurse professional liability exposure claim report: 4th edition: Minimizing risk, achieving excellence.* https://www.nso.com/Learning/Artifacts/Claim-Reports/Minimizing-Risk-Achieving-Excellence

69. Nurses Service Organization (NSO) and CNA Financial Corporation. (2020). *Nurse professional liability exposure claim report: 4th edition: Minimizing risk, achieving excellence.* https://www.nso.com/Learning/Artifacts/Claim-Reports/Minimizing-Risk-Achieving-Excellence

PROVISION OF SERVICES BEYOND SCOPE OF PRACTICE

The second most common allegation related to scope of practice is provision of services beyond one's scope of practice. This category typically involves nurses making changes to clients' prescribed treatments or administering medication that had not been prescribed.

> **Sample Case**
>
> An RN in the ICU was caring for a client with extreme nausea. The nurse made several unsuccessful attempts to reach the provider for an order for Ondansetron. The nurse called the pharmacy and relayed her concern for the client's nausea and her inability to reach the provider. The nurse informed the pharmacist that she believed the situation was urgent, and she would contact the provider for an order. The pharmacy dispensed Ondansetron and the nurse administered the medication. Although the client did not suffer adverse effects from the medication, no order was ever received for the medication. Upon finding the RN violated the Nurse Practice Act by practicing beyond the scope of practice for an RN, the SBON publicly reprimanded the nurse and ordered her to pay a fine of $600. Expenses associated with defending the nurse exceeded $6,100.[70]

Documentation

Over half of the allegations in 2020 regarding documentation were related to fraudulent or falsified client care or billing records. The health care record is a legal document. It should never be altered, deleted, or falsified. Maintaining accurate and timely documentation is a primary professional responsibility of nurses.

> **Sample Case**
>
> In a case involving a nursing student, the preceptor instructed the student to monitor the client's vital signs every 15 minutes for one hour and then every 30 minutes for two hours and then every hour for four hours. The student allegedly documented vital signs every 15 minutes for one hour but did not record any vital signs thereafter. When confronted by her preceptor about the incomplete record, the student stated that she "forgot to do them." Approximately 30 minutes later, the preceptor discovered the missing vital signs were documented in the client's record. The preceptor asked the student about the entries, and the student replied that she "made them up." The student later contended that she meant she charted the vital signs accurately but made up the times the vital signs were taken to match the preceptor's instructions. The SBON considered the student was still learning but viewed documentation as a basic nursing skill. Because the student's conduct involved dishonesty, they imposed a penalty of a one-year suspension followed by one year of probation. The expenses associated with defending the student nurse exceeded $6,900.[71]

---

70. Nurses Service Organization (NSO) and CNA Financial Corporation. (2020). *Nurse professional liability exposure claim report: 4th edition: Minimizing risk, achieving excellence.* https://www.nso.com/Learning/Artifacts/Claim-Reports/Minimizing-Risk-Achieving-Excellence

71. Nurses Service Organization (NSO) and CNA Financial Corporation. (2020). *Nurse professional liability exposure claim report: 4th edition: Minimizing risk, achieving excellence.* https://www.nso.com/Learning/Artifacts/Claim-Reports/Minimizing-Risk-Achieving-Excellence

PROFESSIONAL MISCONDUCT CASE STUDY SCENARIO

Sarah is a registered nurse working in a busy hospital emergency department. One evening, she is assigned to care for Mr. Thompson, a 68-year-old man who was admitted with severe chest pain. The emergency department is understaffed, and Sarah is handling multiple clients at once.

During her shift, Sarah receives a call from her supervisor asking her to assist in another critical case. In her hurry to attend to the other client, Sarah administers Mr. Thompson's medication without double-checking the doctor's orders. Unfortunately, she administers the wrong dosage of a medication, causing Mr. Thompson's condition to worsen significantly.

Upon realizing her mistake, Sarah panics and decides not to report the error to avoid potential disciplinary action. She adjusts Mr. Thompson's medical record to conceal the mistake. Later, Mr. Thompson's condition deteriorates further, requiring intensive care. An investigation reveals the medication error and the altered medical records.

1. Identify the ethical and legal issues present in this case.
2. How does Sarah's behavior constitute professional misconduct?
3. What are the potential consequences for Sarah, both professionally and legally?
4. How might the lack of adequate staffing and supervision have contributed to this incident?
5. What policies should the hospital have in place to prevent such errors and ensure proper reporting?
6. How did Sarah's actions affect Mr. Thompson's safety and overall outcome?
7. What impact might this incident have on the trust between health care professionals and clients?

5.5 PROTECTING YOUR NURSING LICENSE

You have worked hard to obtain a nursing license and it will be your livelihood. See Figure 5.7[72] for an illustration of a nursing license. Protecting your nursing license is vital.

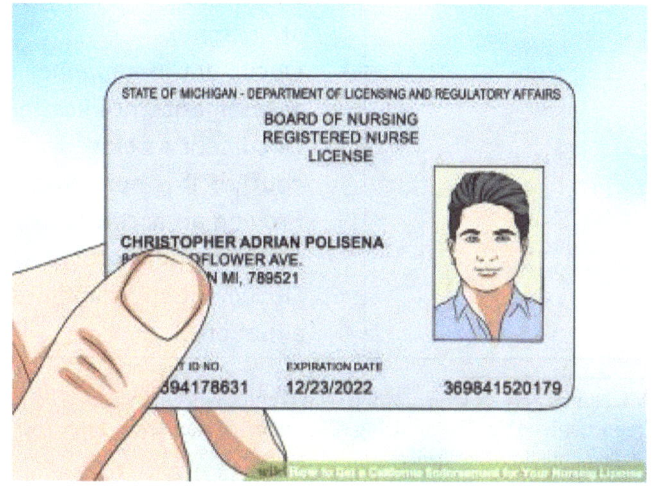

FIGURE 5.7 Nursing License

72. "aid9688616-v4-728px-Get-a-California-Endorsement-for-Your-Nursing-License-Step-11.jpg" by unknown is licensed under CC BY-NC-SA 3.0

Actions to Protect Your License

There are several actions that nurses can take to protect their nursing license, avoid liability, and promote client safety. See Table 5.5 for a summary of recommendations.

TABLE 5.5. Risk Management Recommendations to Protect Your Nursing License

Legal Issues	Recommendations to Protect Your License
Practicing outside one's scope of practice	• Practice within the requirements of your state's Nurse Practice Act, in compliance with organizational policies and procedures, and within the national standard of care. • Maintain basic clinical and specialty competencies by proactively obtaining the professional information, education, and training needed to remain current regarding nursing techniques, clinical practice, biologics, and equipment.[73] • Only accept client care assignments you are trained and competent to perform. Ask for additional training as needed. • Recognize one's limitations and ask for assistance when needed. • If necessary, utilize the chain of command or the risk management or legal departments regarding concerns about client care or practice issues and pursue concerns to resolution.[74]
Failure to assess & monitor	• Ensure that you are following appropriate guidelines for routine assessments and following up appropriately if client condition warrants additional monitoring. • Ensure the client condition aligns to skills and monitoring capabilities of unit/staff. • Escalate changes in client condition via appropriate channels.
Documentation	• Document client care assessments, observations, communications, and actions in an objective, timely, accurate, complete, and appropriate manner. • Document in a manner that permits accurate reconstruction of client assessments, notification of others, and the sequence of events. • Document as close to the time of care provision as possible. (In court, if it is not documented, it is considered not done.) • Provide an accurate documentation of a change in client condition, care provided, providers notified, and orders received. • Document specific times of interventions provided during emergency situations.

73. Nurses Service Organization (NSO) and CNA Financial *Corporation. (2020).* Nurse professional liability exposure claim report: 4th edition: Minimizing risk, achieving excellence. https://www.nso.com/Learning/Artifacts/Claim-Reports/Minimizing-Risk-Achieving-Excellence

74. Nurses Service Organization (NSO) and CNA Financial *Corporation. (2020).* Nurse professional liability exposure claim report: 4th edition: Minimizing risk, achieving excellence. https://www.nso.com/Learning/Artifacts/Claim-Reports/Minimizing-Risk-Achieving-Excellence

TABLE 5.5. Continued...

	• When notifying a provider about a client, document the name of the provider notified, the time of the notification, and the provider's response. Follow through with any nursing actions taken and the client's response. • Never alter, delete, or falsify information. • If there is information that should have been charted but was not, document "late entry," noting the time the charting occurred and the specific time the assessment or intervention actually took place.[75] • When describing a client problem, include the nursing actions taken and the client's response.[76] • Use medical terminology. • Avoid abbreviations. • Review notes from other health care team members to ensure coordination of efforts is occurring.[77] • Maintain your own personal files that can be helpful with respect to your character, such as letters of recommendation, performance evaluations, and continuing education certificates.[78]
Medication errors	• Avoid workarounds. (For example, if an error message is received when scanning a medication with a barcode scanner during med pass, don't assume it is a technology error and "workaround" it by just documenting the medication in the MAR. Instead, investigate error messages because they could be indicating a medication error, not a technology error.) • Always check the "rights of medication administration" three times, even when using barcode scanners and other equipment. (Review information about checking medication rights in the "Administration of Enteral Medications" chapter in Open RN *Nursing Skills, 2e* at https://wtcs.pressbooks.pub/nursingskills.) • Be aware of look alike/sound alike medications. • Double-check dosage calculations, especially for pediatric clients. • Follow agency policies and procedures related to medication administration and documentation. • Clarify prescriptions with prescribing providers if they are unclear or you have concerns. For example, if acetaminophen is prescribed for fever and the client is experiencing pain, clarify the indications in the order before administering it for pain.

75. Brous, E. (2019). The elements of a nursing malpractice case, Part 1: Duty. *American Journal of Nursing, 119*(7), 64–67. https://doi.org/10.1097/01.NAJ.0000569476.17357.f5

76. Brous, E. (2019). The elements of a nursing malpractice case, Part 1: Duty. *American Journal of Nursing, 119*(7), 64–67. https://doi.org/10.1097/01.NAJ.0000569476.17357.f5

77. Brous, E. (2019). The elements of a nursing malpractice case, Part 1: Duty. *American Journal of Nursing, 119*(7), 64–67. https://doi.org/10.1097/01.NAJ.0000569476.17357.f5

78. Nurses Service Organization (NSO) and CNA Financial Corporation. (2020). *Nurse professional liability exposure claim report: 4th edition: Minimizing risk, achieving excellence.* https://www.nso.com/Learning/Artifacts/Claim-Reports/Minimizing-Risk-Achieving-Excellence

TABLE 5.5. Continued...

Medication errors	• Avoid distractions while preparing and administering medications. (Read more information about preventing medication errors in the "Legal/Ethical" chapter in Open RN *Nursing Pharmacology, 2e* at https://wtcs.pressbooks.pub/pharmacology2e.) • Maintain a chain of possession when administering medications. Never administer a medication for which you have not personally done the medication checks. • Never leave medication unattended. • If a medication error occurs, follow agency policy regarding notification and submitting an incident report.
Substance abuse and drug diversion	• Waste controlled substances and document wasting according to agency policy. • Perform accurate counting and documentation of controlled substances per agency policy. • Seek assistance if you are experiencing challenges with substance use. Report impaired professionals regarding suspected substance abuse. (Read more about drug diversion and support for nurses with substance use disorder in the "Legal/Ethical" chapter in Open RN *Nursing Pharmacology, 2e* at https://wtcs.pressbooks.pub/pharmacology2e.) • Report convictions such as drug possession, driving under the influence (DUI), or operating under the influence (OWI) to your State Board of Nursing as required.
Acts that may result in potential or actual client harm	• Participate in accurate and thorough handoff reports according to agency policy. (Read more about handoff reports in the "Communication" chapter of Open RN *Nursing Fundamentals, 2e* at https://wtcs.pressbooks.pub/nursingfundamentals.) • Communicate with other members of the health care team using ISBARR format. (Read more about ISBARR format in the "Communication" chapter of Open RN *Nursing Fundamentals, 2e* at https://wtcs.pressbooks.pub/nursingfundamentals.) • Follow the nursing care plan. Assess appropriateness of interventions according to the client's current condition before implementing them. • Conduct thorough nursing assessments, especially for skin breakdown or pressure injuries. (Read more about assessing skin breakdown and pressure injuries in the "Integumentary" chapter of Open RN *Nursing Fundamentals, 2e* at https://wtcs.pressbooks.pub/nursingfundamentals.) • Advocate for quality client care and speak up regarding concerns about client safety. • Educate clients and encourage them to actively participate in their care and make informed decisions. • Follow National Patient Safety Goals. Implement fall prevention interventions according to agency policy. Report unsafe equipment. (Read more about promoting client safety in the "Safety" chapter in Open RN *Nursing Fundamentals, 2e* "at https://wtcs.pressbooks.pub/nursingfundamentals.) • Document and report unsafe staffing or other workplace safety concerns per agency policy, state policy, or OSHA.

TABLE 5.5. Continued...

Safe-guarding client possessions & valuables	• Encourage client valuables to be sent home. • Document all client possessions upon admission to inpatient facilities and obtain client or family signature or acknowledgement. • Lock up client valuables per agency policy. • Follow agency policy regarding receipt of gifts from clients or family.
Adherence to mandatory reporting responsibilities	• Report suspected abuse of children, elders, and other vulnerable populations. (Read more about mandatory reporting under the "Duty" subsection of the "Understanding the Legal System" section of this chapter.) • Report gunshot wounds, dog bites, and communicable disease per agency and state policy.

Culture of Safety

It can be frightening to think about entering the nursing profession after becoming aware of potential legal actions and risks to your nursing license, especially when realizing even an unintentional error could result in disciplinary or legal action. When seeking employment, it is helpful for nurses to ask questions during the interview process regarding organizational commitment to a culture of safety to reduce errors and enhance client safety.

Many health care agencies have adopted a **culture of safety** that embraces error reporting by employees with the goal of identifying root causes of problems so they may be addressed to improve client safety. One component of a culture of safety is "Just Culture." Just Culture is culture where people feel safe raising questions and concerns and report safety events in an environment that emphasizes a nonpunitive response to errors and near misses. Clear lines are drawn between human error, at-risk, and reckless behaviors.[79]

The American Nurses Association (ANA) officially endorses the Just Culture model. In 2019 the ANA published a position statement on Just Culture. They stated that while our traditional health care culture held individuals accountable for all errors and accidents that happened to clients under their care, the Just Culture model recognizes that individual practitioners should not be held accountable for system failings over which they have no control. The Just Culture model also recognizes that many errors represent predictable interactions between human operators and the systems in which they work. However, the Just Culture model does not tolerate conscious disregard of clear risks to clients or gross misconduct (e.g., falsifying a record or performing professional duties while intoxicated).[80]

The Just Culture model categorizes human behavior into three categories of errors: simple human error, at-risk behavior, or reckless behavior. Consequences of errors are based on these categories.[81] When seeking

79. The Joint Commission. (2017). The essential role of leadership in developing a safety culture. *Sentinel event alert, Issue 57.* https://www.jointcommission.org/-/media/tjc/documents/resources/patient-safety-topics/sentinel-event/sea_57_safety_culture_leadership_0317pdf.pdf
80. American Nursing Association. (2010). *Position statement: Just culture.* https://www.nursingworld.org/~4afe07/globalassets/practiceandpolicy/health-and-safety/just_culture.pdf
81. American Nursing Association. (2010). *Position statement: Just culture.* https://www.nursingworld.org/~4afe07/globalassets/

employment, it is helpful for nurses to determine how an agency implements a culture of safety because of its potential impact on one's professional liability and licensure.

Read more about the Just Culture model in the "Basic Concepts" section of the "Leadership and Management" chapter.

5.6 OTHER LEGAL ISSUES

In addition to being aware of the legal and regulatory frameworks in which one practices nursing, it is also important for nurses to understand the legal concepts of informed consent and advance directives.

INFORMED CONSENT

Informed consent is the fundamental right of a client to accept or reject health care. Nurses have a legal responsibility to provide verbal and/or written information and obtain verbal or written consent for performing nursing care such as bathing, medication administration, and urinary or intravenous catheter insertion. While physicians have the responsibility to provide information and obtain informed consent related to medical procedures, nurses are typically required to verify the presence of a valid, signed informed consent before the procedure is performed. Additionally, if nurses do not believe the client has adequate understanding of a procedure, its risks, benefits, or alternatives to treatment, they should request the provider return to clarify unclear information with the client. Nurses must remain within their scope of practice related to informed consent beyond nursing acts.

Two legal concepts related to informed consent are competence and capacity. **Competence** is a legal term defined as the ability of an individual to participate in legal proceedings. A judge decides if an individual is "competent" or "incompetent." In contrast, **capacity** is "a functional determination that an individual is or is not capable of making a medical decision within a given situation."[82] It is outside the scope of practice for nurses to formally assess capacity, but nurses may initiate the evaluation of client capacity and contribute assessment information. States typically require two health care providers to identify an individual as "incapacitated" and unable to make their own health care decisions. Capacity may be a temporary or permanent state.

practiceandpolicy/health-and-safety/just_culture.pdf
82. Darby, R. R., & Dickerson, B. C. (2017). Dementia, decision making, and capacity. *Harvard Review of Psychiatry, 25*(6), 270–278. https://doi.org/10.1097/HRP.0000000000000163

The following box outlines situations where the nurse may question a client's decision-making capacity.

Triggers for Questioning Capacity and Decision-Making[83]

- Inability to voice a decision
- Blanket acceptance or refusal of care
- Absence of questions about the treatment being offered or provided
- Excessive or inconsistent reasons for refusing care
- New inability to perform activities of daily living
- Hyperactivity, disruptive behavior, or agitation
- Labile emotions or affect
- Hallucinations
- Intoxication

If an individual has an advance directive in place, their designated power of attorney for health care may step in and make medical decisions when the client is deemed incapacitated. In the absence of advance directives, the legal system may take over and appoint a guardian to make medical decisions for an individual. The guardian is often a family member or friend but may be completely unrelated to the incapacitated individual. Nurses are instrumental in encouraging a client to complete an advance directive while they have capacity to do so.

Advance Directives

The Patient Self-Determination Act (PSDA) is a federal law passed by Congress in 1990 following highly publicized cases involving the withdrawal of life-supporting care for incompetent individuals. (Read more about the Karen Quinlan, Nancy Cruzan, and Terri Shaivo cases in the boxes at the end of this section.) The PSDA requires health care institutions, such as hospitals and long-term care facilities, to offer adults written information that advises them "to make decisions concerning their medical care, including the right to accept or refuse medical or surgical treatment and the right to formulate, at the individual's option, advance directives."[84] **Advance directives** are defined as written instructions, such as a living will or durable power of attorney for health care, recognized under state law, relating to the provision of health care when the individual is incapacitated. The PSDA allows clients to record their preferences about do-not-resuscitate (DNR) orders and withdrawing life-sustaining treatment. In the absence of a client's advance directives, the court may assert an "unqualified interest in the preservation of human life to be weighed against the constitutionally protected interests of the individual."[85] For this reason, nurses must educate and support the communities they serve regarding the creation of advanced directives.

Advanced directives vary by state. For example, some states allow lay witness signatures whereas some require a notary signature. Some states place restrictions on family members, doctors, or nurses serving as witnesses. It is important for individuals creating advance directives to follow instructions for state-specific documents to ensure they are legally binding and honored.

83. American Nursing Association. (2010). *Position statement: Just culture.* https://www.nursingworld.org/~4afe07/globalassets/practiceandpolicy/health-and-safety/just_culture.pdf

84. Centers for Medicare & Medicaid Services, Department of Health and Human Services. (2012). *Part 489-Provider agreements and supplier approval, Subpart A-General provisions.* https://www.govinfo.gov/content/pkg/CFR-2012-title42-vol5/pdf/CFR-2012-title42-vol5-chapIV.pdf

85. Nurses Service Organization (NSO) and CNA Financial Corporation. (2020). *Nurse professional liability exposure claim report: 4th edition: Minimizing risk, achieving excellence.* https://www.nso.com/Learning/Artifacts/Claim-Reports/Minimizing-Risk-Achieving-Excellence

Advance directives do not require an attorney to complete. In many organizations, social workers or chaplains assist individuals to complete advance directives following referral from physicians or nurses. Clients should review and update their documents every 10-15 years, as well as with changes in relationship status or if new medical conditions are diagnosed.

Although advanced directive documents vary by state, they generally fall into two categories, referred to as a living will or durable power of attorney for healthcare.

LIVING WILL

A **living will** is a type of advance directive in which an individual identifies what treatments they would like to receive or refuse if they become incapacitated and unable to make decisions. In most states, a living will only goes into effect if an individual meets specific medical criteria.[86] The living will often includes instructions regarding life-sustaining measures, such as cardiopulmonary resuscitation (CPR), mechanical ventilation, and tube feeding.

DURABLE POWER OF ATTORNEY FOR HEALTHCARE

It is impossible for an individual to document their preferences in a living will for every conceivable medical scenario that may occur. For this reason, it is essential for individuals to complete a durable power of attorney for healthcare. A **durable power of attorney for healthcare (DPOAHC)** is a person chosen to speak on one's behalf if one becomes incapacitated. Typically, a primary health care power of attorney (POA) is identified with an alternative individual designated if the primary POA is unable or unwilling to do so. The health care POA is expected to make health care decisions for an individual they believe the person would make for themselves, based on wishes expressed in a living will or during previous conversations.[87]

It is essential for nurses to encourage clients to complete advance directives and have conversations with their designated POA about health care preferences, especially related to possible traumatic or end-of-life events that could require medical treatment decisions. Nurses can also dispel common misconceptions, such as these documents give the health care POA power to manage an individual's finances. (A financial POA performs different functions than a health care POA and should be discussed with an attorney.)

After the advance directives are completed and included in the client's medical record, the nurse has the responsibility to ensure they are appropriately incorporated into their care if they should become incapacitated.

View state-specific advance directives at the American Association of Retired Persons website. Access supplementary digital content in the online book using this QR code.

86. AARP. (2020). *Advance directive forms.* https://www.aarp.org/caregiving/financial-legal/free-printable-advance-directives/#more-advancedirectives
87. AARP. (2020). *Advance directive forms.* https://www.aarp.org/caregiving/financial-legal/free-printable-advance-directives/#more-advancedirectives

Sample Case: Karen Ann Quinlan[88]

Karen Ann Quinlan is an important figure in the United States' history of defining life and death, a client's privacy, and the state's interest in preserving life and preventing murder. In April 1975, Karen Quinlan was 21 years old and became unresponsive after ingesting a combination of valium and alcohol while celebrating a friend's birthday. She experienced respiratory failure, and although resuscitation efforts were successful, she suffered irreversible brain damage. She remained in a persistent vegetative state and became ventilator dependent. Her parents requested her physicians discontinue the ventilator because they believed it constituted extraordinary means to prolong her life. Her physicians denied their request out of concern of possible homicide charges based on New Jersey's law. The Quinlans filed the first "right to die" lawsuit in September of 1975 but were denied by the New Jersey Superior Court in November. In March of 1976, the New Jersey Supreme Court determined the parent's right to determine Karen's medical treatment exceeded that of the state. Karen was discontinued from the ventilator six weeks later. When taken off the ventilator, Karen shocked many by continuing to breathe on her own. She lived in a coma for nine more years and succumbed to pneumonia on June 11, 1985.

Sample Case: Nancy Beth Cruzan[89]

Nancy Cruzan is another important figure in the history of US "right to die" legal cases. At the age of 25, Nancy Cruzan was in a car accident on January 11, 1983. She never regained consciousness. After three years in a rehabilitation hospital, her parents began an eight-year battle in the courts to remove Nancy's feeding tube. Nancy's case was the first "right to die" case heard by the United States Supreme Court. Beyond allowing for the discontinuation of Nancy's feeding tube, the U.S. Supreme Court ruled that all adults have the right to the following:

1) Choose or refuse any medical or surgical intervention, including artificial nutrition and hydration.

2) Make advance directives and name a surrogate to make decisions on their behalf.

3) Surrogates can decide on treatment options even when all concerned are aware that such measures will hasten death, as long as causing death is not their intent. Nancy died nine days after removal of her feeding tube in December 1990. As a result of the Cruzan decision, the Patient Self-Determination Act (PSDA) was passed and took effect December 1, 1991. The act requires facilities to inform clients about their right to refuse treatment and to ask if they would like to prepare an advance directive.

88. Arthur J. Morris Law Library. (n.d.). *Karen Ann Quinlan and the right to die.* https://archives.law.virginia.edu/dengrove/writeup/karen-ann-quinlan-and-right-die
89. Taub, S. (2001). Art of medicine "Departed, Jan 11, 1983; At Peace, Dec 26, 1990." *Virtual Mentor, American Medical Association Journal of Ethics,* 3(7), 231-233. https://journalofethics.ama-assn.org/sites/journalofethics.ama-assn.org/files/2021-05/artm1-0107.pdf

Sample Case: Terri Schaivo[90]

The Terri Schaivo case is a key case in history of advance directives in the United States because of its focus on the importance of having written advance directives to prevent family animosity, pain, and suffering. In 1990 Terri Schaivo was 26 years old. In her Florida home, she experienced a cardiac arrest thought to be a function of a low potassium level resulting from an eating disorder. She experienced severe anoxic brain injury and entered a persistent vegetative state. A PEG tube was inserted to provide medications, nutrition, and hydration. After three years, her husband refused further life-sustaining measures on her behalf, based on a statement Terri had once made, stating, "I don't want to be kept alive on a machine." He expressed interest in obtaining a DNR order, withholding antibiotics for a urinary tract infection, and ultimately requested removal of the PEG tube. However, Terri's parents never accepted the diagnosis of persistent vegetative state and vigorously opposed their son-in-law's decision and requests. Seven years of litigation generated 30 legal opinions, all supporting Michael Schiavo's right to make a decision on his wife's behalf. Terri died on March 31, 2005, following removal of her feeding tube.

5.7 SPOTLIGHT APPLICATION

Sara is a new graduate nurse orienting on the medical floor at a large teaching hospital. She has been working on the floor for two weeks and notices that many of the nurses provide shift handoff reports to one another outside of the client rooms. Sara asks her preceptor why the nurses stand and report client care information in the hallway. Her preceptor responds that this is the standard way staff can meet the agency guidelines for beside handoff reporting without "disturbing" clients while they are resting. Sara has concerns about this action on many levels. What legal repercussions might this "hallway reporting" have?

Sara is smart to identify that discussing client care information in a hallway outside of client rooms may jeopardize client HIPAA protections and confidentiality. Sensitive client information should never be discussed freely where others may overhear care information and details. Additionally, the act of bedside handoff reporting is meant to provide an inclusive environment for clients to participate with care staff in the report and information exchange. Discussing report details outside of the client room does not actively include the client in the bedside reporting procedure.

90. Weijer, C. (2005). A death in the family: Reflections on the Terri Schiavo case. *Canadian Medical Association Journal = journal de l'Association medicale canadienne, 172*(9), 1197–1198. https://doi.org/10.1503/cmaj.050348

5.8 LEARNING ACTIVITIES

Learning Activities

(Answers to "Learning Activities" can be found in the "Answer Key" at the end of the book. Answers to interactive activities are provided as immediate feedback.)

1. In 2006 Nurse Julie Thao was charged with felony criminal negligence in the death of a 16-year-old laboring mother when she mistakenly hung a bag of epidural medication instead of intravenous penicillin. Although the baby was successfully delivered via cesarean section, the client died following aggressive resuscitation attempts as a result of circulatory collapse. Nurse Thao was fired from her job of 16 years. Her felony charge was amended to two misdemeanor counts, and her state's Board of Nursing suspended her license, imposed practice limitations upon return, mandated completion of an education program, and imposed a $2,500 fine. Beyond these sanctions, she stated at her sentencing hearing, "The anguish and remorse are a life sentence that will serve for all time."

View the "Chasing Zero" documentary on YouTube[91] Access supplementary digital content in the online book using this QR code.

Discuss factors that contributed to Nurse Julie Thao's medication error. What reflections on your own nursing practice can be made after viewing this video clip? What actions might have been taken to avoid this error? Do you believe other members of the health care team were culpable in their actions?

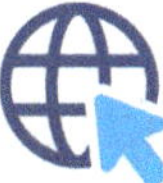

Interactive learning activities have been excluded from the print version of the text. Access free online learning activities in the online book using this QR code.

91. TMIT1. (2012, August 3). *Chasing zero: Winning the war on healthcare harm* [Video]. YouTube. All rights reserved. https://youtu.be/MtSbgUuXdaw

5.9 GLOSSARY

Administrative law: Law made by government agencies that have been granted the authority to pass rules and regulations. For example, each state's Board of Nursing is an example of administrative law.

Advance directives: Written instruction, such as a living will or durable power of attorney for health care, recognized under state law, relating to the provision of health care when the individual is incapacitated.

Assault: Intentionally putting another person in reasonable apprehension of an imminent harmful or offensive contact.[92]

Battery: Intentional causation of harmful or offensive contact with another's person without that person's consent.[93]

Capacity: A functional determination that an individual is or is not capable of making a medical decision within a given situation.

Civil law: Law focusing on the rights, responsibilities, and legal relationships between private citizens.

Commission: Doing something a reasonable nurse would not have done.[94]

Competence: In a legal sense, the ability of an individual to participate in legal proceedings. A judge decides if an individual is "competent" or "incompetent."

Confidentiality: The right of an individual to have personal, identifiable medical information kept private.

Constitutional law: The rights, privileges, and responsibilities established by the U.S. Constitution. For example, the right to privacy is a right established by the constitution.

Contracts: Binding written, verbal, or implied agreements.

Crime: A type of behavior defined by Congress or state legislature as deserving of punishment.

Criminal law: A system of laws concerned with punishment of individuals who commit crimes.

Culture of safety: Culture that embraces error reporting by employees with the goal of identifying root causes of problems so they may be addressed to improve client safety.

Defamation of character: An act of making negative, malicious, and false remarks about another person to damage their reputation. Slander is spoken defamation and libel is written defamation.

Defendants: The parties named in a lawsuit.

Durable power of attorney for healthcare (DPOAHC): Person chosen to speak on one's behalf if one becomes incapacitated.

Duty of reasonable care: Legal obligations nurses have to their clients to adhere to current standards of practice.

Ethics: A system of moral principles that a society uses to identify right from wrong.

False imprisonment: An act of restraining another person causing that person to be confined in a bounded area. Restraints can be physical, verbal, or chemical.

92. Legal Information Institute. (n.d.). Cornell Law School. https://www.law.cornell.edu

93. Legal Information Institute. (n.d.). Cornell Law School. https://www.law.cornell.edu

94. Brous, E. (2019). The elements of a nursing malpractice case, Part 2: Breach. *American Journal of Nursing, 119*(9), 42–46. https://doi.org/10.1097/01.NAJ.0000580256.10914.2e

Felonies: Serious crimes that cause the perpetrator to be imprisoned for greater than one year.

Fraud: An act of deceiving an individual for personal gain.

Good Samaritan Law: State law providing protections against negligence claims to individuals who render aid to people experiencing medical emergencies outside of clinical environments.

Informed consent: The fundamental right of a client to accept or reject health care.

Infractions: Minor offenses, such as speeding tickets, that result in fines but not jail time.

Institutional liability: When the health care institution (e.g., hospital, clinic) is held responsible for the actions of its employees or for failing to implement adequate policies and procedures to prevent harm.

Intentional tort: An act of commission with the intent of harming or causing damage to another person. Examples of intentional torts include assault, battery, false imprisonment, slander, libel, and breach of privacy or client confidentiality.

Laws: Rules and regulations created by society and enforced by courts, statutes, and/or professional licensure boards.

Libel: Written defamation.

Living will: A type of advance directive in which an individual identifies what treatments they would like to receive or refuse if they become incapacitated and unable to make decisions.

Malpractice: A specific term used for negligence committed by a professional with a license.

Misdemeanors: Less serious crimes resulting in fines and/or imprisonment for less than one year.

Negligence: The failure to exercise the ordinary care a reasonable person would use in similar circumstances. Wisconsin civil jury instruction states, "A person is not using ordinary care and is negligent, if the person, without intending to do harm, does something (or fails to do something) that a reasonable person would recognize as creating an unreasonable risk of injury or damage to a person or property."[95]

Omission: Not doing something a reasonable nurse would have done.[96]

Plaintiff: The person bringing the lawsuit.

Private law: Laws that govern the relationships between private entities.

Protected Health Information (PHI): Individually identifiable health information and includes demographic data related to the individual's past, present, or future physical or mental health or condition; the provision of health care to the individual; and the past, present, or future payment for the provision of health care to the individual.

Public law: Law regulating relations of individuals with the government or institutions.

Slander: Spoken defamation.

Statutory law: Written laws enacted by the federal or state legislature. For example, the Nurse Practice Act in each state is an example of statutory law that is enacted by the state government.

Student liability: When the student nurse is held responsible for their own actions that cause harm to clients or violate protocols.

---

95. Wis. JI—Civil 1005. (2016). https://wilawlibrary.gov/jury/civil/instruction.php?n=1005

96. Brous, E. (2019). The elements of a nursing malpractice case, Part 2: Breach. *American Journal of Nursing, 119*(9), 42–46. https://doi.org/10.1097/01.NAJ.0000580256.10914.2e

Supervisory liability: When a clinical supervisor or preceptor is held responsible for the actions of the student nurse or for failing to properly supervise them.

Tort: An act of commission or omission that causes injury or harm to another person for which the courts impose liability. In the context of torts, "injury" describes the invasion of any legal right, whereas "harm" describes a loss or detriment the individual suffers. Torts are classified as intentional or unintentional.

Unintentional tort: Acts of omission (not doing something a person has a responsibility to do) or inadvertently doing something causing unintended accidents leading to injury, property damage, or financial loss. Examples of unintentional torts impacting nurses include negligence and malpractice.

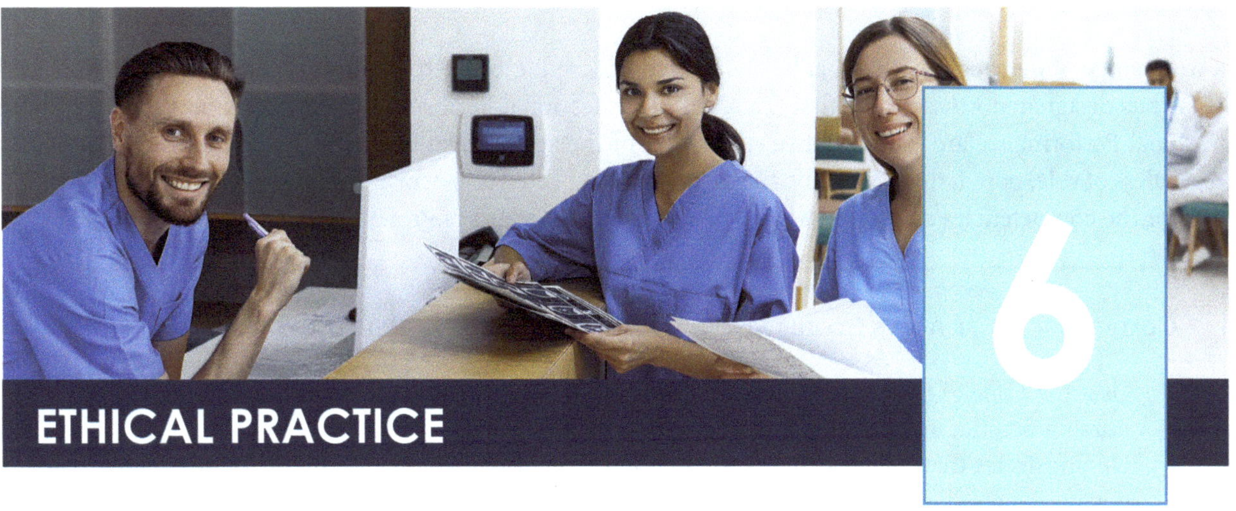

6.1 ETHICAL PRACTICE INTRODUCTION

LEARNING OBJECTIVES

- Compare theories of ethical decision-making
- Examine resources to resolve ethical dilemmas
- Examine competent practice within the ethical framework of health care
- Apply the ANA Code of Ethics to diverse situations in health care
- Analyze the impact of cultural diversity in ethical decision-making
- Explain advocacy as part of the nursing role when responding to ethical dilemmas

The nursing profession is guided by a code of ethics. As you practice nursing, how will you determine "right" from "wrong" actions? What is the difference between morality, values, and ethical principles? What additional considerations impact your ethical decision-making? What are ethical dilemmas and how should nurses participate in resolving them? This chapter answers these questions by reviewing concepts related to ethical nursing practice and describing how nurses can resolve ethical dilemmas. By the end of this chapter, you will be able to describe how to make ethical decisions using the Code of Ethics established by the American Nurses Association.

6.2 BASIC ETHICAL CONCEPTS

The American Nurses Association (ANA) defines **morality** as "personal values, character, or conduct of individuals or groups within communities and societies," whereas **ethics** is the formal study of morality from a wide range of perspectives.[1] Ethical behavior is considered to be such an important aspect of nursing the ANA has designated *Ethics* as the first Standard of Professional Performance. The ANA Standards of Professional Performance are "authoritative statements of the actions and behaviors that all registered nurses, regardless of role, population, specialty, and setting, are expected to perform competently." See the following box for the competencies associated with the ANA *Ethics* Standard of Professional Performance[2]:

Competencies of ANA's Ethics Standard of Professional Performance[3]

- Uses the *Code of Ethics for Nurses With Interpretive Statements* as a moral foundation to guide nursing practice and decision-making.
- Demonstrates that every person is worthy of nursing care through the provision of respectful, person-centered, compassionate care, regardless of personal history or characteristics (Beneficence).
- Advocates for health care consumer perspectives, preferences, and rights to informed decision-making and self-determination (Respect for autonomy).
- Demonstrates a primary commitment to the recipients of nursing and health care services in all settings and situations (Fidelity).
- Maintains therapeutic relationships and professional boundaries.
- Safeguards sensitive information within ethical, legal, and regulatory parameters (Nonmaleficence).
- Identifies ethics resources within the practice setting to assist and collaborate in addressing ethical issues.
- Integrates principles of social justice in all aspects of nursing practice (Justice).
- Refines ethical competence through continued professional education and personal self-development activities.
- Depicts one's professional nursing identity through demonstrated values and ethics, knowledge, leadership, and professional comportment.
- Engages in self-care and self-reflection practices to support and preserve personal health, well-being, and integrity.
- Contributes to the establishment and maintenance of an ethical environment that is conducive to safe, quality health care.
- Collaborates with other health professionals and the public to protect human rights, promote health diplomacy, enhance cultural sensitivity and congruence, and reduce health disparities.
- Represents the nursing perspective in clinic, institutional, community, or professional association ethics discussions.

Reflective Questions

1. What *Ethics* competencies have you already demonstrated during your nursing education?
2. What *Ethics* competencies are you most interested in mastering?
3. What questions do you have about the ANA's *Ethics* competencies?

1. American Nurses Association. (2015). *Code of ethics for nurses with interpretive statements.* American Nurses Association. https://www.nursingworld.org/practice-policy/nursing-excellence/ethics/code-of-ethics-for-nurses/coe-view-only/
2. American Nurses Association. (2021). *Nursing: Scope and standards of practice* (4th ed.). American Nurses Association.
3. American Nurses Association. (2021). *Nursing: Scope and standards of practice* (4th ed.). American Nurses Association.

The ANA's *Code of Ethics for Nurses With Interpretive Statements* is an ethical standard that guides nursing practice and ethical decision-making.[4] This section will review several basic ethical concepts related to the ANA's *Ethics* Standard of Professional Performance, such as values, morals, ethical theories, ethical principles, and the ANA *Code of Ethics for Nurses*.

Values

Values are individual beliefs that motivate people to act one way or another and serve as guides for behavior considered "right" and "wrong." People tend to adopt the values with which they were raised and believe those values are "right" because they are the values of their culture. Some personal values are considered sacred and moral imperatives based on an individual's religious beliefs.[5] See Figure 6.1[6] for an image depicting choosing right from wrong actions.

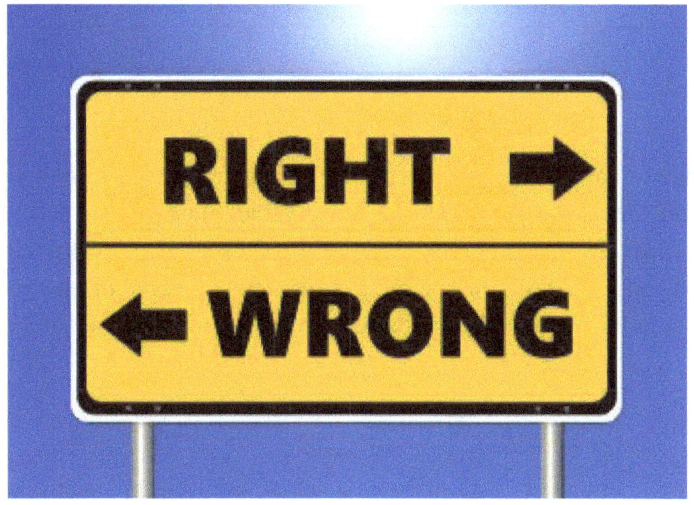

FIGURE 6.1 Values

In addition to personal values, organizations also establish values. The American Nurses Association (ANA) Professional Nursing Model states that nursing is based on values such as caring, compassion, presence, trustworthiness, diversity, acceptance, and accountability. These values emerge from nursing practice beliefs, such as the importance of relationships, service, respect, willingness to bear witness, self-determination, and the pursuit of health.[7] As a result of these traditional values and beliefs by nurses, Americans have ranked nursing as the most ethical and honest profession in Gallup polls since 1999, with the exception of 2001, when firefighters earned the honor after the attacks on September 11.[8]

4. American Nurses Association. (2015). *Code of ethics for nurses with interpretive statements.* American Nurses Association. https://www.nursingworld.org/practice-policy/nursing-excellence/ethics/code-of-ethics-for-nurses/coe-view-only/
5. Ethics Unwrapped - McCombs School of Business. (n.d.). *Ethics defined (a glossary).* University of Texas at Austin. https://ethicsunwrapped.utexas.edu/glossary
6. "ethics-2991600_1920" by Tumisu is licensed under CC0 1.0
7. American Nurses Association. (2021). *Nursing: Scope and standards of practice* (4th ed.). American Nurses Association.
8. Walker, A. (2025). *Nurses ranked most trusted profession for 23rd years in a row.* Nurse.org. https://nurse.org/articles/nursing-ranked-most-honest-profession

The National League of Nursing (NLN) has also established four core values for nursing education: caring, integrity, diversity, and excellence[9]:

- **Caring:** Promoting health, healing, and hope in response to the human condition.
- **Integrity:** Respecting the dignity and moral wholeness of every person without conditions or limitations.
- **Diversity:** Affirming the uniqueness of and differences among persons, ideas, values, and ethnicities.
- **Excellence:** Cocreating and implementing transformative strategies with daring ingenuity.

View the McCombs School of Business "Values" video on YouTube.[10] Access supplementary digital content in the online book using this QR code.

Morals

Morals are the prevailing standards of behavior of a society that enable people to live cooperatively in groups. "Moral" refers to what societies sanction as right and acceptable. Most people tend to act morally and follow societal guidelines, and most laws are based on the morals of a society. Morality often requires that people sacrifice their own short-term interests for the benefit of society. People or entities that are indifferent to right and wrong are considered "amoral," while those who do evil acts are considered "immoral."[11]

Ethical Theories

There are two major types of ethical theories that guide values and moral behavior referred to as deontology and consequentialism.

Deontology is an ethical theory based on rules that distinguish right from wrong. See Figure 6.2[12] for a word cloud illustration of deontology. Deontology is based on the word *deon* that refers to "duty." It is associated with philosopher Immanuel Kant. Kant believed that ethical actions follow universal moral laws, such as, "Don't lie. Don't steal. Don't cheat."[13] Deontology is simple to apply because it just requires people to follow the rules and do their duty. It doesn't require weighing the costs and benefits of a situation, thus avoiding subjectivity and uncertainty.[14,15,16]

9. National League for Nursing. *Core values.* https://www.nln.org/about/about/core-values
10. McCombs School of Business. (2018, December 18). *Values | Ethics defined* [Video]. YouTube. All rights reserved. https://youtu.be/SCjYaatMJuY
11. Ethics Unwrapped - McCombs School of Business. (n.d.). *Ethics defined (a glossary).* University of Texas at Austin. https://ethicsunwrapped.utexas.edu/glossary
12. "ethics-947572_1920" by rdaconnect at Pixabay.com is licensed under CC0 1.0
13. Ethics Unwrapped - McCombs School of Business. (n.d.). *Ethics defined (a glossary).* University of Texas at Austin. https://ethicsunwrapped.utexas.edu/glossary
14. Alexander, L., & Moore, M. (2024). *Deontological ethics.* Stanford Encyclopedia of Psychology. https://plato.stanford.edu/entries/ethics-deontological/
15. Ethics Unwrapped - McCombs School of Business. (n.d.). *Ethics defined (a glossary).* University of Texas at Austin. https://ethicsunwrapped.utexas.edu/glossary
16. American Nurses Association. (2021). *Nursing: Scope and standards of practice* (4th ed.). American Nurses Association.

The nurse-client relationship is deontological in nature because it is based on the ethical principles of beneficence and maleficence that drive clinicians to "do good" and "avoid harm."[17] Ethical principles will be discussed further in this chapter.

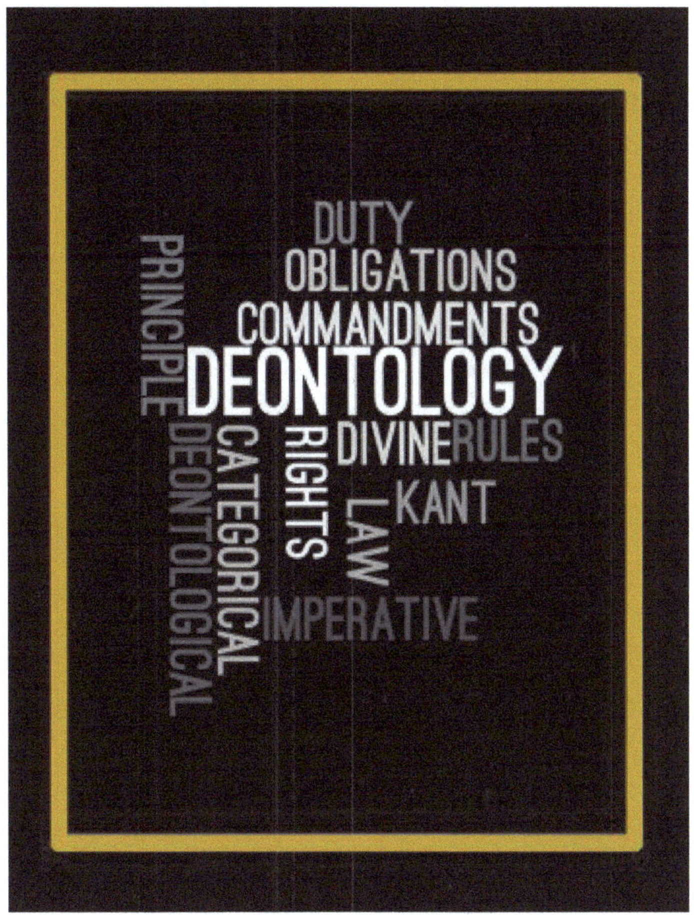

FIGURE 6.2 Deontology

View the McCombs School of Business "Deontology" video on YouTube.[18] Access supplementary digital content in the online book using this QR code.

17. Mandal, J., Ponnambath, D. K., & Parija, S. C. (2016). Utilitarian and deontological ethics in medicine. *Tropical Parasitology, 6*(1), 5–7. https://pubmed.ncbi.nlm.nih.gov/26998430/
18. McCombs School of Business. (2018, December 18). *Deontology | Ethics defined* [Video]. YouTube. All rights reserved. https://youtu.be/wWZi-8Wji7M

Consequentialism is an ethical theory used to determine whether or not an action is right by the consequences of the action. See Figure 6.3[19] for an illustration of weighing the consequences of an action in consequentialism. For example, most people agree that lying is wrong, but if telling a lie would help save a person's life, consequentialism says it's the right thing to do. One type of consequentialism is utilitarianism. **Utilitarianism** determines whether or not actions are right based on their consequences with the standard being achieving the greatest good for the greatest number of people.[20,21,22] For this reason, utilitarianism tends to be society-centered. When applying utilitarian ethics to health care resources, money, time, and clinician energy are considered finite resources that should be appropriately allocated to achieve the best health care for society.[23]

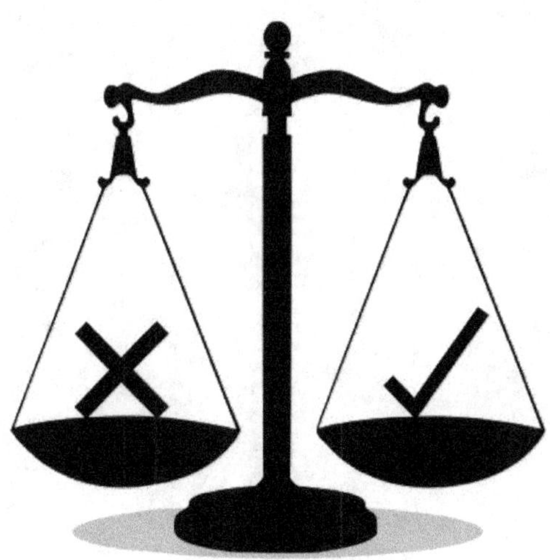

FIGURE 6.3 Consequentialism

Utilitarianism can be complicated when accounting for values such as justice and individual rights. For example, assume a hospital has four clients whose lives depend upon receiving four organ transplant surgeries for a heart, lung, kidney, and liver. If a healthy person without health insurance or family support experiences a life-threatening accident and is considered brain dead but is kept alive on life-sustaining equipment in the ICU, the utilitarian framework might suggest the organs be harvested to save four lives at the expense of one life.[24] This action could arguably produce the greatest good for the greatest number of people, but the deontological approach could argue this action would be unethical because it does not follow the rule of "do no harm."

---

19. "balance-6097898_1280" by mohamed_hassan is licensed under CC0 1.0
20. Alexander, L., & Moore, M. (2024). *Deontological ethics.* Stanford Encyclopedia of Psychology. https://plato.stanford.edu/entries/ethics-deontological/
21. Ethics Unwrapped - McCombs School of Business. (n.d.). *Ethics defined (a glossary).* University of Texas at Austin. https://ethicsunwrapped.utexas.edu/glossary
22. American Nurses Association. (2021). *Nursing: Scope and standards of practice* (4th ed.). American Nurses Association.
23. Mandal, J., Ponnambath, D. K., & Parija, S. C. (2016). Utilitarian and deontological ethics in medicine. *Tropical Parasitology,* 6(1), 5–7. https://pubmed.ncbi.nlm.nih.gov/26998430/
24. Ethics Unwrapped - McCombs School of Business. (n.d.). *Ethics defined (a glossary).* University of Texas at Austin. https://ethicsunwrapped.utexas.edu/glossary

Watch McCombs School of Business "Consequentialism" video on YouTube.[25] Access supplementary digital content in the online book using this QR code.

Read more about decision-making on organ donation: The dilemmas of relatives of potential brain dead donors. Access supplementary digital content in the online book using this QR code.

Interestingly, deontological and utilitarian approaches to ethical issues may result in the same outcome, but the rationale for the outcome or decision is different because it is focused on duty (deontologic) versus consequences (utilitarian).

Societies and cultures have unique ethical frameworks that may be based upon either deontological or consequentialist ethical theory. Culturally derived deontological rules may apply to ethical issues in health care. For example, a traditional Chinese philosophy based on Confucianism results in a culturally acceptable practice of family members (rather than the client) receiving information from health care providers about life-threatening medical conditions and making treatment decisions. As a result, cancer diagnoses and end-of-life treatment options may not be disclosed to the client in an effort to alleviate the suffering that may arise from knowledge of their diagnosis. In this manner, a client's family and the health care provider may ethically prioritize a client's psychological well-being over their autonomy and self-determination.[26] However, in the United States, this ethical decision may conflict with HIPAA Privacy Rules and the ethical principle of client autonomy. As a result, a nurse providing client care in this type of situation may experience an ethical dilemma. Ethical dilemmas are further discussed in the "Ethical Dilemmas" section of this chapter.

See Table 6.2 comparing common ethical issues in health care viewed through the lens of deontological and consequential ethical frameworks.

25. McCombs School of Business. (2018, December 18). *Consequentialism | Ethics defined* [Video]. YouTube. All rights reserved. https://youtu.be/51DZteag74A
26. Wang, H., Zhao, F., Wang, X., & Chen, X. (2018). To tell or not: The Chinese doctors' dilemma on disclosure of a cancer diagnosis to the patient. *Iranian Journal of Public Health, 47*(11), 1773–1774. https://www.ncbi.nlm.nih.gov/pubmed/30581799

TABLE 6.2. Ethical Issues Through the Lens of Deontological or Consequential Ethical Frameworks

Ethical Issue	Deontological View	Consequential View
Abortion	Abortion is unacceptable based on the rule of preserving life.	Abortion may be acceptable in cases of an unwanted pregnancy, rape, incest, or risk to the mother.
Bombing an area with known civilians	Killing civilians is not acceptable due to the loss of innocent lives.	The loss of innocent lives may be acceptable if the bombing stops a war that could result in significantly more deaths than the civilian casualties.
Stealing	Taking something that is not yours is wrong.	Taking something to redistribute resources to others in need may be acceptable.
Killing	It is never acceptable to take another human being's life.	It may be acceptable to take another human life in self-defense or to prevent additional harm they could cause others.
Euthanasia/physician-assisted suicide	It is never acceptable to assist another human to end their life prematurely.	End-of-life care can be expensive and emotionally upsetting for family members. If a competent, capable adult wishes to end their life, medically supported options should be available.
Vaccines	Vaccination is a personal choice based on religious practices or other beliefs.	Recommended vaccines should be mandatory for everyone (without a medical contraindication) because of its greater good for all of society.

Ethical Principles and Obligations

Ethical principles are used to define nurses' moral duties and aid in ethical analysis and decision-making.[27] Although there are many ethical principles that guide nursing practice, foundational ethical principles include autonomy (self-determination), beneficence (do good), nonmaleficence (do no harm), justice (fairness), fidelity (keep promises), and veracity (tell the truth).

Autonomy

The ethical principle of **autonomy** recognizes each individual's right to self-determination and decision-making based on their unique values, beliefs, and preferences. See Figure 6.4[28] for an illustration of autonomy. The American Nurses Association (ANA) defines autonomy as the "capacity to determine one's own

27. American Nurses Association. (2021). *Nursing: Scope and standards of practice* (4th ed.). American Nurses Association.
28. "Autonomy and Self-Determination.png" by Meredith Pomietlo for Chippewa Valley Technical College is licensed under CC BY 4.0

actions through independent choice, including demonstration of competence."[29] The nurse's primary ethical obligation is client autonomy.[30] Based on autonomy, clients have the right to refuse nursing care and medical treatment. An example of autonomy in health care is advance directives. Advance directives allow clients to specify health care decisions if they become incapacitated and unable to do so.

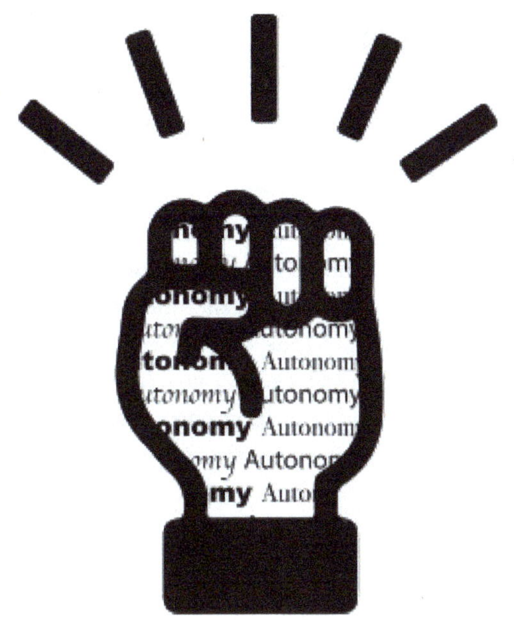

FIGURE 6.4 Autonomy and Self-Determination

Read more about advance directives and determining capacity and competency in the "Legal Implications" chapter.

NURSES AS ADVOCATES: SUPPORTING AUTONOMY

Nurses have a responsibility to act in the interest of those under their care, referred to as advocacy. The American Nurses Association (ANA) defines advocacy as "the act or process of pleading for, supporting, or recommending a cause or course of action. Advocacy may be for persons (whether an individual, group, population, or society) or for an issue, such as potable water or global health."[31] See Figure 6.5[32] for an illustration of advocacy.

29. American Nurses Association. (2021). *Nursing: Scope and standards of practice* (4th ed.). American Nurses Association.
30. American Nurses Association. (2015). *Code of ethics for nurses with interpretive statements.* American Nurses Association. https://www.nursingworld.org/practice-policy/nursing-excellence/ethics/code-of-ethics-for-nurses/coe-view-only/
31. American Nurses Association. (2015). *Code of ethics for nurses with interpretive statements.* American Nurses Association. https://www.nursingworld.org/practice-policy/nursing-excellence/ethics/code-of-ethics-for-nurses/coe-view-only/
32. "Advocacy" by Meredith Pomietlo for Chippewa Valley Technical College is licensed under CC BY 4.0

FIGURE 6.5 Advocacy

Advocacy includes providing education regarding client rights, supporting autonomy and self-determination, and advocating for client preferences to health care team members and family members. Nurses do not make decisions for clients, but instead support them in making their own informed choices. At the core of making informed decisions is knowledge. Nurses serve an integral role in client education. Clarifying unclear information, translating medical terminology, and making referrals to other health care team members (within their scope of practice) ensures that clients have the information needed to make treatment decisions aligned with their personal values.

At times, nurses may find themselves in a position of supporting a client's decision they do not agree with and would not make for themselves or for the people they love. However, self-determination is a human right that honors the dignity and well-being of individuals. The nursing profession, rooted in caring relationships, demands that nurses have nonjudgmental attitudes and reflect "unconditional positive regard" for every client. Nurses must suspend personal judgement and beliefs when advocating for their clients' preferences and decision-making.[33]

Beneficence

Beneficence is defined by the ANA as "the bioethical principle of benefiting others by preventing harm, removing harmful conditions, or affirmatively acting to benefit another or others, often going beyond what is required by law."[34] See Figure 6.6[35] for an illustration of beneficence. Put simply, beneficence is acting for the good and welfare of others, guided by compassion. An example of beneficence in daily nursing care is when a nurse sits with a dying client and holds their hand to provide presence.

---

33. American Nurses Association. (2021). *Nursing: Scope and standards of practice* (4th ed.). American Nurses Association.
34. American Nurses Association. (2015). *Code of ethics for nurses with interpretive statements.* American Nurses Association. https://www.nursingworld.org/practice-policy/nursing-excellence/ethics/code-of-ethics-for-nurses/coe-view-only/
35. "Air_Force_special_operations_medical_team_saves_lives,_helps_shape_future_of_Afghan_medicine_111010-F-QW942-082.jpg" by Senior Airman Tyler Placie is in the Public Domain

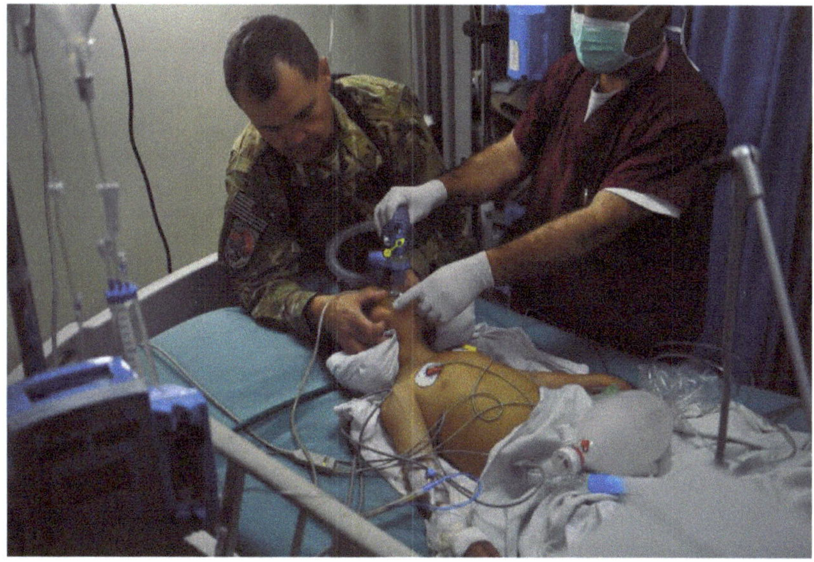

FIGURE 6.6 Beneficence

Nursing advocacy extends beyond direct client care to advocating for beneficence in communities. Vulnerable populations such as children, older adults, cultural minorities, and the homeless often benefit from nurse advocacy in promoting health equity. **Cultural humility** is a humble and respectful attitude towards individuals of other cultures and an approach to learning about other cultures as a lifelong goal and process.[36] Nurses, the largest segment of the health care community, have a powerful voice when addressing community beneficence issues, such as health disparities and social determinants of health, and can serve as the conduit for advocating for change.

Nonmaleficence

Nonmaleficence is defined by the ANA as "the bioethical principle that specifies a duty to do no harm and balances avoidable harm with benefits of good achieved."[37] An example of doing no harm in nursing practice is reflected by nurses checking medication rights three times before administering medications. In this manner, medication errors can be avoided, and the duty to do no harm is met. Another example of nonmaleficence is when a nurse assists a client with a serious, life-threatening condition to participate in decision-making regarding their treatment plan. By balancing the potential harm with potential benefits of various treatment options, while also considering quality of life and comfort, the client can effectively make decisions based on their values and preferences.

Justice

Justice is defined by the ANA as "a moral obligation to act on the basis of equality and equity and a standard linked to fairness for all in society."[38] The principle of justice requires health care to be provided in a fair and equitable way. Nurses provide quality care for all individuals with the same level of fairness despite many

36. American Nurses Association. (2021). *Nursing: Scope and standards of practice* (4th ed.). American Nurses Association.
37. American Nurses Association. (2015). *Code of ethics for nurses with interpretive statements.* American Nurses Association. https://www.nursingworld.org/practice-policy/nursing-excellence/ethics/code-of-ethics-for-nurses/coe-view-only/
38. American Nurses Association. (2021). *Nursing: Scope and standards of practice* (4th ed.). American Nurses Association.

characteristics, such as the individual's financial status, culture, religion, gender, or sexual orientation. Nurses have a social contract to "provide compassionate care that addresses the individual's needs for protection, advocacy, empowerment, optimization of health, prevention of illness and injury, alleviation of suffering, comfort, and well-being."[39] An example of a nurse using the principle of justice in daily nursing practice is effective prioritization based on client needs.

Read more about prioritization models in the "Prioritization" chapter.

Other Ethical Principles

Additional ethical principles commonly applied to health care include **fidelity** (keeping promises) and **veracity** (telling the truth). An example of fidelity in daily nursing practice is when a nurse tells a client, "I will be back in an hour to check on your pain level." This promise is kept. An example of veracity in nursing practice is when a nurse honestly explains potentially uncomfortable side effects of prescribed medications. Determining how truthfulness will benefit the client and support their autonomy is dependent on a nurse's clinical judgment, self-reflection, knowledge of the client and their cultural beliefs, and other factors.[40]

A principle historically associated with health care is paternalism. **Paternalism** is defined as the interference by the state or an individual with another person, defended by the claim that the person interfered with will be better off or protected from harm.[41] Paternalism is the basis for legislation related to drug enforcement and compulsory wearing of seatbelts.

In health care, paternalism has been used as rationale for performing treatment based on what the provider believes is in the client's best interest. In some situations, paternalism may be appropriate for individuals who are unable to comprehend information in a way that supports their informed decision-making, but it must be used cautiously to ensure vulnerable individuals are not misused and their autonomy is not violated.

Nurses may find themselves acting paternalistically when performing nursing care to ensure client health and safety. For example, repositioning clients to prevent skin breakdown is a preventative intervention commonly declined by clients when they prefer a specific position for comfort. In this situation, the nurse should explain the benefits of the preventative intervention and the risks if the intervention is not completed. If the client continues to decline the intervention despite receiving this information, the nurse should document the education provided and the client's decision to decline the intervention. The process of reeducating the client and reminding them of the importance of the preventative intervention should be continued at regular intervals and documented.

39. American Nurses Association. (2021). *Nursing: Scope and standards of practice* (4th ed.). American Nurses Association.
40. American Nurses Association. (2021). *Nursing: Scope and standards of practice* (4th ed.). American Nurses Association.
41. Dworkin, G. (2020, September 9). Paternalism. *Stanford Encyclopedia of Philosophy*. https://plato.stanford.edu/entries/paternalism/

Care-Based Ethics

Nurses use a client-centered, care-based ethical approach to client care that focuses on the specific circumstances of each situation. This approach aligns with nursing concepts such as caring, holism, and a nurse-client relationship rooted in dignity and respect through virtues such as kindness and compassion.[42,43] This care-based approach to ethics uses a holistic, individualized analysis of situations rather than the prescriptive application of ethical principles to define ethical nursing practice. This care-based approach asserts that ethical issues cannot be handled deductively by applying concrete and prefabricated rules, but instead require social processes that respect the multidimensionality of problems.[44] Frameworks for resolving ethical situations are discussed in the "Ethical Dilemmas" section of this chapter.

Nursing Code of Ethics

Many professions and institutions have their own set of ethical principles, referred to as a **code of ethics,** designed to govern decision-making and assist individuals to distinguish right from wrong. The American Nurses Association (ANA) provides a framework for ethical nursing care and guides nurses during decision-making in its formal document titled *Code of Ethics for Nurses With Interpretive Statements (Nursing Code of Ethics).* The *Nursing Code of Ethics* serves the following purposes[45]:

- It is a succinct statement of the ethical values, obligations, duties, and professional ideals of nurses individually and collectively.
- It is the profession's nonnegotiable ethical standard.
- It is an expression of nursing's own understanding of its commitment to society.

The preface of the ANA's *Nursing Code of Ethics* states, "Individuals who become nurses are expected to adhere to the ideals and moral norms of the profession and also to embrace them as a part of what it means to be a nurse. The ethical tradition of nursing is self-reflective, enduring, and distinctive. A code of ethics makes explicit the primary goals, values, and obligations of the profession."[46]

The *Nursing Code of Ethics* contains nine provisions. Each provision contains several clarifying or "interpretive" statements. Read a summary of the nine provisions in the following box.

42. Fry, S. T. (1989). The role of caring in a theory of nursing ethics. *Hypatia, 4*(2), 87-103. https://doi.org/10.1111/j.1527-2001.1989.tb00575.x
43. Taylor, C. (1993). Nursing ethics: The role of caring. *Awhonn's Clinical Issues in Perinatal and Women's Health Nursing, 4*(4), 552-560. https://pubmed.ncbi.nlm.nih.gov/8220369/
44. Schuchter, P., & Heller, A. (2018). The care dialog: The "ethics of care" approach and its importance for clinical ethics consultation. *Medicine, Health Care, and Philosophy, 21*(1), 51–62. https://doi.org/10.1007/s11019-017-9784-z
45. American Nurses Association. (2015). *Code of ethics for nurses with interpretive statements.* American Nurses Association. https://www.nursingworld.org/practice-policy/nursing-excellence/ethics/code-of-ethics-for-nurses/coe-view-only/
46. American Nurses Association. (2015). *Code of ethics for nurses with interpretive statements.* American Nurses Association. https://www.nursingworld.org/practice-policy/nursing-excellence/ethics/code-of-ethics-for-nurses/coe-view-only/

Nine Provisions of the ANA *Nursing Code of Ethics*

- **Provision 1:** The nurse practices with compassion and respect for the inherent dignity, worth, and unique attributes of every person.
- **Provision 2:** The nurse's primary commitment is to the client, whether an individual, family, group, community, or population.
- **Provision 3:** The nurse promotes, advocates for, and protects the rights, health, and safety of the client.
- **Provision 4:** The nurse has authority, accountability, and responsibility for nursing practice; makes decisions; and takes action consistent with the obligation to promote health and to provide optimal care.
- **Provision 5:** The nurse owes the same duties to self as to others, including the responsibility to promote health and safety, preserve wholeness of character and integrity, maintain competence, and continue personal and professional growth.
- **Provision 6:** The nurse, through individual and collective effort, establishes, maintains, and improves the ethical environment of the work setting and conditions of employment that are conducive to safe, quality health care.
- **Provision 7:** The nurse, in all roles and settings, advances the profession through research and scholarly inquiry, professional standards development, and the generation of both nursing and health policy.
- **Provision 8**: The nurse collaborates with other health professionals and the public to protect human rights, promote health diplomacy, and reduce health disparities.
- **Provision 9:** The profession of nursing, collectively through its professional organizations, must articulate nursing values, maintain the integrity of the profession, and integrate principles of social justice into nursing and health policy.

Read the free, online full version of the *ANA's Code of Ethics for Nurses With Interpretive Statements*. Access supplementary digital content in the online book using this QR code.

In addition to the *Nursing Code of Ethics,* the ANA established the Center for Ethics and Human Rights to help nurses navigate ethical conflicts and life-and-death decisions common to everyday nursing practice.

Read more about the ANA Center for Ethics and Human Rights. Access supplementary digital content in the online book using this QR code.

Specialty Organization Code of Ethics

Many specialty nursing organizations have additional codes of ethics to guide nurses practicing in settings such as the emergency department, home care, or hospice care. These documents are unique to the specialty discipline but mirror the statements from the ANA's *Nursing Code of Ethics.* View examples of ethical statements of specialty nursing organizations using the information in the following box.

Sample Ethical Statements of Selected Specialty Nursing Organizations

- American College of Nurse-Midwives
- National Association of Neonatal Nurses

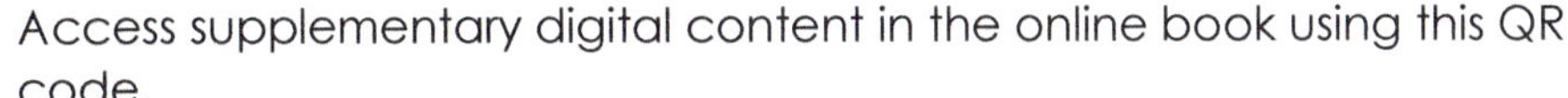

Access supplementary digital content in the online book using this QR code.

6.3 ETHICAL DILEMMAS

Nurses frequently find themselves involved in conflicts during client care related to opposing values and ethical principles. These conflicts are referred to as ethical dilemmas. An **ethical dilemma** results from conflict of competing values and requires a decision to be made from equally desirable or undesirable options.

An ethical dilemma can involve conflicting client's values, nurse values, health care provider's values, organizational values, and societal values associated with unique facts of a specific situation. For this reason, it can be challenging to arrive at a clearly superior solution for all stakeholders involved in an ethical dilemma. Nurses may also encounter moral dilemmas where the right course of action is known but the nurse is limited by forces outside their control. See Table 6.3a for an example of ethical dilemmas a nurse may experience in their nursing practice.

TABLE 6.3A. Examples of Ethical Issues Involving Nurses

Workplace	Organizational Processes	Client Care
• High client acuity • Inadequate staffing • Overuse of agency staff • Improper use of assistive personnel • Practicing beyond one's scope of practice • Floating to other units without appropriate orientation • Horizontal violence/ workplace bullying • Impaired coworkers • Violation of client privacy on social media	• Paperwork and administrative task requirements • Substituting outpatient for inpatient care • Spending limits on care based on reimbursement codes for medical conditions • Discharging clients too soon and expecting family members to provide care	• Reproduction Issues – Abortion – Birth control methods – Sterilization – Alternative conception • End-of-Life Issues – Physician-assisted suicide – Withdrawal of food/fluids – Withdrawal of life support – DNR/DNI – Full code despite a persistent vegetative state • Genetics – Screening – Stem cell research – Cloning • Organ transplantation • Client refusal of medications or treatments

Read more about ethics topics and articles on the ANA website. Access supplementary digital content in the online book using this QR code.

According to the American Nurses Association (ANA), a nurse's ethical competence depends on several factors[47]:

- Continuous appraisal of personal and professional values and how they may impact interpretation of an issue and decision-making
- An awareness of ethical obligations as mandated in the *Code of Ethics for Nurses With Interpretive Statements*[48]
- Knowledge of ethical principles and their application to ethical decision-making
- Motivation and skills to implement an ethical decision

47. American Nurses Association. (2021). *Nursing: Scope and standards of practice* (4th ed.). American Nurses Association.
48. American Nurses Association. (2015). *Code of ethics for nurses with interpretive statements.* American Nurses Association. https://www.nursingworld.org/practice-policy/nursing-excellence/ethics/code-of-ethics-for-nurses/coe-view-only/

Nurses and nursing students must have **moral courage** to address the conflicts involved in ethical dilemmas with "the willingness to speak out and do what is right in the face of forces that would lead us to act in some other way."[49] See Figure 6.7[50] for an illustration of nurses' moral courage.

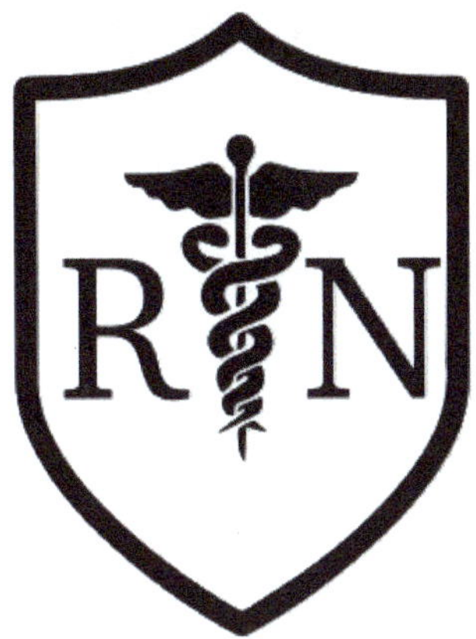

FIGURE 6.7 Moral Courage

Nurse leaders and organizations can support moral courage by creating environments where nurses feel safe and supported to speak up.[51] Nurses may experience **moral conflict** when they are uncertain about what values or principles should be applied to an ethical issue that arises during client care. Moral conflict can progress to **moral distress** when the nurse identifies the correct ethical action but feels constrained by competing values of an organization or other individuals. Nurses may also feel **moral outrage** when witnessing immoral acts or practices they feel powerless to change. For this reason, it is essential for nurses and nursing students to be aware of frameworks for solving ethical dilemmas that consider ethical theories, ethical principles, personal values, societal values, and professionally sanctioned guidelines such as the ANA *Nursing Code of Ethics.*

Moral injury felt by nurses and other health care workers in response to the COVID-19 pandemic has gained recent public attention. **Moral injury** refers to the distressing psychological, behavioral, social, and sometimes spiritual aftermath of exposure to events that contradict deeply held moral beliefs and expectations.[52] Health care workers may not have the time or resources to process their feelings of moral injury caused by the pandemic, which can result in burnout. Organizations can assist employees in processing these feelings of moral injury with expanded employee assistance programs or other structured support programs.[53]

Read more about self-care strategies to address feelings of burnout in the "Burnout and Self-Care" chapter.

49. American Nurses Association (ANA). (2025). *Ethics topics and articles.* https://www.nursingworld.org/practice-policy/nursing-excellence/ethics/ethics-topics-and-articles/
50. "Moral courage.png" by Meredith Pomietlo for Chippewa Valley Technical College is licensed under CC BY 4.0
51. American Nurses Association. (2021). *Nursing: Scope and standards of practice* (4th ed.). American Nurses Association.
52. Norman, S. & Maguen, S. (2024). *Moral injury.* PTSD: National Center for PTSD, U.S. Department of Veterans Affairs. https://www.ptsd.va.gov/professional/treat/cooccurring/moral_injury.asp
53. Dean, W., Jacobs, B., & Manfredi, R. A. (2020). Moral injury: The invisible epidemic in COVID health care workers. *Annals of Emergency Medicine, 76*(4), 385–386. https://doi.org/10.1016/j.annemergmed.2020.05.023

Frameworks for Solving Ethical Dilemmas

Systematically working through an ethical dilemma is key to identifying a solution. Many frameworks exist for solving an ethical dilemma, including the nursing process, four-quadrant approach, the MORAL model, and the organization-focused PLUS Ethical Decision-Making model.[54] When nurses use a structured, systematic approach to resolving ethical dilemmas with appropriate data collection, identification and analysis of options, and inclusion of stakeholders, they have met their legal, ethical, and moral responsibilities, even if the outcome is less than ideal.

Nursing Process Model

The nursing process is a structured problem-solving approach that nurses may apply in ethical decision-making to guide data collection and analysis. See Table 6.3b for suggestions on how to use the nursing process model during an ethical dilemma.[55]

TABLE 6.3B. Using the Nursing Process in Ethical Situations[56]

Nursing Process Stage	Considerations
Assessment/Data Collection	• What is the issue? • Who is involved? • What are the facts (health status, pain, treatment)? • What are the stakeholder (client, family, health care team, community) concerns? • What ethics resources exist (such as an organization's ethics committee)?
Assessment/Analysis	• Analyze the facts and stakeholder values using ethical principles, ethical theories, the ANA *Nursing Code of Ethics*, or another ethical framework model. • Document the ethics resources consulted.
Diagnosis	• Determine the care context and issues, including areas of agreement and conflict. • Consider the entire context, including the client, family, health care team, and institutional circumstances.
Outcome Identification	• Establish a goal based on client autonomy.
Planning	• Identify a range of options, realizing there may only be "best available" options when possibilities are limited.

54. American Nurses Association. (2021). *Nursing: Scope and standards of practice* (4th ed.). American Nurses Association.
55. American Nurses Association. (2021). *Nursing: Scope and standards of practice* (4th ed.). American Nurses Association.
56. American Nurses Association. (2021). *Nursing: Scope and standards of practice* (4th ed.). American Nurses Association.

TABLE 6.3B. Continued...

Implementation	• Ensure the option chosen is right, suitable, and appropriate. Be aware that not all options are appropriate in all contexts. • Implement the plan in collaboration with the client, family, and other stakeholders.
Evaluation	• Evaluate what happened and what can be learned after every ethical dilemma.

Four-Quadrant Approach

The four-quadrant approach integrates ethical principles (e.g., beneficence, nonmaleficence, autonomy, and justice) in conjunction with health care indications, individual and family preferences, quality of life, and contextual features.[57] See Table 6.3c for sample questions used during the four-quadrant approach.

TABLE 6.3C. Four-Quadrant Approach[58]

Health Care Indications (Beneficence and Nonmaleficence) • What is the diagnosis/prognosis? • What are the goals of treatment/care? • What is the likelihood of success of treatment? • Will the proposed treatment plan benefit the client and avoid harm?	**Individual and Family Preferences (Respect for Autonomy)** • What are the client's preferences? • Does the client understand their condition? • Has the client provided informed consent, and do they understand the risks and benefits of the proposed treatment? • Is the client competent and capacitated to make decisions? If not, are there advance directives in place?
Quality of Life (Beneficence, Nonmaleficence, and Respect for Autonomy) • What is the probability of the client's return to normal life with or without treatment? • Would the person experience any physical, mental, or social deficits even if the treatment succeeds? • Do the health care providers have any biases that might prejudice their evaluation of the client's quality of life? • Has forgoing treatment been discussed? • Are there plans for comfort and/or palliative care?	**Contextual Features (Justice and Fairness)** • Are there family or provider issues, such as implicit bias, that might influence treatment decisions? • Are there religious, financial, social, racial, or legal issues that might affect treatment decisions? • Are there issues related to allocation of resources that might affect treatment?

57. American Nurses Association. (2021). *Nursing: Scope and standards of practice* (4th ed.). American Nurses Association.
58. American Nurses Association. (2021). *Nursing: Scope and standards of practice* (4th ed.). American Nurses Association.

MORAL Model

The MORAL model is a nurse-generated, decision-making model originating from research on nursing-specific moral dilemmas involving client autonomy, quality of life, distributing resources, and maintaining professional standards. The model provides guidance for nurses to systematically analyze and address real-life ethical dilemmas. The steps in the process may be remembered by using the mnemonic MORAL. See Table 6.3d for a description of each step of the MORAL model.[59,60]

TABLE 6.3D. MORAL Model

M: Massage the dilemma	Collect data by identifying the interests and perceptions of those involved, defining the dilemma, and describing conflicts. Establish a goal.
O: Outline options	Generate several effective alternatives to reach the goal.
R: Review criteria and resolve	Identify moral criteria and select the course of action.
A: Affirm position and act	Implement action based on knowledge from the previous steps (M-O-R).
L: Look back	Evaluate each step and the decision made.

PLUS Ethical Decision-Making Model

The PLUS Ethical Decision-Making model was created by the Ethics and Compliance Initiative to help organizations empower employees to make ethical decisions in the workplace. This model uses four filters throughout the ethical decision-making process, referred to by the mnemonic PLUS:

- **P:** Policies, procedures, and guidelines of an organization
- **L:** Laws and regulations
- **U:** Universal values and principles of an organization
- **S:** Self-identification of what is good, right, fair, and equitable[61]

The seven steps of the PLUS Ethical Decision-Making model are as follows[62]:

- Define the problem using PLUS filters
- Seek relevant assistance, guidance, and support
- Identify available alternatives
- Evaluate the alternatives using PLUS to identify their impact
- Make the decision

59. American Nurses Association. (2021). *Nursing: Scope and standards of practice* (4th ed.). American Nurses Association.
60. Crisham, P. (1985). Moral: How can I do what is right? *Nursing Management, 16*(3), 44. https://journals.lww.com/nursingmanagement/citation/1985/03000/moral__how_can_i_do_what_s_right_.6.aspx
61. Ethics & Compliance Initiative. (2021). *The PLUS Ethical Decision Making Model.* https://www.ethics.org/resources/free-toolkit/decision-making-model/
62. Ethics & Compliance Initiative. (2021). *The PLUS Ethical Decision Making Model.* https://www.ethics.org/resources/free-toolkit/decision-making-model/

- Implement the decision
- Evaluate the decision using PLUS filters

6.4 ETHICS COMMITTEES

In addition to using established frameworks to resolve ethical dilemmas, nurses can also consult their organization's ethics committee for ethical guidance in the workplace. **Ethics committees** are typically composed of interdisciplinary team members such as physicians, nurses, allied health professionals, administrators, social workers, and clergy to problem-solve ethical dilemmas. See Figure 6.8[63] for an illustration of an ethics committee. Hospital ethics committees were created in response to legal controversies regarding the refusal of life-sustaining treatment, such as the Karen Quinlan case.[64]

Read more about the Karen Quinlan case and controversies surrounding life-sustaining treatment in the "Legal Implications" chapter.

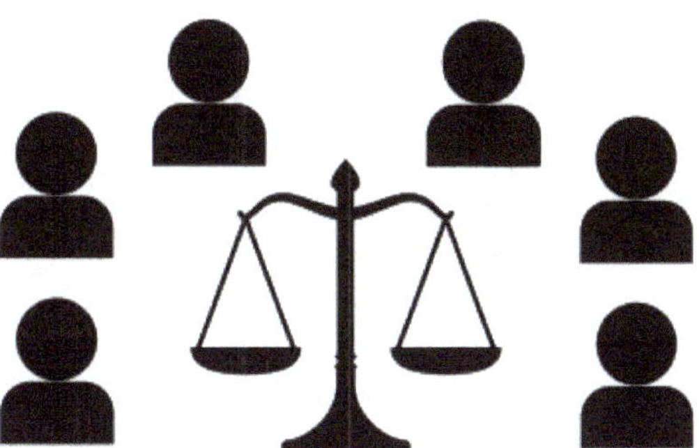

FIGURE 6.8 Ethics Committee

After the passage of the Patient Self-Determination Act in 1991, all health care institutions receiving Medicare or Medicaid funding are required to form ethics committees. The Joint Commission (TJC) also requires organizations to have a formalized mechanism of dealing with ethical issues. Nurses should be aware of the process for requesting guidance and support from ethics committees at their workplace for ethical issues affecting clients or staff.[65]

Institutional Review Boards and Ethical Research

Other types of ethics committees have been formed to address the ethics of medical research on clients. Historically, there are examples of medical research causing harm to clients. For example, an infamous research

63. "Ethics Committee.png" by Meredith Pomietlo for Chippewa Valley Technical College is licensed under CC BY 4.0
64. Annas, G., & Grodin, M. (2016). Hospital ethics committees, consultants, and courts. *AMA Journal of Ethics, 18*(5), 554-559. https://journalofethics.ama-assn.org/article/hospital-ethics-committees-consultants-and-courts/2016-05
65. Aulisio, M. (2016). Why did hospital ethics committees emerge in the US? *AMA Journal of Ethics, 18*(5), 546-553. https://journalofethics.ama-assn.org/article/why-did-hospital-ethics-committees-emerge-us/2016-05

study called the "Tuskegee Study" raised concern regarding ethical issues in research such as informed consent, paternalism, maleficence, truth-telling, and justice.

In 1932 the Tuskegee Study began a 40-year study looking at the long-term progression of syphilis. Over 600 Black men were told they were receiving free medical care, but researchers only treated men diagnosed with syphilis with aspirin, even after it was discovered that penicillin was a highly effective treatment for the disease. The institute allowed the study to go on, even when men developed long-stage neurological symptoms of the disease and some wives and children became infected with syphilis. In 1972 these consequences of the Tuskegee Study were leaked to the media and public outrage caused the study to shut down.[66]

Potential harm to clients participating in research studies like the Tuskegee Study was rationalized based on the utilitarian view that potential harm to individuals was outweighed by the benefit of new scientific knowledge resulting in greater good for society. As a result of public outrage over ethical concerns related to medical research, Congress recognized that an independent mechanism was needed to protect research subjects. In 1974 regulations were established requiring research with human subjects to undergo review by an **institutional review board (IRB)** to ensure it meets ethical criteria. An IRB is a group that has been formally designated to review and monitor biomedical research involving human subjects.[67] The IRB review ensures the following criteria are met when research is performed:

- The benefits of the research study outweigh the potential risks.
- Individuals' participation in the research is voluntary.
- Informed consent is obtained from research participants who have the ability to decline participation.
- Participants are aware of the potential risks of participating in the research.[68]

View a YouTube video "Henrietta Lacks, the Tuskegee Experiment, ethics and research.[69] Access supplementary digital content in the online book using this QR code.

6.5 ETHICS AND THE NURSING STUDENT

Nursing students may encounter ethical dilemmas when in clinical practice settings. Read more about research regarding ethical dilemmas experienced by students as described in the box.

66. Centers for Disease Control and Prevention. (2021). *The Untreated Syphilis Study at Tuskegee Timeline.* https://www.cdc.gov/tuskegee/about/timeline.html?CDC_AAref_Val=https://www.cdc.gov/tuskegee/timeline.htm

67. U.S. Food & Drug Administration. (2019). *Institutional review boards (IRBs) and protection of human subjects in clinical trials.* U.S. Department of Health & Human Services. https://www.fda.gov/about-fda/center-drug-evaluation-and-research-cder/institutional-review-boards-irbs-and-protection-human-subjects-clinical-trials

68. Annas, G., & Grodin, M. (2016). Hospital ethics committees, consultants, and courts. *AMA Journal of Ethics, 18*(5), 554-559. https://journalofethics.ama-assn.org/article/hospital-ethics-committees-consultants-and-courts/2016-05

69. CrashCourse. (2018, April 18). *Henrietta Lacks, the Tuskegee experiment, and ethical data collection: Crash course statistics #1* [Video]. YouTube. All rights reserved. https://youtu.be/CzNANZnoiRs

Nursing Students and Ethical Dilemmas[70]

An integrative literature review performed by Albert, Younas, and Sana in 2020 identified ethical dilemmas encountered by nursing students in clinical practice settings. Three themes were identified:

1. Applying learned ethical values vs. accepting unethical practice

Students observed unethical practices of nurses and physicians, such as breach of client privacy, confidentiality, respect, rights, duty to provide information, and physical and psychological mistreatment, that opposed the ethical values learned in nursing school. Students experienced ethical conflict due to their sense of powerlessness, low status as students, dependence on staff nurses for learning experiences, and fear of offending health care providers.

2. Desiring to provide ethical care but lacking autonomous decision-making

Students reported a lack of moral courage in questioning unethical practices. The hierarchy of health care environments left students feeling disregarded, humiliated, and intimidated by professional nurses and managers. Students also reported a sense of loss of identity in feeling forced to conform their personal identity to that of the clinical environment.

3. Whistleblowing vs. silence regarding client care and neglect

Students observed nurses performing unethical nursing practices, such as ignoring client needs, disregarding pain, being verbally abusive, talking inappropriately about clients, and not providing a safe or competent level of care. Most students reported remaining silent regarding these observations due to a lack of confidence, feeling it was not their place to report, or the fear of negative consequences. Organizational power dynamics influenced student confidence in reporting unethical practices to faculty or nurse managers.

The researchers concluded that nursing students feel moral distress when experiencing these kinds of conflicts:

- Providing ethical care as learned in their program of study or accepting unethical practices
- Staying silent about client care neglect or confronting it and reporting it
- Providing quality, ethical care or adapting to organizational culture due to lack of autonomous decision-making

These ethical conflicts can be detrimental to students' professional learning and mental health. Researchers recommended that nurse educators should develop educational programs to support students as they develop ethical competence and moral courage to confront ethical dilemmas.[71]

---

70. Albert, J. S., Younas, A., & Sana, S. (2020). Nursing students' ethical dilemmas regarding patient care: An integrative review. *Nurse Education Today, 88*, 104389. https://doi.org/10.1016/j.nedt.2020.104389
71. Albert, J. S., Younas, A., & Sana, S. (2020). Nursing students' ethical dilemmas regarding patient care: An integrative review. *Nurse Education Today, 88*, 104389. https://doi.org/10.1016/j.nedt.2020.104389

Read more about ethics education in nursing in the *ANA's Online Journal of Issues in Nursing* article. Access supplementary digital content in the online book using this QR code.

COVID-19 and the Nursing Profession

The COVID-19 pandemic has highlighted the importance of nurses' foundational knowledge of ethical principles and the *Nursing Code of Ethics*. Scarce resources in an overwhelmed health care system resulted in ethical dilemmas and moral injury for nurses involved in balancing conflicting values, rights, and ethical principles. Many nurses were forced to weigh their duty to clients and society against their duty to themselves and their families. Challenging ethical issues occurred related to the ethical principle of justice, such as fair distribution of limited ICU beds and ventilators, and ethical dilemmas related to end-of-life issues such as withdrawing or withholding life-prolonging treatment became common.[72]

Regardless of their practice setting or personal contact with clients affected by COVID-19, nurses have been forced to reflect on the essence of ethical professional nursing practice through the lens of personal values and morals. Nursing students must be knowledgeable about ethical theories, ethical principles, and strategies for resolving ethical dilemmas as they enter the nursing profession that will continue to experience long-term consequences as a result of COVID-19.[73]

6.6 SPOTLIGHT APPLICATION

A True Story of a New Nurse's Introduction to Ethical Dilemmas

A new nurse graduate meets Mary, a 70-year-old woman who was living alone at home with Amyotrophic Lateral Sclerosis (ALS or also referred to as "Lou Gehrig's disease"). Mary's husband died many years ago and they did not have children. She had a small support system, including relatives who lived out of state and friends with whom she had lost touch since her diagnosis. Mary was fiercely independent and maintained her nutrition and hydration through a gastrostomy tube to avoid aspiration.

As Mary's disease progressed, the new nurse discussed several safety issues related to Mary living alone. As the new nurse shared several alternative options related to skilled nursing care with Mary, Mary shared her own plan. Mary said her plan included a combination of opioids, benzodiazepines, and a plastic bag to suffocate herself and be found by a nurse during a scheduled visit. In addition to safety issues and possible suicide ideation, the new nurse recognized she was in the midst of an ethical dilemma in terms of the treatment plan, her values and what she felt was best for Mary, and Mary's preferences.

72. McKenna, H. (2020). Covid-19: Ethical issues for nurses. *International Journal of Nursing Studies, 110*, 103673. https://doi.org/10.1016/j.ijnurstu.2020.103673

73. McKenna, H. (2020). Covid-19: Ethical issues for nurses. *International Journal of Nursing Studies, 110*, 103673. https://doi.org/10.1016/j.ijnurstu.2020.103673

Applying the MORAL Ethical Decision-Making Model to Mary's Case

<table>
<tr><td>Massage the Dilemma</td><td>Data: Mary lives alone and does not want to go to a nursing home. She lacks social support. She has a progressive and incurable disease that affects her ability to swallow, talk, walk, and eventually breathe. She has made statements to staff indicating she prefers to die rather than leave her home to receive total care in a long-term care setting.

Ethical Conflicts: According to the deontological theory, suicide is always wrong. According to the consequentialism ethical theory, an action's morality depends on the consequences of that action. Mary has a progressive, incurable illness that requires total care that will force her to leave the home. She wishes to stay in her home until she dies.

Ethical Goals: To honor Mary's dignity and respect her autonomy in making treatment decisions. For Mary to experience a "good" death as she defines it, and neither hasten nor prolong her dying process through illegal or amoral interventions.</td></tr>
<tr><td>Outline the Options</td><td>• Allow Mary to implement her plan for suicide.
• Admit Mary to the hospital due to suicidal ideation with a clearly expressed plan and means to implement her plan.
• Talk Mary into being admitted to a nursing home.
• Call distant family members or friends to see if they could care for Mary.
• Remove all available means that Mary could use to end her life prematurely (including medications for symptom management that could be used to end her life, resulting in untreated pain).
• Discontinue tube feeding and limit hydration to only that necessary for medication to provide comfort and symptom management.
• Facilitate Mary's ideas regarding physician-assisted suicide. Although illegal in Mary's state of residence, Mary discussed travelling to a state where it was legal.</td></tr>
<tr><td>Review Criteria and Resolve</td><td>Mary was assessed to be rational and capable of decision-making by a psychiatrist. Mary defined a "good" death as one occurring in her home and not in a hospital or long-term care setting. Mary did not want her life to be prolonged through the use of technology such as a ventilator.

Resolution: Mary elected to discontinue tube feeding and limit hydration to only that necessary for medication to provide comfort care and symptom management.</td></tr>
</table>

Affirm Position and Act	Although some health care members did not personally believe in discontinuing food and fluids through the g-tube based on their interpretation of the deontological ethical theory, Mary's decision was acceptable both legally and ethically, based on the consequentialism ethical theory that the decision best supported Mary's goals and respected her autonomy. Daily visits were scheduled with hospice staff, including the nurse, nursing assistant, social worker, chaplain, and volunteers. Hired caregivers supplemented visits and in the last couple of days were scheduled around the clock. Mary died comfortably in her bed seven days after implementation of the agreed-upon plan.
Look Back	The health care team evaluated what happened during Mary's situation and what could be learned from this ethical dilemma and applied to future client-care scenarios.

6.7 LEARNING ACTIVITIES

Learning Activities

(Answers to "Learning Activities" can be found in the "Answer Key" at the end of the book. Answers to interactive activities are provided as immediate feedback.)

Ethical Application & Reflection Activity

Case A

Filmmaker Lulu Wang first shared a story about her grandmother on *This American Life* podcast and later turned it into the 2019 movie *The Farewell* starring Awkwafina. Both share the challenges of a Chinese-born but U.S.-raised woman returning to China and a family who has chosen to not disclose that the grandmother has been given a Stage IV lung cancer diagnosis and three months to live. Listen to the podcast and then answer the following questions:

Listen to the This American Life podcast entitled, "585: In Defense of Ignorance Act One: What You Don't Know." Access supplementary digital content in the online book using this QR code.

1. Reflect on the similarities and differences of your family culture with that of the Billi family. Consider things such as what family gatherings, formal and informal, look like and spoken and unspoken rules related to communication and behavior.

2. The idea of "good" lies and "bad" lies is introduced in the podcast. Nai Nai's family supports the decision to not tell her about her Stage IV lung cancer, stage a wedding as the excuse to visit and say their good-byes, and even alter a medical report as good lies necessary to support her mental health, well-being, and happiness. Is the family applying deontological or utilitarian ethics to the situation? Defend your response.

3. Define the following ethical principles and identify examples from this story:

   - Autonomy
   - Beneficence
   - Nonmaleficence
   - Paternalism

4. Imagine this story is happening in the United States rather than China and you are the nurse admitting Nai Nai to an inpatient oncology unit. Using the ethical problem-solving model of your choice, identify and support your solution to the ethical dilemma posed when her family requests that Nai Nai not be told that she has cancer.

Ethical Application & Reflection Activity

Case B

You are caring for a 32-year-old client who has been in a persistent vegetative state for many years. There is an outdated advanced directive that is confusing on the issue of food and fluids, though clear about not wanting to be on a ventilator if she were in a coma. Her husband wants the feeding tube removed but is unable to say that it would have been the client's wish. He says that it is his decision for her. Her two adult siblings and parents reject this as a possibility because they say that "human life is sacred" and that the daughter believed this. They say their daughter is alive and should receive nursing care, including feeding. The health care team does not know what to do ethically and fear being sued by either the husband, siblings, or the parents. What do you need to know about this clinical situation? What are the values and obligations at stake in this case? What values or obligations should be affirmed and why? How might that be done

1. Define the problem.

2. List what facts/information you have.

3. What are the stakeholders' positions?

   - Client:
   - Spouse:
   - Family:
   - Health Care Team:
   - Facility:
   - Community:

4. How might the stakeholders' values differ?
5. What are your values in this situation?
6. Do your values conflict with those of the client? Describe.

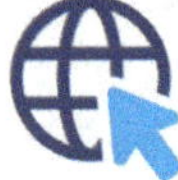

Interactive learning activities have been excluded from the print version of the text. Access free online learning activities in the online book using this QR code.

6.8 GLOSSARY

Advocacy: The act or process of pleading for, supporting, or recommending a cause or course of action. Advocacy may be for persons (whether an individual, group, population, or society) or for an issue, such as potable water or global health.[74]

Autonomy: The capacity to determine one's own actions through independent choice, including demonstration of competence.[75]

Beneficence: The bioethical principle of benefiting others by preventing harm, removing harmful conditions, or affirmatively acting to benefit another or others, often going beyond what is required by law.[76]

Code of ethics: A set of ethical principles established by a profession that is designed to govern decision-making and assist individuals to distinguish right from wrong.

Consequentialism: An ethical theory used to determine whether or not an action is right by the consequences of the action. For example, most people agree that lying is wrong, but if telling a lie would help save a person's life, consequentialism says it's the right thing to do.

Cultural humility: A humble and respectful attitude towards individuals of other cultures and an approach to learning about other cultures as a lifelong goal and process.

Deontology: An ethical theory based on rules that distinguish right from wrong.

Ethical dilemma: Conflict resulting from competing values that requires a decision to be made from equally desirable or undesirable options.

Ethical principles: Principles used to define nurses' moral duties and aid in ethical analysis and decision-making.[77] Foundational ethical principles include autonomy (self-determination), beneficence (do good), nonmaleficence (do no harm), justice (fairness), and veracity (tell the truth).

Ethics: The formal study of morality from a wide range of perspectives.[78]

Ethics committee: A formal committee established by a health care organization to problem-solve ethical dilemmas.

Fidelity: An ethical principle meaning keeping promises.

Institutional Review Board (IRB): A group that has been formally designated to review and monitor biomedical research involving human subjects.

Justice: A moral obligation to act on the basis of equality and equity and a standard linked to fairness for all in society.[79]

Moral conflict: Feelings occurring when an individual is uncertain about what values or principles should be applied to an ethical issue.[80]

---

74. American Nurses Association. (2015). *Code of ethics for nurses with interpretive statements.* American Nurses Association. https://www.nursingworld.org/practice-policy/nursing-excellence/ethics/code-of-ethics-for-nurses/coe-view-only/
75. American Nurses Association. (2021). *Nursing: Scope and standards of practice* (4th ed.). American Nurses Association
76. American Nurses Association. (2015). *Code of ethics for nurses with interpretive statements.* American Nurses Association. https://www.nursingworld.org/practice-policy/nursing-excellence/ethics/code-of-ethics-for-nurses/coe-view-only/
77. American Nurses Association. (2021). *Nursing: Scope and standards of practice* (4th ed.). American Nurses Association
78. American Nurses Association. (2015). *Code of ethics for nurses with interpretive statements.* American Nurses Association. https://www.nursingworld.org/practice-policy/nursing-excellence/ethics/code-of-ethics-for-nurses/coe-view-only/
79. American Nurses Association. (2021). *Nursing: Scope and standards of practice* (4th ed.). American Nurses Association.
80. American Nurses Association (ANA). *Ethics topics and articles.* https://www.nursingworld.org/practice-policy/nursing-excellence/ethics/ethics-topics-and-articles/

Moral courage: The willingness of an individual to speak out and do what is right in the face of forces that would lead us to act in some other way.[81]

Moral distress: Feelings occurring when correct ethical action is identified but the individual feels constrained by competing values of an organization or other individuals.[82]

Moral injury: The distressing psychological, behavioral, social, and sometimes spiritual aftermath of exposure to events that contradict deeply held moral beliefs and expectations.

Morality: Personal values, character, or conduct of individuals or groups within communities and societies.[83]

Moral outrage: Feelings occurring when an individual witnesses immoral acts or practices they feel powerless to change.[84]

Morals: The prevailing standards of behavior of a society that enable people to live cooperatively in groups.[85]

Nonmaleficence: The bioethical principle that specifies a duty to do no harm and balances avoidable harm with benefits of good achieved.[86]

Paternalism: The interference by the state or an individual with another person, defended by the claim that the person interfered with will be better off or protected from harm.[87]

Utilitarianism: A type of consequentialism that determines whether or not actions are right based on their consequences, with the standard being achieving the greatest good for the greatest number of people.

Values: Individual beliefs that motivate people to act one way or another and serve as a guide for behavior.[88]

Veracity: An ethical principle meaning telling the truth.

---

81. American Nurses Association (ANA). *Ethics topics and articles.* https://www.nursingworld.org/practice-policy/nursing-excellence/ethics/ethics-topics-and-articles/

82. American Nurses Association (ANA). *Ethics topics and articles.* https://www.nursingworld.org/practice-policy/nursing-excellence/ethics/ethics-topics-and-articles/

83. American Nurses Association. (2015). *Code of ethics for nurses with interpretive statements.* American Nurses Association. https://www.nursingworld.org/practice-policy/nursing-excellence/ethics/code-of-ethics-for-nurses/coe-view-only/

84. American Nurses Association (ANA). *Ethics topics and articles.* https://www.nursingworld.org/practice-policy/nursing-excellence/ethics/ethics-topics-and-articles/

85. Ethics Unwrapped - McCombs School of Business. (n.d.). *Ethics defined (a glossary).* University of Texas at Austin. https://ethicsunwrapped.utexas.edu/glossary

86. American Nurses Association. (2015). *Code of ethics for nurses with interpretive statements.* American Nurses Association. https://www.nursingworld.org/practice-policy/nursing-excellence/ethics/code-of-ethics-for-nurses/coe-view-only/

87. Dworkin, G. (2020). *Paternalism.* Stanford Encyclopedia of Philosophy. https://plato.stanford.edu/entries/paternalism/

88. Ethics Unwrapped - McCombs School of Business. (n.d.). *Ethics defined (a glossary).* University of Texas at Austin. https://ethicsunwrapped.utexas.edu/glossary

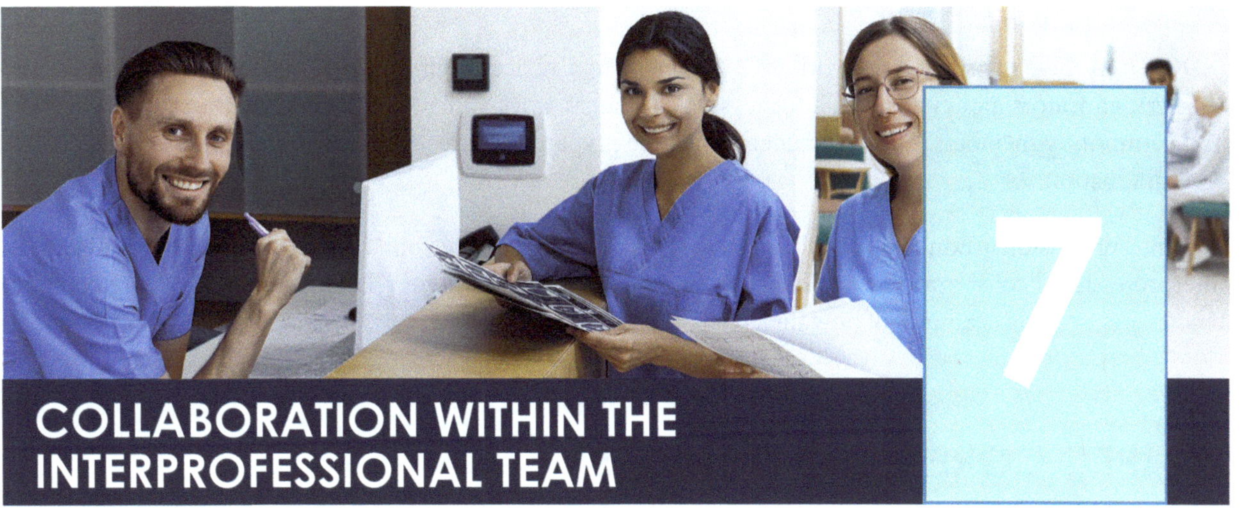

COLLABORATION WITHIN THE INTERPROFESSIONAL TEAM

7.1 COLLABORATION WITHIN THE INTERPROFESSIONAL TEAM INTRODUCTION

LEARNING OBJECTIVES

- Describe how nurses collaborate with the health care team to coordinate appropriate health care services for clients
- Describe collegial and professional practice within the health care team
- Identify members of the team and describe their contributions to optimize client outcomes
- Explore community resources to maximize a client's functional abilities
- Describe procedures used to safely admit, transfer, and/or discharge clients

All health care students must prepare to deliberately work together in clinical practice with a common goal of building a safer, more effective, client-centered health care system. The World Health Organization (WHO) defines **interprofessional collaborative practice** as multiple health workers from different professional backgrounds working together with clients, families, caregivers, and communities to deliver the highest quality of care.[1]

Effective teamwork and communication have been proven to reduce medical errors, promote a safety culture, and improve client outcomes.[2] The importance of effective interprofessional collaboration has become even more important as nurses advocate to reduce health disparities related to social determinants of health

1. World Health Organization. (2010). *Framework for action on interprofessional education & collaborative practice.* https://www.who.int/publications/i/item/framework-for-action-on-interprofessional-education-collaborative-practice
2. AHRQ. (2015). *TeamSTEPPS: National implementation research/evidence base.* https://www.ahrq.gov/teamstepps/evidence-base/safety-culture-improvement.html

(SDOH). In these efforts, nurses work with people from a variety of professions, such as physicians, social workers, educators, policy makers, attorneys, faith leaders, government employees, community advocates, and community members. Nursing students must be prepared to effectively collaborate interprofessionally after graduation.[3]

The Interprofessional Education Collaborative (IPEC) has identified four core competencies for effective interprofessional collaborative practice. This chapter will review content related to these four core competencies and provide examples of how they relate to nursing.

7.2 IPEC CORE COMPETENCIES

The Interprofessional Education Collaborative (IPEC) established standard core competencies for effective interprofessional collaborative practice. The competencies guide the education of future health professionals with the necessary knowledge, skills, values, and attitudes to collaboratively work together in providing client care. See Table 7.2 for a description of the four IPEC core competencies.[4] Each of these competencies will be further discussed in the following sections of this chapter.

TABLE 7.2. IPEC Core Competencies[5]

Competency 1: Values/Ethics for Interprofessional Practice
Work with individuals of other professions to maintain a climate of mutual respect and shared values.
Competency 2: Roles/Responsibilities
Use the knowledge of one's own role and those of other professions to appropriately assess and address the health care needs of clients and to promote and advance the health of populations.
Competency 3: Interprofessional Communication
Communicate with clients, families, communities, and professionals in health and other fields in a responsive and responsible manner that supports a team approach to the promotion and maintenance of health and the prevention and treatment of disease.
Competency 4: Teams and Teamwork
Apply relationship-building values and the principles of team dynamics to perform effectively in different team roles to plan, deliver, and evaluate client/population-centered care and population health programs and policies that are safe, timely, efficient, effective, and equitable.

3. National Academies of Sciences, Engineering, and Medicine. (2021). *The future of nursing 2020-2030: Charting a path to achieve health equity.* The National Academies Press. https://doi.org/10.17226/25982
4. Interprofessional Education Collaborative. (2023). *IPEC core competencies.* https://www.ipecollaborative.org/ipec-core-competencies
5. Interprofessional Education Collaborative. (2023). *IPEC core competencies.* https://www.ipecollaborative.org/ipec-core-competencies

7.3 VALUES AND ETHICS FOR INTERPROFESSIONAL PRACTICE

The first IPEC competency is related to values and ethics and states, "Work with individuals of other professions to maintain a climate of mutual respect and shared values."[6] See the box below for the components related to this competency. Notice how these interprofessional competencies are very similar to the Standards of Professional Performance established by the American Nurses Association related to *Ethics, Advocacy, Respectful and Equitable Practice, Communication*, and *Collaboration*.[7]

Components of IPEC's Values/Ethics for Interprofessional Practice Competency[8]

- Place interests of clients and populations at the center of interprofessional health care delivery and population health programs and policies, with the goal of promoting health and health equity across the life span.
- Respect the dignity and privacy of clients while maintaining confidentiality in the delivery of team-based care.
- Embrace the cultural diversity and individual differences that characterize clients, populations, and the health team.
- Respect the unique cultures, values, roles/responsibilities, and expertise of other health professions and the impact these factors can have on health outcomes.
- Work in cooperation with those who receive care, those who provide care, and others who contribute to or support the delivery of prevention and health services and programs.
- Develop a trusting relationship with clients, families, and other team members.
- Demonstrate high standards of ethical conduct and quality of care in contributions to team-based care.
- Manage ethical dilemmas specific to interprofessional client/population-centered care situations.
- Act with honesty and integrity in relationships with clients, families, communities, and other team members.
- Maintain competence in one's own profession appropriate to scope of practice.

Nursing, medical, and other health professional programs typically educate students in "silos" with few opportunities to collaboratively work together in the classroom or in clinical settings. However, after being hired for their first job, these graduates are thrown into complex clinical situations and expected to function as part of the team. One of the first steps in learning how to function as part of an effective interprofessional team is to value each health care professional's contribution to quality, client-centered care. Mutual respect and trust are foundational to effective interprofessional working relationships for collaborative care delivery across the health professions. Collaborative care also honors the diversity reflected in the individual expertise each profession brings to care delivery.[9]

6. Interprofessional Education Collaborative. (2023). *IPEC core competencies.* https://www.ipecollaborative.org/ipec-core-competencies
7. American Nurses Association. (2021). *Nursing: Scope and standards of practice* (4th ed.). American Nurses Association.
8. Interprofessional Education Collaborative. (2023). *IPEC core competencies.* https://www.ipecollaborative.org/ipec-core-competencies
9. Interprofessional Education Collaborative. (2023). *Core competencies for interprofessional collaborative practice: Version 3.* Interprofessional Education Collaborative. https://www.ipecollaborative.org/assets/core-competencies/IPEC_Core_Competencies_Version_3_2023.pd

Cultural diversity is a term used to describe cultural differences among clients, family members, and health care team members. While it is useful to be aware of specific traits of a culture, it is just as important to understand that each individual is unique, and there are always variations in beliefs among individuals within a culture. Nurses should, therefore, refrain from making assumptions about the values and beliefs of members of specific cultural groups.[10] Instead, a better approach is recognizing that culture is not a static, uniform characteristic but instead realizing there is diversity within every culture and in every person. The American Nurses Association (ANA) defines **cultural humility** as, "A humble and respectful attitude toward individuals of other cultures that pushes one to challenge their own cultural biases, realize they cannot possibly know everything about other cultures, and approach learning about other cultures as a lifelong goal and process."[11] It is imperative for nurses to integrate culturally responsive care into their nursing practice and interprofessional collaborative practice.

Read more about cultural diversity, cultural humility, and integrating culturally responsive care in the "Diverse Patients" chapter of Open RN *Nursing Fundamentals, 2e*. Access supplementary digital content in the online book using this QR code.

Nurses value the expertise of interprofessional team members and integrate this expertise when providing client-centered care. Some examples of valuing and integrating the expertise of interprofessional team members include the following:

- A nurse is caring for a client admitted with chronic heart failure to a medical-surgical unit. During the shift the client's breathing becomes more labored and the client states, "My breathing feels worse today." The nurse ensures the client's head of bed is elevated, oxygen is applied according to the provider orders, and the appropriate scheduled and PRN medications are administered, but the client continues to complain of dyspnea. The nurse calls the respiratory therapist and requests a STAT consult. The respiratory therapist assesses the client and recommends implementation of BiPAP therapy. The provider is notified and an order for BiPAP is received. The client reports later in the shift the dyspnea is resolved with the BiPAP therapy.
- A nurse is working in the Emergency Department when an adolescent client arrives via ambulance experiencing a severe asthma attack. The paramedic provides a handoff report with the client's current vital signs, medications administered, and intravenous (IV) access established. The paramedic also provides information about the home environment, including information about vaping products and a cat in the adolescent's bedroom. The nurse thanks the paramedic for sharing these observations and plans to use information about the home environment to provide client education about asthma triggers and tobacco cessation after the client has been stabilized.
- A nurse is working in a long-term care environment with several unlicensed assistive personnel (UAP) who work closely with the residents providing personal cares and have excellent knowledge regarding their baseline status. Today, after helping Mrs. Smith with her morning bath, one of the UAPs tells the nurse, "Mrs. Smith doesn't seem like herself today. She was very tired and kept falling asleep while I was talking to her, which is not her normal behavior." The nurse immediately assesses Mrs. Smith and

10. Interprofessional Education Collaborative. (2023). *Core competencies for interprofessional collaborative practice: Version 3.* Interprofessional Education Collaborative. https://www.ipecollaborative.org/assets/core-competencies/IPEC_Core_Competencies_Version_3_2023.pd

11. American Nurses Association. (2021). *Nursing: Scope and standards of practice* (4th ed.). American Nurses Association.

confirms her somnolescence and confirms her vital signs are within her normal range. The nurse reviews Mrs. Smith's chart and notices that a new prescription for furosemide was started last month but no potassium supplements were ordered. The nurse notifies the provider of the client's change in status and receives an order for lab work, including an electrolyte panel. The results indicate that Mrs. Smith's potassium level has dropped to an abnormal level, which is the likely cause of her fatigue and somnolescence. The provider is notified, and an order is received for a potassium supplement. The nurse thanks the UAP for recognizing and reporting Mrs. Smith's change in status and successfully preventing a poor client outcome such as a life-threatening cardiac dysrhythmia.

Effective client-centered, interprofessional collaborative practice improves client outcomes. View supplementary material and reflective questions in the following box.[12]

View the "How does interprofessional collaboration impact care: The patient's perspective?" video on YouTube regarding clients' perspectives about the importance of interprofessional collaboration.

Read "Ten Lessons in Collaboration." Although this is an older publication, it provides ten lessons to consider in collaborative relationships and practice. The discussion reflects many components of collaboration that have been integral to nursing practice in interprofessional teamwork and leadership.

Reflective Questions

1. What is the difference between client-centered care and disease-centered care?
2. Why is it important for health professionals to collaborate?

Access supplementary digital content in the online book using this QR code.

7.4 ROLES AND RESPONSIBILILITES OF HEALTH CARE PROFESSIONALS

The second IPEC competency relates to the roles and responsibilities of health care professionals and states, "Use the knowledge of one's own role and those of other professions to appropriately assess and address the health care needs of clients and to promote and advance the health of populations."[13]

See the following box for the components of this competency. It is important to understand the roles and responsibilities of the other health care team members; recognize one's limitations in skills, knowledge, and abilities; and ask for assistance when needed to provide quality, client-centered care.

12. Leadership and Influencing Change in Nursing by Joan Wagner is licensed under CC BY 4.0
13. Interprofessional Education Collaborative. (2023). *IPEC core competencies.* https://www.ipecollaborative.org/ipec-core-competencies

Components of IPEC's Roles/Responsibilities Competency[14]

- Communicate one's roles and responsibilities clearly to clients, families, community members, and other professionals.
- Recognize one's limitations in skills, knowledge, and abilities.
- Engage with diverse professionals who complement one's own professional expertise, as well as associated resources, to develop strategies to meet specific health and health care needs of clients and populations.
- Explain the roles and responsibilities of other providers and the manner in which the team works together to provide care, promote health, and prevent disease.
- Use the full scope of knowledge, skills, and abilities of professionals from health and other fields to provide care that is safe, timely, efficient, effective, and equitable.
- Communicate with team members to clarify each member's responsibility in executing components of a treatment plan or public health intervention.
- Forge interdependent relationships with other professions within and outside of the health system to improve care and advance learning.
- Engage in continuous professional and interprofessional development to enhance team performance and collaboration.
- Use unique and complementary abilities of all members of the team to optimize health and client care.
- Describe how professionals in health and other fields can collaborate and integrate clinical care and public health interventions to optimize population health.

Nurses communicate with several individuals during a typical shift. For example, during inpatient care, nurses may communicate with clients and their family members; pharmacists and pharmacy technicians; providers from different specialties; physical, speech, and occupational therapists; dietary aides; respiratory therapists; chaplains; social workers; case managers; nursing supervisors, charge nurses, and other staff nurses; assistive personnel; nursing students; nursing instructors; security guards; laboratory personnel; radiology and ultrasound technicians; and surgical team members. Providing holistic, quality, safe, and effective care means every team member taking care of clients must work collaboratively and understand the knowledge, skills, and scope of practice of the other team members. Table 7.4 provides examples of the roles and responsibilities of common health care team members that nurses frequently work with when providing client care. To fully understand the roles and responsibilities of the multiple members of the complex health care delivery system, it is beneficial to spend time shadowing those within these roles.

14. Interprofessional Education Collaborative. (2023). *IPEC core competencies.* https://www.ipecollaborative.org/ipec-core-competencies

TABLE 7.4. Roles and Responsibilities of Members of the Health Care Team

Member	Role/Responsibilities
Unlicensed Assistive Personnel (UAP) (e.g., certified nursing assistants [CNA], patient-care technicians [PCT], certified medical assistants [CMA], certified medication aides, and home health aides)	Work under the direct supervision of the RN. (Read more about Unlicensed Assistive Personnel (UAP) in the "Delegation and Supervision" chapter.)
Licensed Practical/Vocational Nurses (LPN/VN)	Assist the RN by performing routine, basic nursing care with predictable outcomes. (Read more details in the "Delegation and Supervision" chapter.)
Registered Nurses (RN)	Use the nursing process to assess, diagnose, identify expected outcomes, plan and implement interventions, and evaluate care according to the Nurse Practice Act of the state they are employed.
Charge Nurses or Nursing Supervisors	Supervise members of the nursing team and overall client care on the unit (or organization) to ensure quality, safe care is delivered.
Directors of Nursing (DON), Chief Nursing Officer (CNO), or Vice President of Patient Services	Ensure federal and state regulations and standards are being followed and are accountable for all aspects of client care.
Clinical Nurse Specialist (CNS)	Practice in a variety of health care environments and participate in mentoring other nurses, case management, research, designing and conducting quality improvement programs, and serving as educators and consultants.
Nurse Practitioners (NP) or Advanced Practice Registered Nurses (APRN)	Work in a variety of settings and complete physical examinations, diagnose and treat common acute illness, manage chronic illness, order laboratory and diagnostic tests, prescribe medications and other therapies, provide health teaching and supportive counseling with an emphasis on prevention of illness and health maintenance, and refer clients to other health professionals and specialists as needed. NPs have advanced knowledge with a graduate degree and national certification.
Certified Registered Nurse Anesthetists (CRNA)	Administer anesthesia and related care before, during, and after surgical, therapeutic, diagnostic, and obstetrical procedures, as well as provide airway management during medical emergencies.

TABLE 7.4. Continued...

Certified Nurse Midwives (CNM)	Provide gynecological exams, family planning guidance, prenatal care, management of low-risk labor and delivery, and neonatal care.
Medical Doctors (MD)	Licensed providers who diagnose, treat, and direct medical care. There are many types of physician specialists such as surgeons, pulmonologists, neurologists, cardiologists, nephrologists, pediatricians, and ophthalmologists.
Physician Assistants (PA)	Work under the direct supervision of a medical doctor as licensed and certified professionals following protocols based on the state in which they practice.
Doctors of Osteopathy (DO)	Licensed providers similar to medical physicians but with different educational preparation and licensing exams. They provide care, prescribe, and can perform surgeries.
Dieticians	Assess, plan, implement, and evaluate interventions related to specific dietary needs of clients, including regular or therapeutic diets. Formulate diets for clients with dysphagia or other physical disorders and provide dietary education such as diabetes education.
Physical Therapists (PT)	Develop and implement a plan of care as a licensed professional for clients with dysfunctional physical abilities, including joints, strength, mobility, gait, balance, and coordination.
Occupational Therapists (OT)	Plan, provide, and evaluate care for clients with dysfunction affecting their independence and ability to complete activities of daily living (ADLs). Assist clients in using adaptive devices to reach optimal levels of functioning and provide home safety assessments.
Speech Therapists (ST)	Develop and initiate a plan of care for clients diagnosed with communication and swallowing disorders.
Respiratory Therapists (RT)	Specialize in treating clients with respiratory disorders or conditions in collaboration with providers. Provide treatments such as CPAP, BiPAP, respiratory treatments and medications like aerosol nebulizers, chest physiotherapy, and postural drainage. They also intubate clients, assist with bronchoscopies, manage mechanical ventilation, and perform pulmonary function tests.
Social Workers (SW)	Provide a liaison between the community and the health care setting to ensure continuity of care after discharge. Assist clients with establishing community resources, health insurance, and advance directives.

TABLE 7.4. Continued...

Psychologists and Psychiatrists	Provide mental health services to clients in both acute and long-term settings. As physician specialists, psychiatrists prescribe medications and perform other medical treatments for mental health disorders. Psychologists focus on counseling.
Nurse Case Managers or Discharge Planners	Ensure clients are provided with effective and efficient medical care and services, during inpatient care and post-discharge, while also managing the cost of these services.

The coordination and delivery of safe, quality client care demands reliable teamwork and collaboration across the organizational and community boundaries. Clients often have multiple visits across multiple providers working in different organizations. Communication failures between health care settings, departments, and team members is the leading cause of client harm.[15] The health care system is becoming increasingly complex requiring collaboration among diverse health care team members. For example, when a COPD exacerbation client is discharged from the acute care setting, their condition may necessitate home resources or care in order to optimize their recovery. This may require the coordination of home oxygen resources, a walker, or home visits in order to assess their transition and recovery. Nurses must understand that community resources are individualized to their regional area and advocating for client needs and resource gaps is an important part of their role.

The goal of good interprofessional collaboration is improved client outcomes, as well as increased job satisfaction of health care team professionals. Clients receiving care with poor teamwork are almost five times as likely to experience complications or death. Hospitals in which staff report higher levels of teamwork have lower rates of workplace injuries and illness, fewer incidents of workplace harassment and violence, and lower turnover.[16]

Valuing and understanding the roles of team members are important steps toward establishing good interprofessional teamwork. Another step is learning how to effectively communicate with interprofessional team members.

Community Resource Care Coordination Case Scenario

Patient Background

Name: Mr. Gerald Hermso

Age: 72

Medical History: Chronic Heart Failure (CHF), Hypertension, Type 2 Diabetes, Hyperlipidemia

Recent Hospitalization: Mr. Hermso was admitted to the hospital due to a CHF exacerbation characterized by shortness of breath, fatigue, and fluid retention. After stabilization with diuretics, beta-blockers, and lifestyle adjustments, Mr. Hermso is ready for discharge.

15. Rosen, M. A., DiazGranados, D., Dietz, A. S., Benishek, L. E., Thompson, D., Pronovost, P. J., & Weaver, S. J. (2018). Teamwork in healthcare: Key discoveries enabling safer, high-quality care. *The American Psychologist, 73*(4), 433-450. https://doi.org/10.1037/amp0000298

16. Rosen, M. A., DiazGranados, D., Dietz, A. S., Benishek, L. E., Thompson, D., Pronovost, P. J., & Weaver, S. J. (2018). Teamwork in healthcare: Key discoveries enabling safer, high-quality care. *The American Psychologist, 73*(4), 433-450. https://doi.org/10.1037/amp0000298

Discharge Planning Goals:

1. Ensure Mr. Hermso's safe transition from hospital to home.
2. Minimize the risk of readmission.
3. Provide ongoing support for managing CHF at home.

Discharge Coordinator's Role:

The discharge coordinator plays a crucial role in organizing Mr. Hermso's transition from the hospital to his home. This includes identifying and coordinating community resources that can support his ongoing care.

- **Assessment of Needs:** The coordinator reviews Mr. Hermso's medical records and discharge plan, including prescribed medications, follow-up appointments, dietary restrictions, and physical activity recommendations. The coordinator assesses Mr. Hermso's living situation. Does he live alone? Does he have any support systems such as family or friends who can assist him? Identify any potential barriers to Mr. Hermso managing his condition at home, such as mobility issues, medication management challenges, or limited access to transportation.
- **Collaboration with Nursing Staff:** The discharge coordinator collaborates with the nurse assigned to Mr. Hermso to ensure all his needs are met. The nurse provides insights into Mr. Hermso's physical and psychological readiness for discharge. Together, they develop a plan to address his needs post-discharge.
- **Community Resources Identification:** The discharge coordinator arranges for a home health nurse to visit Mr. Hermso several times a week to monitor his vital signs, administer medications, and provide education on CHF management. The coordinator sets up a service with a local pharmacy for medication delivery and synchronization, ensuring that Mr. Hermso receives his prescriptions on time. The nurse will teach Mr. Hermso how to use a pill organizer. A referral is made to a community dietician who specializes in CHF to provide Mr. Hermso with personalized meal planning that aligns with his dietary restrictions. The coordinator arranges for Mr. Hermso to receive telehealth equipment, including a scale and blood pressure monitor, so that his weight and blood pressure can be monitored remotely. The nurse will educate Mr. Hermso on using this equipment. The coordinator refers Mr. Hermso to a local cardiac rehab program, where he can receive supervised exercise and education on heart health. If Mr. Hermso lacks transportation, the coordinator connects him with local transportation services that can take him to follow-up appointments and rehab sessions. The coordinator links Mr. Hermso with a local CHF support group where he can connect with others who have similar experiences, providing emotional and social support.

Nurse's Role:

- **Patient Education:** The nurse provides detailed education on CHF management, including recognizing early signs of exacerbation, the importance of medication adherence, dietary restrictions (e.g., low-sodium diet), and the need for regular physical activity. The nurse teaches Mr. Hermso how to use his new telehealth equipment and ensures he understands how to log and report his readings.
- **Care Coordination:** The nurse ensures that all community resources are in place before discharge. This includes confirming home health services, medication delivery, and transportation arrangements. The nurse reviews the discharge plan with Mr. Hermso and his family (if applicable) to ensure they understand the follow-up schedule and how to access the resources provided.

- **Follow-up:** The nurse schedules a follow-up call within 48 hours of discharge to check on Mr. Hermso's progress, answer any questions, and address any emerging issues.

Outcome:

- **Immediate Post-Discharge:** Mr. Hermso transitions home with a solid support system in place. He has access to home health services, medication management, dietary support, and telehealth monitoring.
- **Long-term Monitoring:** Through consistent follow-up and engagement with community resources, Mr. Hermso is better equipped to manage his CHF at home, reducing the likelihood of readmission and improving his overall quality of life.

7.5 INTERPROFESSIONAL COMMUNICATION

The third IPEC competency focuses on interprofessional communication and states, "Communicate with clients, families, communities, and professionals in health and other fields in a responsive and responsible manner that supports a team approach to the promotion and maintenance of health and the prevention and treatment of disease."[17] See Figure 7.1[18] for an image of interprofessional communication supporting a team approach. This competency also aligns with The Joint Commission's National Patient Safety Goal for improving staff communication.[19] See the following box for the components associated with the Interprofessional Communication competency.

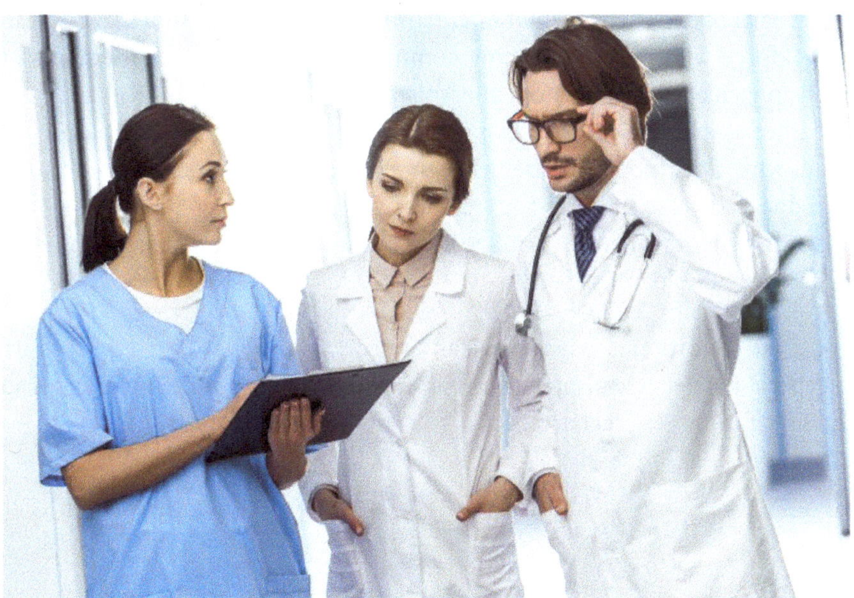

FIGURE 7.1 Image from Nursing Fundamentals

17. Interprofessional Education Collaborative. (2023). *IPEC core competencies.* https://www.ipecollaborative.org/ipec-core-competencies
18. "1322557028-huge.jpg" by LightField Studios is used under license from Shutterstock.com
19. The Joint Commission. (2025). *Hospital national patient safety goals.* https://www.jointcommission.org/standards/national-patient-safety-goals/hospital-national-patient-safety-goals/

Components of IPEC's Interprofessional Communication Competency[20]

- Choose effective communication tools and techniques, including information systems and communication technologies, to facilitate discussions and interactions that enhance team function.
- Communicate information with clients, families, community members, and health team members in a form that is understandable, avoiding discipline-specific terminology when possible.
- Express one's knowledge and opinions to team members involved in client care and population health improvement with confidence, clarity, and respect, working to ensure common understanding of information, treatment, care decisions, and population health programs and policies.
- Listen actively and encourage ideas and opinions of other team members.
- Give timely, sensitive, constructive feedback to others about their performance on the team, responding respectfully as a team member to feedback from others.
- Use respectful language appropriate for a given difficult situation, crucial conversation, or conflict.
- Recognize how one's uniqueness (experience level, expertise, culture, power, and hierarchy within the health care team) contributes to effective communication, conflict resolution, and positive interprofessional working relationships.
- Communicate the importance of teamwork in client-centered care and population health programs and policies.

Transmission of information among members of the health care team and facilities is ongoing and critical to quality care. However, information that is delayed, inefficient, or inadequate creates barriers for providing quality of care. Communication barriers continue to exist in health care environments due to interprofessional team members' lack of experience when interacting with other disciplines. For instance, many novice nurses enter the workforce without experiencing communication with other members of the health care team (e.g., providers, pharmacists, respiratory therapists, social workers, surgical staff, dieticians, physical therapists, etc.). Additionally, health care professionals tend to develop a professional identity based on their educational program with a distinction made between groups. This distinction can cause tension between professional groups due to diverse training and perspectives on providing quality client care. In addition, a health care organization's environment may not be conducive to effectively sharing information with multiple staff members across multiple units.

In addition to potential educational, psychological, and organizational barriers to sharing information, there can also be general barriers that impact interprofessional communication and collaboration. See the following box for a list of these general barriers.[21]

20. Interprofessional Education Collaborative. (2023). *IPEC core competencies.* https://www.ipecollaborative.org/ipec-core-competencies

21. O'Daniel, M., & Rosenstein, A. H. (2011). Professional communication and team collaboration. In: Hughes R.G. (Ed.). *Patient safety and quality: An evidence-based handbook for nurses.* Agency for Healthcare Research and Quality (US); Chapter 33. https://www.ncbi.nlm.nih.gov/books/NBK2637

General Barriers to Interprofessional Communication and Collaboration[22]

- Personal values and expectations
- Personality differences
- Organizational hierarchy
- Lack of cultural humility
- Generational differences
- Historical interprofessional and intraprofessional rivalries
- Differences in language and medical jargon
- Differences in schedules and professional routines
- Varying levels of preparation, qualifications, and status
- Differences in requirements, regulations, and norms of professional education
- Fears of diluted professional identity
- Differences in accountability and reimbursement models
- Diverse clinical responsibilities
- Increased complexity of client care
- Emphasis on rapid decision-making

There are several national initiatives that have been developed to overcome barriers to communication among interprofessional team members. These initiatives are summarized in Table 7.5a.[23]

TABLE 7.5A. Initiatives to Overcome Barriers to Interprofessional Communication and Collaboration[24]

Action	Description
Teach structured interprofessional communication strategies	Structured communication strategies, such as ISBARR, handoff reports, I-PASS reports, and closed-loop communication, should be taught to all health professionals.
Train interprofessional teams together	Teams that work together should train together.
Train teams using simulation	Simulation creates a safe environment to practice communication strategies and increase interdisciplinary understanding.

22. O'Daniel, M., & Rosenstein, A. H. (2011). Professional communication and team collaboration. In: Hughes R.G. (Ed.). *Patient safety and quality: An evidence-based handbook for nurses.* Agency for Healthcare Research and Quality (US); Chapter 33. https://www.ncbi.nlm.nih.gov/books/NBK2637

23. Weller, J., Boyd, M., & Cumin, D. (2014). Teams, tribes and patient safety: Overcoming barriers to effective teamwork in healthcare. *Postgraduate Medical Journal, 90*(1061), 149-154. https://doi.org/10.1136/postgradmedj-2012-131168

24. Weller, J., Boyd, M., & Cumin, D. (2014). Teams, tribes and patient safety: Overcoming barriers to effective teamwork in healthcare. *Postgraduate Medical Journal, 90*(1061), 149-154. https://doi.org/10.1136/postgradmedj-2012-131168

TABLE 7.5A. Continued...

Define cohesive interprofessional teams	Interprofessional health care teams should be defined within organizations as a cohesive whole with common goals and not just a collection of disciplines.
Create democratic teams	All members of the health care team should feel valued. Creating democratic teams (instead of establishing hierarchies) encourages open team communication.
Support teamwork with protocols and procedures	Protocols and procedures encouraging information sharing across the whole team include checklists, briefings, huddles, and debriefing. Technology and informatics should also be used to promote information sharing among team members.
Develop an organizational culture supporting health care teams	Agency leaders must establish a safety culture and emphasize the importance of effective interprofessional collaboration for achieving good client outcomes.

Communication Strategies

Several communication strategies have been implemented nationally to ensure information is exchanged among health care team members in a structured, concise, and accurate manner to promote safe client care. Examples of these initiatives are ISBARR, handoff reports, closed-loop communication, and I-PASS. Documentation that promotes sharing information interprofessionally to promote continuity of care is also essential. These strategies are discussed in the following subsections.

ISBARR

A common format used by health care team members to exchange client information is **ISBARR**, a mnemonic for the components of **I**ntroduction, **S**ituation, **B**ackground, **A**ssessment, **R**equest/Recommendations, and **R**epeat back.[25,26]

- **Introduction:** Introduce your name, role, and the agency from which you are calling.
- **Situation:** Provide the client's name and location, the reason you are calling, recent vital signs, and the status of the client.
- **Background:** Provide pertinent background information about the client such as admitting medical diagnoses, code status, recent relevant lab or diagnostic results, and allergies.
- **Assessment:** Share abnormal assessment findings and your evaluation of the current client situation.
- **Request/Recommendations:** State what you would like the provider to do, such as reassess the client, order a lab/diagnostic test, prescribe/change medication, etc.
- **Repeat back:** If you are receiving new orders from a provider, repeat them to confirm accuracy. Be sure to document communication with the provider in the client's chart.

25. Institute for Healthcare Improvement (n.d.). *ISBAR trip tick.* https://www.ihi.org/resources/tools/sbar-tool-situation-background-assessment-recommendation
26. Grbach, W., Vincent, L., & Struth, D. (2008). *Curriculum developer for simulation education.* QSEN Institute. https://qsen.org/reformulating-sbar-to-i-sbar-r/

Nursing Considerations

Before using ISBARR to call a provider regarding a changing client condition or concern, it is important for nurses to prepare and gather appropriate information. See the following box for considerations when calling the provider.

Communication Guidelines for Nurses[27]

- Have I assessed this client before I call?
- Have I reviewed the current orders?
- Are there related standing orders or protocols?
- Have I read the most recent provider and nursing progress notes?
- Have I discussed concerns with my charge nurse, if necessary?
- When ready to call, have the following information on hand:
  - Admitting diagnosis and date of admission
  - Code status
  - Allergies
  - Most recent vital signs
  - Most recent lab results
  - Current meds and IV fluids
  - If receiving oxygen therapy, current device and L/min
- Before calling, reflect on what you expect to happen as a result of this call and if you have any recommendations or specific requests.
- Repeat back any new orders to confirm them.
- Immediately after the call, document with whom you spoke, the exact time of the call, and a summary of the information shared and received.

Read an example of an ISBARR report in the following box.

Sample ISBARR Report From a Nurse to a Health Care Provider

I: "Hello Dr. Smith, this is Jane Smith, RN from the Med-Surg unit."

S: "I am calling to tell you about Ms. White in Room 210, who is experiencing an increase in pain, as well as redness at her incision site. Her recent vital signs were BP 160/95, heart rate 90, respiratory rate 22, O2 sat 96% on room air, and temperature 38 degrees Celsius. She is stable but her pain is worsening."

27. Studer Group. (2007). *Patient safety toolkit – Practical tactics that improve both patient safety and patient perceptions of care.* Studer Group. https://www.ncbi.nlm.nih.gov/books/NBK2637/table/ch33.t4/

B: "Ms. White is a 65-year-old female, admitted yesterday post hip surgical replacement. She has been rating her pain at 3 or 4 out of 10 since surgery with her scheduled medication, but now she is rating the pain as a 7, with no relief from her scheduled medication of Vicodin 5/325 mg administered an hour ago. She is scheduled for physical therapy later this morning and is stating she won't be able to participate because of the pain this morning."

A: "I just assessed the surgical site, and her dressing was clean, dry, and intact, but there is 4 cm redness surrounding the incision, and it is warm and tender to the touch. There is moderate sero-sanguinous drainage. Her lungs are clear, and her heart rate is regular. She has no allergies. I think she has developed a wound infection."

R: "I am calling to request an order for a CBC and increased dose of pain medication."

R: "I am repeating back the order to confirm that you are ordering a STAT CBC and an increase of her Vicodin to 10/325 mg."

View or print an ISBARR reference card. Access supplementary digital content in the online book using this QR code.

Handoff Reports

Handoff reports are defined by The Joint Commission as "a transfer and acceptance of client care responsibility achieved through effective communication. It is a real-time process of passing client specific information from one caregiver to another, or from one team of caregivers to another, for the purpose of ensuring the continuity and safety of the client's care."[28] In 2017 The Joint Commission issued a sentinel alert about inadequate handoff communication that has resulted in client harm such as wrong-site surgeries, delays in treatment, falls, and medication errors.[29]

The Joint Commission encourages the standardization of critical content to be communicated by interprofessional team members during a handoff report both verbally (preferably face to face) and in written form. Critical content to communicate to the receiver in a handoff report includes the following components[30]:

- Sender contact information
- Illness assessment, including severity

---

28. Starmer, A. J., Spector, N. D., Srivastava, R., Allen, A. D., Landrigan, C. P., Sectish, T. C., & I-Pass Study Group. (2012). I-PASS, a Mnemonic to Standardize Verbal Handoffs. *Pediatrics, 129*(2), 201-204. https://www.ipassinstitute.com/hubfs/I-PASS-mnemonic.pdf
29. The Joint Commission. (2017). *Sentinel event alert 58: Inadequate hand-off reports.* https://www.jointcommission.org/resources/patient-safety-topics/sentinel-event/sentinel-event-alert-newsletters/sentinel-event-alert-58-inadequate-hand-off-communication/
30. The Joint Commission. (2017). *Sentinel event alert 58: Inadequate hand-off reports.* https://www.jointcommission.org/resources/patient-safety-topics/sentinel-event/sentinel-event-alert-newsletters/sentinel-event-alert-58-inadequate-hand-off-communication/

- Client summary, including events leading up to illness or admission, hospital course, ongoing assessment, and plan of care
- To-do action list
- Contingency plans
- Allergy list
- Code status
- Medication list
- Recent laboratory tests
- Recent vital signs

Several strategies for improving handoff communication have been implemented nationally, such as the Bedside Handoff Report Checklist, closed-loop communication, and I-PASS.

Bedside Handoff Report Checklist

See Figure 7.2[31] for an example of a Bedside Handoff Report Checklist to improve nursing handoff reports by the Agency for Healthcare Research and Quality (AHRQ).[32] Although a bedside handoff report is similar to an ISBARR report, it contains additional information to ensure continuity of care across nursing shifts.

Print a copy of the AHRQ Bedside Shift Report Checklist.[33] Access supplementary digital content in the online book using this QR code.

View a video example of bedside handoff reporting. Access supplementary digital content in the online book using this QR code.

31. "Strat3_Tool_2_Nurse_Chklst_508.pdf" by AHRQ is licensed under CC0
32. AHRQ. (n.d.). *Bedside shift report checklist.* https://www.ahrq.gov/sites/default/files/wysiwyg/professionals/systems/hospital/engagingfamilies/strategy3/Strat3_Tool_2_Nurse_Chklst_508.pdf
33. AHRQ. (n.d.). *Bedside shift report checklist.* https://www.ahrq.gov/sites/default/files/wysiwyg/professionals/systems/hospital/engagingfamilies/strategy3/Strat3_Tool_2_Nurse_Chklst_508.pdf

Bedside Shift Report Checklist

- ❑ Introduce the nursing staff to the patient and family. Invite the patient and family to take part in the bedside shift report.
- ❑ Open the medical record or access the electronic work station in the patient's room.
- ❑ Conduct a verbal SBAR report with the patient and family. Use words that the patient and family can understand.

  S = **Situation**. What is going on with the patient? What are the current vital signs?

  B = **Background**. What is the pertinent patient history?

  A = **Assessment**. What is the patient's problem now?

  R = **Recommendation**. What does the patient need?

- ❑ Conduct a focused assessment of the patient and a safety assessment of the room.
  - Visually inspect all wounds, incisions, drains, IV sites, IV tubings, catheters, etc.
  - Visually sweep the room for any physical safety concerns.
- ❑ Review tasks that need to be done, such as:
  - Labs or tests needed
  - Medications administered
  - Forms that need to be completed (e.g., admission, patient intake, vaccination, allergy review, etc.)
  - Other tasks: ______________________________
- ❑ Identify the patient's and family's needs or concerns.
  - Ask the patient and family:
    - *"What could have gone better during the last 12 hours?"*
    - *"Tell us how your pain is."*
    - *"Tell us how much you walked today."*
    - *"Do you have any concerns about safety?"*
    - *"Do you have any worries you would like to share?"*
  - Ask the patient and family what the goal is for the next shift. This is the patient's goal — not the nursing staff's goal for the patient.
    - *"What do you want to happen during the next 12 hours?"*
    - Follow up to see if the goal was met during the verbal SBAR at the next bedside shift report.

Adapted from the Emory University Bedside Shift Report Bundle.

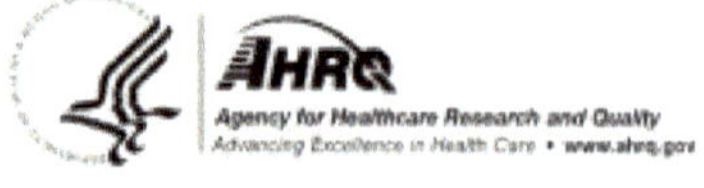

Guide to Patient and Family Engagement

FIGURE 7.2 Bedside Handoff Report Checklist

Closed-Loop Communication

The **closed-loop communication** strategy is used to ensure that information conveyed by the sender is heard by the receiver and completed. Closed-loop communication is especially important during emergency situations when verbal orders are being provided as treatments are immediately implemented. See Figure 7.3[34] for an illustration of closed-loop communication.

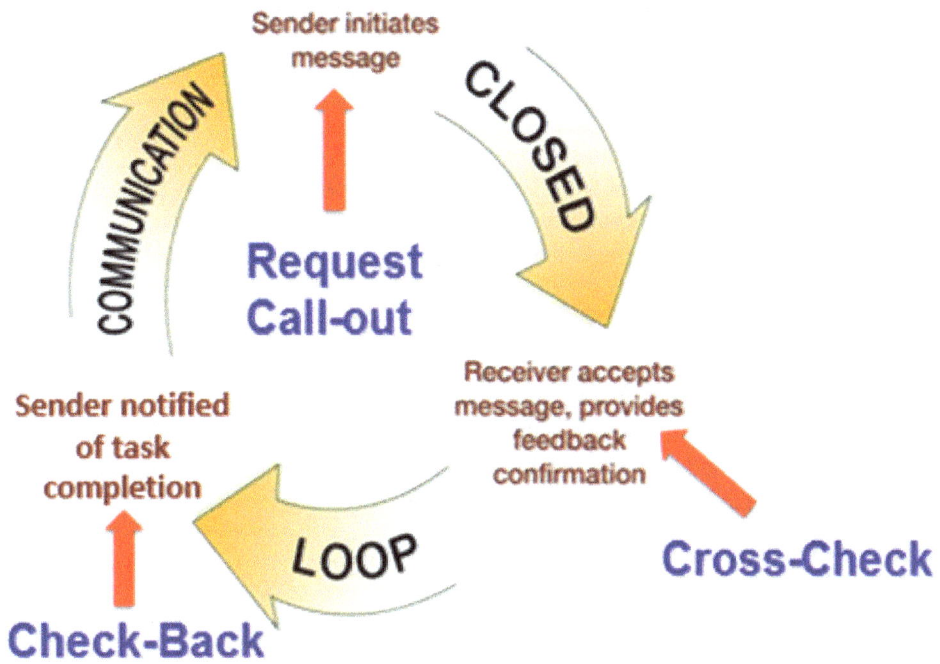

FIGURE 7.3 Closed-Loop Communication

1. The sender initiates the message.
2. The receiver accepts the message and repeats back the message to confirm it (i.e., "Cross-Check").
3. The sender confirms the message.
4. The receiver notified the sender the task was completed (i.e., "Check-Back").

See an example of closed-loop communication during an emergent situation in the following box.

34. Image is derivative of "close-loop.png" by unknown and is licensed under CC0. Access for free at https://www.ahrq.gov/teamstepps/instructor/essentials/pocketguide.html

Closed-Loop Communication Example

Doctor: "Administer 25 mg Benadryl IV push STAT."

Nurse: "Give 25 mg Benadryl IV push STAT?"

Doctor: "That's correct."

Nurse: "Benadryl 25 mg IV push given at 1125."

I-PASS

I-PASS is a mnemonic used to provide structured communication among interprofessional team members. I-PASS stands for the following components[35]:

I: Illness severity
P: Patient summary
A: Action list
S: Situation awareness and contingency plans
S: Synthesis by receiver (i.e., closed-loop communication)

See a sample I-PASS Handoff in Table 7.5b.[36]

TABLE 7.5B. Sample I-PASS Verbal Handoff[37]

I	**Illness Severity**	This is our sickest client on the unit, and he's a full code.
P	**Patient Summary**	AJ is a 4-year-old boy admitted with hypoxia and respiratory distress secondary to left lower lobe pneumonia. He presented with cough and high fevers for two days before admission, and on the day of admission to the emergency department, he had worsening respiratory distress. In the emergency department, he was found to have a sodium level of 130 mg/dL likely due to volume depletion. He received a fluid bolus, and oxygen administration was started at 2.5 L/min per nasal cannula. He is on ceftriaxone.
A	**Action List**	Assess him at midnight to ensure his vital signs are stable. Check to determine if his blood culture is positive tonight.

35. The Joint Commission. (2017). *Sentinel event alert 58: Inadequate hand-off reports.* https://www.jointcommission.org/resources/patient-safety-topics/sentinel-event/sentinel-event-alert-newsletters/sentinel-event-alert-58-inadequate-hand-off-communication/
36. Starmer, A. J., Spector, N. D., Srivastava, R., Allen, A. D., Landrigan, C. P., Sectish, T. C., & I-Pass Study Group. (2012). I-PASS, a Mnemonic to Standardize Verbal Handoffs. *Pediatrics, 129*(2), 201-204. https://www.ipassinstitute.com/hubfs/I-PASS-mnemonic.pdf
37. Starmer, A. J., Spector, N. D., Srivastava, R., Allen, A. D., Landrigan, C. P., Sectish, T. C., & I-Pass Study Group. (2012). I-PASS, a Mnemonic to Standardize Verbal Handoffs. *Pediatrics, 129*(2), 201-204. https://www.ipassinstitute.com/hubfs/I-PASS-mnemonic.pdf

TABLE 7.5B. Continued...

S	**Situations Awareness & Contingency Planning**	If his respiratory distress worsens, get another chest radiograph to determine if he is developing an effusion.
S	**Synthesis by Receiver**	Ok, so AJ is a 4-year-old admitted with hypoxia and respiratory distress secondary to a left lower lobe pneumonia receiving ceftriaxone, oxygen, and fluids. I will assess him at midnight to ensure he is stable and check on his blood culture. If his respiratory status worsens, I will repeat a radiograph to look for an effusion.

Listening Skills

Effective team communication includes both the delivery and receipt of the message. Listening skills are a fundamental element of the communication loop. For nursing staff, this involves listening to clients, families, and coworkers. Active listening involves not just hearing the individual words that someone states, but also understanding the emotions and concerns behind the words. Employing active listening reflects an empathetic approach and can improve client outcomes and foster teamwork.

Nurses often serve as the communication bridge between clients, families, and other health care team members. By listening attentively to colleagues, nurses can ensure that important information is accurately conveyed, reducing the risk of misunderstandings and enhancing the overall efficiency of care delivery. This collaborative environment fosters a culture of mutual respect and support, ultimately leading to better health care outcomes.

In order to develop active listening skills, individuals should practice mindfulness and practice their communication techniques. Listening skills can be cultivated with eye contact, actions such as nodding, and demonstration of other nonverbal strategies to demonstrate engagement. Maintaining an open posture, smiling, and attentiveness are all nonverbal strategies that can facilitate communication. It is important to take measures to avoid distractions, offer a summation of the communication, and ask clarifying questions to further develop the communication.

Documentation

Accurate, timely, concise, and thorough documentation by interprofessional team members ensures continuity of care for their clients. It is well-known by health care team members that in a court of law the rule of thumb is, "If it wasn't documented, it wasn't done." Any type of documentation in the electronic health record (EHR) is considered a legal document. Abbreviations should be avoided in legal documentation and some abbreviations are prohibited. Please see a list of error prone abbreviations in the box below.

Read the current list of error-prone abbreviations by the Institute of Safe Medication Practices. These abbreviations should never be used when communicating medical information verbally, electronically, and/or in handwritten applications. Abbreviations included on The Joint Commission's "Do Not Use" list are identified with a double asterisk (**) and must be included on an organization's "Do Not Use" list. Access supplementary digital content in the online book using this QR code.

Nursing staff access the electronic health record (EHR) to help ensure accuracy in medication administration and document the medication administration to help ensure client safety. Please see Figure 7.4[38] for an image of a nurse accessing a client's EHR.

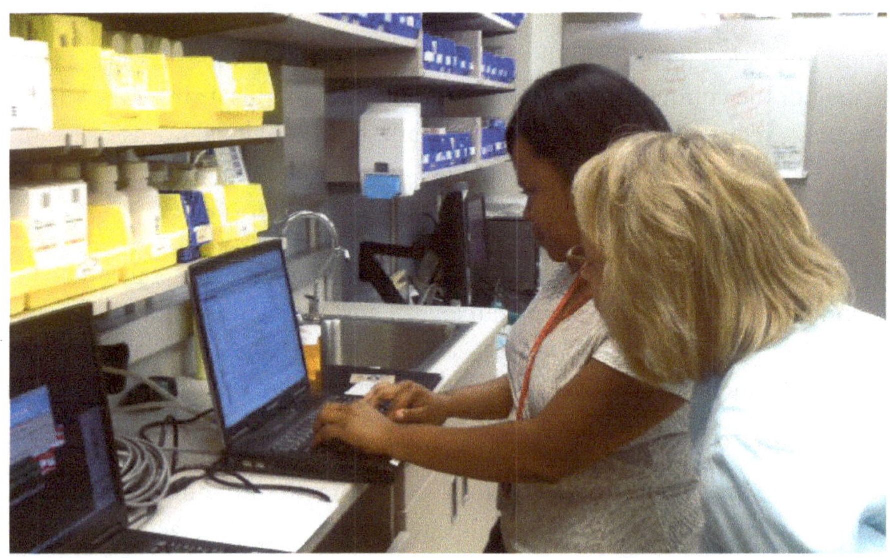

FIGURE 7.4 Documenting in the EHR

Electronic Health Record

The electronic health record (EHR) contains the following important information:

- **History and Physical (H&P):** A history and physical (H&P) is a specific type of documentation created by the health care provider when the client is admitted to the facility. An H&P includes important information about the client's current status, medical history, and the treatment plan in a concise format that is helpful for the nurse to review. Information typically includes the reason for admission, health history, surgical history, allergies, current medications, physical examination findings, medical diagnoses, and the treatment plan.

38. "Winn_Army_Community_Hospital_Pharmacy_Stays_Online_During_Power_Outage.jpg" by Flickr user MC4 Army is licensed under CC BY 2.0

- **Provider orders:** This section includes the prescriptions, or medical orders, that the nurse must legally implement or appropriately communicate according to agency policy if not implemented.
- **Medication Administration Records (MARs):** Medications are charted through electronic medication administration records (MARs). These records interface the medication orders from providers with pharmacists and are also the location where nurses document medications administered.
- **Treatment Administration Records (TARs):** In many facilities, treatments are documented on a treatment administration record.
- **Laboratory results:** This section includes results from blood work and other tests performed in the lab.
- **Diagnostic test results:** This section includes results from diagnostic tests ordered by the provider such as X-rays, ultrasounds, etc.
- **Progress notes:** This section contains notes created by nurses, providers, and other interprofessional team members regarding client care. It is helpful for the nurse to review daily progress notes by all team members to ensure continuity of care.
- **Nursing care plans:** Nursing care plans are created by registered nurses (RNs). Documentation of individualized nursing care plans is legally required in long-term care facilities by the Centers for Medicare and Medicaid Services (CMS) and in hospitals by The Joint Commission. Nursing care plans are individualized to meet the specific and unique needs of each client. They contain expected outcomes and planned interventions to be completed by nurses and other members of the interprofessional team. As part of the nursing process, nurses routinely evaluate the client's progress toward meeting the expected outcomes and modify the nursing care plan as needed.

Access supplementary digital content in the online book using this QR code.

Read the American Nurses Association's "Principles for Nursing Documentation." Access supplementary digital content in the online book using this QR code.

7.6 TEAMS AND TEAMWORK

Now that we have reviewed the first three IPEC competencies related to valuing team members, understanding team members' roles and responsibilities, and using structured interprofessional communication strategies, let's discuss strategies that promote effective teamwork. The fourth IPEC competency states, "Apply relationship-building values and the principles of team dynamics to perform effectively in different team roles to plan, deliver, and evaluate client/population-centered care and population health programs and policies that are safe, timely, efficient, effective, and equitable."[39] See the following box for the components of this IPEC competency.

Components of IPEC's Teams and Teamwork Competency[40]

- Describe the process of team development and the roles and practices of effective teams.
- Develop consensus on the ethical principles to guide all aspects of teamwork.
- Engage health and other professionals in shared client-centered and population-focused problem-solving.
- Integrate the knowledge and experience of health and other professions to inform health and care decisions, while respecting client and community values and priorities/preferences for care.
- Apply leadership practices that support collaborative practice and team effectiveness.
- Engage self and others to constructively manage disagreements about values, roles, goals, and actions that arise among health and other professionals and with clients, families, and community members.
- Share accountability with other professions, clients, and communities for outcomes relevant to prevention and health care.
- Reflect on individual and team performance for individual, as well as team, performance improvement.
- Use process improvement to increase effectiveness of interprofessional teamwork and team-based services, programs, and policies.
- Use available evidence to inform effective teamwork and team-based practices.
- Perform effectively on teams and in different team roles in a variety of settings.

Developing effective teams is critical for providing health care that is client-centered, safe, timely, effective, efficient, and equitable.[41] See Figure 7.5[42] for an image illustrating interprofessional teamwork.

39. Interprofessional Education Collaborative. (2023). *IPEC core competencies.* https://www.ipecollaborative.org/ipec-core-competencies
40. Interprofessional Education Collaborative. (2023). *IPEC core competencies.* https://www.ipecollaborative.org/ipec-core-competencies
41. Interprofessional Education Collaborative Expert Panel. (2011). *Core competencies for interprofessional collaborative practice: Report on an expert panel.* Interprofessional Education Collaborative. https://ipec.memberclicks.net/assets/2011-Original.pdf
42. "400845937-huge.jpg" by Flamingo Images is used under license from Shutterstock.com

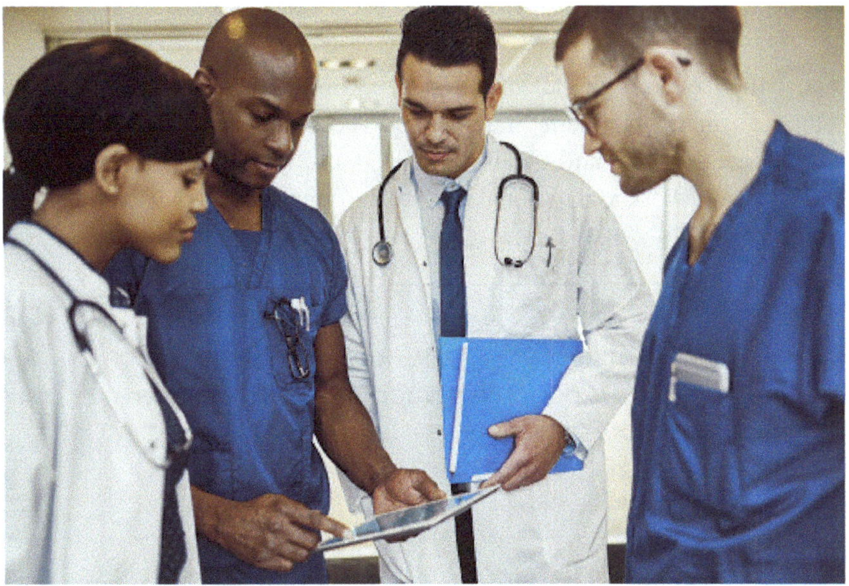

FIGURE 7.5 Interprofessional Teamwork

Nurses collaborate with the interprofessional team by not only assigning and coordinating tasks, but also by promoting solid teamwork in a positive environment. A nursing leader, such as a charge nurse, identifies gaps in workflow, recognizes when task overload is occurring, and promotes the adaptability of the team to respond to evolving client conditions. Qualities of a successful team are described in the following box.[43]

Qualities of a Successful Team[44]

- Promote a respectful atmosphere
- Define clear roles and responsibilities for team members
- Regularly and routinely share information
- Encourage open communication
- Implement a culture of safety
- Provide clear directions
- Share responsibility for team success
- Balance team member participation based on the current situation
- Acknowledge and manage conflict
- Enforce accountability among all team members
- Communicate the decision-making process
- Facilitate access to needed resources
- Evaluate team outcomes and adjust as needed

43. O'Daniel, M., & Rosenstein, A. H. (2011). Professional communication and team collaboration. In: Hughes R.G. (Ed.). *Patient safety and quality: An evidence-based handbook for nurses.* Agency for Healthcare Research and Quality (US); Chapter 33. https://www.ncbi.nlm.nih.gov/books/NBK2637
44. O'Daniel, M., & Rosenstein, A. H. (2011). Professional communication and team collaboration. In: Hughes R.G. (Ed.). *Patient safety and quality: An evidence-based handbook for nurses.* Agency for Healthcare Research and Quality (US); Chapter 33. https://www.ncbi.nlm.nih.gov/books/NBK2637

TeamSTEPPS®

TeamSTEPPS® is an evidence-based framework used to optimize team performance across the health care system. It is a mnemonic standing for Team Strategies and Tools to Enhance Performance and Patient Safety. The Agency for Healthcare Research and Quality (AHRQ) and the Department of Defense (DoD) developed the TeamSTEPPS® framework as a national initiative to improve client safety by improving teamwork skills and communication.[45]

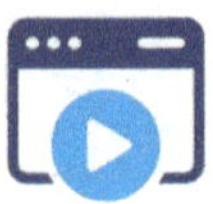

View this video about the TeamSTEPPS® framework[46]: https://wtcs.pressbooks.pub/nursingmpc/?p=1032#oembed-1. Access supplementary digital content in the online book using this QR code.

TeamSTEPPS® is based on establishing team structure and four teamwork skills: communication, leadership, situation monitoring, and mutual support.[47] See Figure 7.6[48] for an image of the TeamSTEPPS® framework followed by a description of each TeamSTEPPS® skill. The components of this model are described in the following subsections.

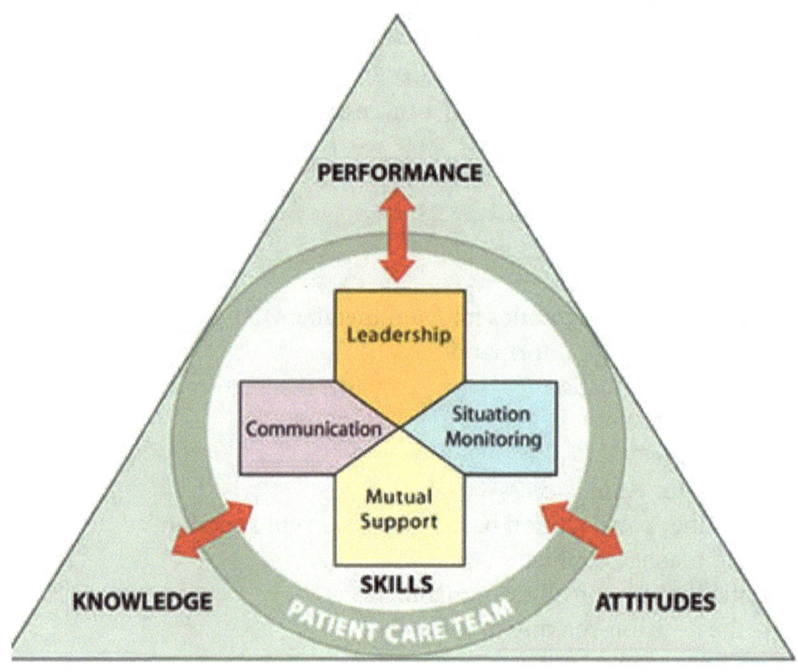

FIGURE 7.6 TeamSTEPPS® Framework

45. AHRQ. (2024). *TeamSTEPPS 3.0.* https://www.ahrq.gov/teamstepps/instructor/index.html
46. AHRQ Patient Safety. (2015, April 29). *TeamSTEPPS overview* [Video]. YouTube. All rights reserved. https://youtu.be/p4n9xPRtSuU
47. AHRQ. (2024). *TeamSTEPPS: 3.0 Pocket guide.* https://www.ahrq.gov/teamstepps-program/resources/pocket-guide/index.html
48. "tslogo1med.jpg" by unknown author is licensed under Public Domain. Access for free at https://www.ahrq.gov/teamstepps/instructor/essentials/pocketguide.html

Team Structure

A nursing leader establishes team structure by assigning or identifying team members' roles and responsibilities, holding team members accountable, and including clients and families as part of the team.

Communication

Communication is the first skill of the TeamSTEPPS® framework. As previously discussed, it is defined as a "structured process by which information is clearly and accurately exchanged among team members." All team members should use these skills to ensure accurate interprofessional communication:

- Provide brief, clear, specific, and timely information to other team members.
- Seek information from all available sources.
- Use ISBARR and handoff techniques to communicate effectively with team members.
- Use closed-loop communication to verify information is communicated, understood, and completed.
- Document appropriately to facilitate continuity of care across interprofessional team members.

These communication strategies are further described in the "Interprofessional Communication" section of this chapter.

Leadership

Leadership is the second skill of the TeamSTEPPS® framework. As previously discussed, it is defined as the "ability to maximize the activities of team members by ensuring that team actions are understood, changes in information are shared, and team members have the necessary resources." An example of a nursing team leader in an inpatient setting is the charge nurse.

Effective team leaders demonstrate the following responsibilities[49]:

- Organize the team.
- Identify and articulate clear goals (i.e., share the plan).
- Assign tasks and responsibilities.
- Monitor and modify the plan and communicate changes.
- Review the team's performance and provide feedback when needed.
- Manage and allocate resources.
- Facilitate information sharing.
- Encourage team members to assist one another.
- Facilitate conflict resolution in a learning environment.
- Model effective teamwork.

Three major leadership tasks include sharing a plan, monitoring and modifying the plan according to situations that occur, and reviewing team performance. Tools to perform these tasks are discussed in the following subsections.

49. AHRQ. (2024). *TeamSTEPPS: 3.0 Pocket guide.* https://www.ahrq.gov/teamstepps-program/resources/pocket-guide/index.html

SHARING THE PLAN

Nursing team leaders identify and articulate clear goals to the team at the start of the shift during inpatient care using a "brief." The **brief** is a short session to share a plan, discuss team formation, assign roles and responsibilities, establish expectations and climate, and anticipate outcomes and contingencies. See a Brief Checklist in the following box with questions based on TeamSTEPPS®.[50]

> **Brief Checklist**
>
> During the brief, the team should address the following questions[51]:
>
> ___ Who is on the team?
> ___ Do all members understand and agree upon goals?
> ___ Are roles and responsibilities understood?
> ___ What is our plan of care?
> ___ What are staff and provider's availability throughout the shift?
> ___ How is workload shared among team members?
> ___ Who are the sickest clients on the unit?
> ___ Which clients have a high fall risk or require 1:1?
> ___ Do any clients have behavioral issues requiring consistent approaches by the team?
> ___ What resources are available?

MONITORING AND MODIFYING THE PLAN

Throughout the shift, it is often necessary for the nurse leader to modify the initial plan as client situations change on the unit. A **huddle** is a brief meeting before and/or during a shift to establish situational awareness, reinforce plans already in place, and adjust the teamwork plan as needed. Read more about situational awareness in the "Situation Monitoring" subsection below.

REVIEWING THE TEAM'S PERFORMANCE

When a significant or emergent event occurs during a shift, such as a "code," it is important to later review the team's performance and reflect on lessons learned by holding a "debrief" session. A **debrief** is an informal information exchange session designed to improve team performance and effectiveness through reinforcement of positive behaviors and reflection on lessons learned.[52] See the following box for a Debrief Checklist.

50. AHRQ. (2024). *TeamSTEPPS: 3.0 Pocket guide.* https://www.ahrq.gov/teamstepps-program/resources/pocket-guide/index.html
51. AHRQ. (2024). *TeamSTEPPS: 3.0 Pocket guide.* https://www.ahrq.gov/teamstepps-program/resources/pocket-guide/index.html
52. AHRQ. (2024). *TeamSTEPPS: 3.0 Pocket guide.* https://www.ahrq.gov/teamstepps-program/resources/pocket-guide/index.html

Debrief Checklist[53]

The team should address the following questions during a debrief:

___ Was communication clear?
___ Were roles and responsibilities understood?
___ Was situation awareness maintained?
___ Was workload distribution equitable?
___ Was task assistance requested or offered?
___ Were errors made or avoided?
___ Were resources available?
___ What went well?
___ What should be improved?

Situation Monitoring

Situation monitoring is the third skill of the TeamSTEPPS® framework and defined as the "process of actively scanning and assessing situational elements to gain information or understanding, or to maintain awareness to support team functioning." **Situation monitoring** refers to the process of continually scanning and assessing the situation to gain and maintain an understanding of what is going on around you. **Situation awareness** refers to a team member knowing what is going on around them. The team leader creates a **shared mental model** to ensure all team members have situation awareness and know what is going on as situations evolve. The STEP tool is used by team leaders to assist with situation monitoring.[54]

STEP

The **STEP tool** is a situation monitoring tool used to know what is going on with you, your clients, your team, and your environment. **STEP** stands for **S**tatus of the clients, **T**eam members, **E**nvironment, and **P**rogress toward goal. See an illustration of STEP in Figure 7.7.[55] The components of the STEP tool are described in the following box.[56]

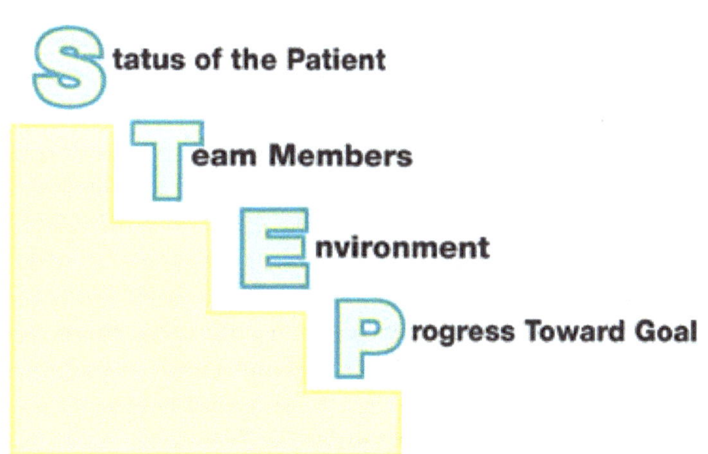

FIGURE 7.7 STEP Tool

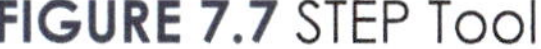

53. AHRQ. (2024). *TeamSTEPPS: 3.0 Pocket guide.* https://www.ahrq.gov/teamstepps-program/resources/pocket-guide/index.html
54. AHRQ. (2024). *TeamSTEPPS: 3.0 Pocket guide.* https://www.ahrq.gov/teamstepps-program/resources/pocket-guide/index.html
55. "stepfig1.jpg" by unknown author is licensed under Public Domain. Access for free at https://www.ahrq.gov/teamstepps/instructor/essentials/pocketguide.html
56. AHRQ. (2024). *TeamSTEPPS: 3.0 Pocket guide.* https://www.ahrq.gov/teamstepps-program/resources/pocket-guide/index.html

STEP Tool[57]

Status of Clients: "What is going on with your clients?"

__ Patient History
__ Vital Signs
__ Medications
__ Physical Exam
__ Plan of Care
__ Psychosocial Issues

Team Members: "What is going on with you and your team?"(See the "I'M SAFE Checklist" below.)

__ Fatigue
__ Workload
__ Task Performance
__ Skill
__ Stress

Environment: Knowing Your Resources

__ Facility Information
__ Administrative Information
__ Human Resources
__ Triage Acuity
__ Equipment

Progression Towards Goal:

__ Status of the Team's Clients
__ Established Goals of the Team
__ Tasks/Actions of the Team
__ Appropriateness of the Plan and are Modifications Needed?

CROSS-MONITORING

As the STEP tool is implemented, the team leader continues to cross monitor to reduce the incidence of errors. Cross-monitoring includes the following[58]:

- Monitoring the actions of other team members.
- Providing a safety net within the team.
- Ensuring that mistakes or oversights are caught quickly and easily.
- Supporting each other as needed.

57. AHRQ. (2024). *TeamSTEPPS: 3.0 Pocket guide.* https://www.ahrq.gov/teamstepps-program/resources/pocket-guide/index.html
58. AHRQ. (2024). *TeamSTEPPS: 3.0 Pocket guide.* https://www.ahrq.gov/teamstepps-program/resources/pocket-guide/index.html

I'M SAFE CHECKLIST

The **I'M SAFE** mnemonic is a tool used to assess one's own safety status, as well as that of other team members in their ability to provide safe client care. See the I'M SAFE Checklist in the following box.[59] If a team member feels their ability to provide safe care is diminished because of one of these factors, they should notify the charge nurse or other nursing supervisor. In a similar manner, if a nurse notices that another member of the team is impaired or providing care in an unsafe manner, it is an ethical imperative to protect clients and report their concerns according to agency policy.[60]

I'M SAFE CHECKLIST[61]

__ **I**: Illness
__**M**: Medication
__**S**: Stress
__**A**: Alcohol and Drugs
__**F**: Fatigue
__**E**: Eating and Elimination

Read an example of a nursing team leader performing situation monitoring using the STEP tool in the following box.

EXAMPLE OF SITUATION MONITORING

Two emergent situations occur simultaneously on a busy medical-surgical hospital unit as one client codes and another develops a postoperative hemorrhage. The charge nurse is performing situation monitoring by continually scanning and assessing the status of all clients on the unit and directing additional assistance where it is needed. Each nursing team member maintains situation awareness by being aware of what is happening on the unit, in addition to caring for the clients they have been assigned. The charge nurse creates a shared mental model by ensuring all team members are aware of their evolving responsibilities as the situation changes. The charge nurse directs additional assistance to the emergent clients while also ensuring appropriate coverage for the other clients on the unit to ensure all clients receive safe and effective care.

For example, as the "code" is called, the charge nurse directs two additional nurses and two additional assistive personnel to assist with the emergent clients while the other nurses and unlicensed assistive personnel are directed to "cover" the remaining clients, answer call lights, and assist clients to the bathroom to prevent falls. Additionally, the charge nurse is aware that after performing a few rounds of CPR for the coding client, the unlicensed assistive personnel must be switched with another team member to maintain effective chest compressions. As the situation progresses, the charge nurse evaluates the status of all clients and makes adjustments to the plan as needed.

59. AHRQ. (2024). *TeamSTEPPS: 3.0 Pocket guide.* https://www.ahrq.gov/teamstepps-program/resources/pocket-guide/index.html
60. AHRQ. (2024). *TeamSTEPPS: 3.0 Pocket guide.* https://www.ahrq.gov/teamstepps-program/resources/pocket-guide/index.html
61. AHRQ. (2024). *TeamSTEPPS: 3.0 Pocket guide.* https://www.ahrq.gov/teamstepps-program/resources/pocket-guide/index.html

Mutual Support

Mutual support is the fourth skill of the TeamSTEPPS® framework and defined as the "ability to anticipate and support team members' needs through accurate knowledge about their responsibilities and workload." Mutual support includes providing task assistance, giving feedback, and advocating for client safety by using assertive statements to correct a safety concern. Managing conflict is also a component of supporting team members' needs.

TASK ASSISTANCE

Helping other team members with tasks builds a strong team. Task assistance includes the following components[62]:

- Team members protect each other from work-overload situations.
- Effective teams place all offers and requests for assistance in the context of client safety.
- Team members foster a climate where it is expected that assistance will be actively sought and offered.

> **Example of Task Assistance**
>
> In a previous example, one client on the unit was coding while another was experiencing a postoperative hemorrhage. After the emergent care was provided and the hemorrhaging client was stabilized, Sue, the nurse caring for the hemorrhaging client, finds many scheduled medications for her other clients are past due. Sue reaches out to Sam, another nurse on the team, and requests assistance. Sam agrees to administer a scheduled IV antibiotic to a stable third client so Sue can administer oral medications to her remaining clients. Sam knows that on an upcoming shift, he may need to request assistance from Sue when unexpected situations occur. In this manner, team members foster a climate where assistance is actively sought and offered to maintain client safety.

FEEDBACK

Feedback is provided to a team member for the purpose of improving team performance. Effective feedback should follow these parameters[63]:

- *Timely:* Provided soon after the target behavior has occurred.
- *Respectful:* Focused on behaviors, not personal attributes.
- *Specific:* Related to a specific task or behavior that requires correction or improvement.
- *Directed towards improvement:* Suggestions are made for future improvement.
- *Considerate:* Team members' feelings should be considered and privacy provided. Negative information should be delivered with fairness and respect.

62. AHRQ. (2024). *TeamSTEPPS: 3.0 Pocket guide.* https://www.ahrq.gov/teamstepps-program/resources/pocket-guide/index.html
63. AHRQ. (2024). *TeamSTEPPS: 3.0 Pocket guide.* https://www.ahrq.gov/teamstepps-program/resources/pocket-guide/index.html

ADVOCATING FOR SAFETY WITH ASSERTIVE STATEMENTS

When a team member perceives a potential client safety concern, they should assertively communicate with the decision-maker to protect client safety. This strategy holds true for ALL team members, no matter their position within the hierarchy of the health care environment. The message should be communicated to the decision-maker in a firm and respectful manner using the following steps[64]:

- Make an opening.
- State the concern.
- State the problem (real or perceived).
- Offer a solution.
- Reach agreement on next steps.

> **EXAMPLES OF USING ASSERTIVE STATEMENTS TO PROMOTE CLIENT SAFETY**
>
> A nurse notices that a team member did not properly wash their hands during client care. Feedback is provided immediately in a private area after the team member left the client room: *"I noticed you didn't wash your hands when you entered the client's room. Can you help me understand why that didn't occur?" (Wait for an answer.) "Performing hand hygiene is essential for protecting our clients from infection. It is also hospital policy, and we are audited for compliance to this policy. Let me know if you have any questions and I will check back with you later in the shift." (Monitor the team member for appropriate hand hygiene for the remainder of the shift.)*

Two-Challenge Rule

When an assertive statement is ignored by the decision-maker, the team member should assertively voice their concern at least two times to ensure that it has been heard by the decision-maker. This strategy is referred to as the **two-challenge rule**. When this rule is adopted as a policy by a health care organization, it empowers all team members to pause care if they sense or discover an essential safety breach. The decision-maker being challenged is expected to acknowledge the concern has been heard.[65]

CUS Assertive Statements

During emergent situations, when stress levels are high or when situations are charged with emotion, the decision-maker may not "hear" the message being communicated, even when the two-challenge rule is implemented. It is helpful for agencies to establish assertive statements that are well-recognized by all staff as implementation of the two-challenge rule. These assertive statements are referred to as the CUS mnemonic: "I am **C**oncerned – I am **U**ncomfortable – This is a **S**afety issue!"[66] See Figure 7.8[67] for an illustration of CUS assertive statements.

---

64. AHRQ. (2024). *TeamSTEPPS: 3.0 Pocket guide.* https://www.ahrq.gov/teamstepps-program/resources/pocket-guide/index.html
65. AHRQ. (2024). *TeamSTEPPS: 3.0 Pocket guide.* https://www.ahrq.gov/teamstepps-program/resources/pocket-guide/index.html
66. AHRQ. (2024). *TeamSTEPPS: 3.0 Pocket guide.* https://www.ahrq.gov/teamstepps-program/resources/pocket-guide/index.html
67. "cusfig1.jpg" by unknown author is licensed under Public Domain. Access for free at https://www.ahrq.gov/teamstepps/instructor/essentials/pocketguide.html

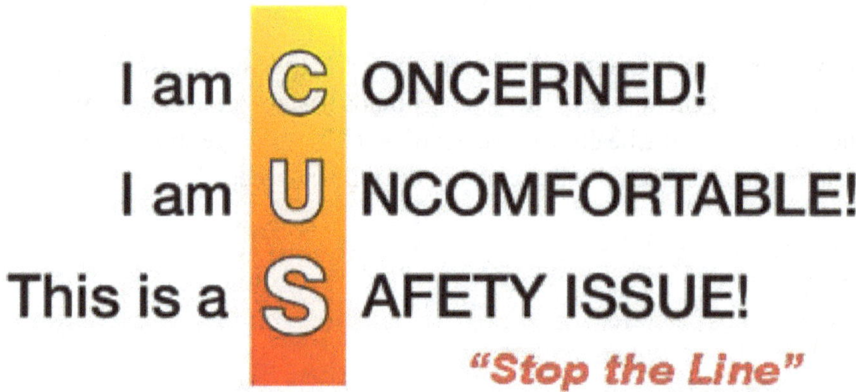

FIGURE 7.8 CUS Assertive Statements

Using these scripted messages may effectively catch the attention of the decision-maker. However, if the safety issue still isn't addressed after the second statement or the use of "CUS" assertive statements, the team member should take a stronger course of action and utilize the agency's chain of command. For the two-challenge rule and CUS assertive statements to be effective within an agency, administrators must support a culture of safety and emphasize the importance of these initiatives to promote client safety.

Read an example of a nurse using assertive statements in the following box.

Assertive Statement Example

A nurse observes a new physician resident preparing to insert a central line at a client's bedside. The nurse notes the resident has inadvertently contaminated the right sterile glove prior to insertion.

Nurse: "Dr. Smith, I noticed that you contaminated your sterile gloves when preparing the sterile field for central line insertion. I will get a new set of sterile gloves for you."

Dr. Smith: (Ignores nurse and continues procedure.)

Nurse: "Dr. Smith, please pause the procedure. I noticed that you contaminated your right sterile glove by touching outside the sterile field. I will get a new set of sterile gloves for you."

Dr. Smith: "My gloves are fine." (Prepares to initiate insertion.)

Nurse: "Dr. Smith – I am concerned! I am uncomfortable! This is a safety issue!"

Dr. Smith: (Stops procedure, looks up, and listens to the nurse.) "I'll wait for that second pair of gloves."

MANAGING CONFLICT

Conflict is not uncommon on interprofessional teams, especially when there are diverse perspectives from multiple staff regarding client care. Nurse leaders must be prepared to manage conflict to support the needs of their team members.

When conflict occurs, the **DESC tool** can be used to help resolve conflict by using "I statements." DESC is a mnemonic that stands for the following[68]:

- **D:** Describe the specific situation or behavior; provide concrete data.
- **E:** Express how the situation makes you feel/what your concerns are using "I" statements.
- **S:** Suggest other alternatives and seek agreement.
- **C:** Consequences stated in terms of impact on established team goals while striving for consensus.

The DESC tool should be implemented in a private area with a focus on WHAT is right, not WHO is right. Read an example of a nurse using the DESC tool in the following box.

> ### Example of Using the DESC Tool[69]
>
> **Situation:** A physician became angry at a nurse who was inserting a client's Foley catheter and yelled at the nurse in front of the client and other team members. The nurse later addressed the physician in a private area outside the client's room using the DESC tool and "I statements":
>
> **D:** "I noticed you got angry at me when I inserted the client's Foley catheter."
>
> **E:** "I'm concerned how you addressed that issue in front of the client and three other staff members. It made me feel bad in front of the client and my colleagues."
>
> **S:** "In the future, if you have an issue with how I do things, please pull me aside privately to discuss your concern."
>
> **C:** "Our organization has a policy for managing communication challenges among team members if we can't agree on this alternative."

Managing interpersonal conflict resolution is described further in the "Conflict Resolution" section.

View a supplementary detailed video webinar from AHRQ describing the TeamSTEPPS® principles at youtu.be/fxlRtpzsUug.[70] Access supplementary digital content in the online book using this QR code.

68. AHRQ. (2024). *TeamSTEPPS: 3.0 Pocket guide.* https://www.ahrq.gov/teamstepps-program/resources/pocket-guide/index.html
69. AHRQ. (2024). *TeamSTEPPS: 3.0 Pocket guide.* https://www.ahrq.gov/teamstepps-program/resources/pocket-guide/index.html
70. AHRQ Patient Safety. (2017, July 26). *Introduction to the fundamentals of TeamSTEPPS® concepts and tools* [Video]. YouTube. Video in the Public Domain. https://youtu.be/fxlRtpzsUug

Team Qualitities Case Application (*Answers can be found at the end of book*)

Mary is recovering from a stroke and requires comprehensive care involving multiple disciplines. Her care team has scheduled interdisciplinary team meetings twice a week to discussion Mary's progress, adjust her care plan, and address any concerns. Dr. Patel is Mary's primary physician and consults with Chris (physical therapist) and Emily (speech therapist) before making any changes to Mary's medication that might affect her therapy sessions. Chris and Emily coordinate their therapy schedules to help maximize Mary's participation and avoid conflicting sessions and fatigue. Laura is Mary's social worker and has a large roster of clients. Laura struggles to include Mary's family in the discharge planning discussions but feels that she has identified an appropriate facility that Mary and her family will be receptive to for discharge. She moves forward with the client placement paperwork. Lisa is Mary's dietician, and she has identified a dietary plan that will best contribute to Mary's nutritional needs and healing. She acknowledges that Mary's dietary preferences are much different than what she has selected in her dietary plan, but Lisa knows that she has identified the best dietary plan to meet Mary's energy needs.

Identify which team members are demonstrating team success strategies and how they are demonstrated?

Which team members are not demonstrating team success strategies? How could these team members modify their approach?

7.7 CONFLICT RESOLUTION

Conflicts are inevitable when working on a team composed of members with different personalities, roles, and responsibilities. It is essential for all nurses to develop conflict resolution skills.

Common Sources of Interpersonal Conflict

Common sources of interpersonal conflict in health care settings are passive-aggressiveness, horizontal aggression, defensiveness, peer informer behavior, and victimization behaviors.[71]

Passive-Aggressiveness

Passive-aggressiveness is a behavior that shows disconnection between what a person says and does. Many times, a passive-aggressive person will agree with another person's request, but later express feelings of frustration or anger to others and not comply with the request.

71. Elizabeth, A. (2019). Managing interpersonal conflict: Steps for success. *Nursing Management, 50*(6), 22-28. https://journals.lww.com/nursingmanagement/Fulltext/2019/06000/Managing_interpersonal_conflict__Steps_for_success.7.aspx

As an example, a charge nurse informs the team of RNs in a team meeting that a new policy requires bedside rounding. A nurse responds enthusiastically during the meeting but then complains to others about the policy and refuses to do it. The best method of managing passive-aggressive behavior is to confront it calmly and directly. For this example, it would be helpful for the charge nurse to say, "*I was disappointed to hear you are upset about the new bedside rounding policy because you didn't express any concerns directly to me. It would be helpful for you to directly communicate concerns to me so we can discuss them and make a plan for going forward.*"[72]

Horizontal Aggression

The nursing literature describes diffuse incivility, lateral/horizontal violence, and bullying among nurses in the workplace.[73] **Horizontal aggression** refers to hostile behavior among one's peers. It is not acceptable and should be directly confronted in a constructive manner or it will get worse. A suggested approach to a peer displaying horizontal aggression is to respond calmly and sincerely, "*I value your expertise and experience and am looking for your help and support.*" If the negative behavior continues after an attempt to address the individual directly, the nurse supervisor should be notified according to the agency's chain of command.[74]

Defensiveness

It can be difficult to receive negative feedback. Some people respond by becoming defensive. Defensiveness puts the blame for one's shortcomings on another person to make oneself appear better.

As an example, a charge nurse addresses a nurse about not turning on the bed alarm after repositioning a client and leaving the room. The nurse responds defensively by inaccurately blaming others, stating, "*The nursing assistants are always sloppy with their responsibilities.*" It is helpful to confront defensiveness by restating the facts in a calm manner and redirecting the conversation to the problem, its resolution, and the risk of jeopardizing client safety. For example, the charge nurse could reply, "*In this situation, I saw you leave the room after repositioning the client, and when I went into the room to answer the client's call light, the bed alarm was off.*"[75]

Peer Informer Behavior

Peer informer behavior is similar to gossip. Peer informers relay information about fellow team members to the nurse leader, and this information often lacks objective evidence. It is often best to respond to the informer by asking them to speak to their team member directly about their concerns unless it is an urgent matter that must be dealt with immediately. However, keep in mind that if concerns are shared about a staff member by more than one team member, it may be a pattern of behavior, and the nurse leader should follow up with that staff member.[76]

---

72. Elizabeth, A. (2019). Managing interpersonal conflict: Steps for success. *Nursing Management, 50*(6), 22-28. https://journals.lww.com/nursingmanagement/Fulltext/2019/06000/Managing_interpersonal_conflict__Steps_for_success.7.aspx
73. Bambi, S., Guazzini, A., De Felippis, C., Lucchini, A., & Rasero, L. (2017). Preventing workplace incivility, lateral violence and bullying between nurses. A narrative literature review. *Acta bio-medica: Atenei Parmensis, 88*(5S), 39–47. https://www.ncbi.nlm.nih.gov/pmc/articles/PMC6357576/
74. Elizabeth, A. (2019). Managing interpersonal conflict: Steps for success. *Nursing Management, 50*(6), 22-28. https://journals.lww.com/nursingmanagement/Fulltext/2019/06000/Managing_interpersonal_conflict__Steps_for_success.7.aspx
75. Elizabeth, A. (2019). Managing interpersonal conflict: Steps for success. *Nursing Management,* 50(6), 22-28. https://journals.lww.com/nursingmanagement/Fulltext/2019/06000/Managing_interpersonal_conflict__Steps_for_success.7.aspx
76. Elizabeth, A. (2019). Managing interpersonal conflict: Steps for success. *Nursing Management, 50*(6), 22-28. https://journals.lww.com/nursingmanagement/Fulltext/2019/06000/Managing_interpersonal_conflict__Steps_for_success.7.aspx

As an example, a nurse approaches the charge nurse and says, *"Everyone is concerned about how much time Nancy is spending in the room with her clients. She gets behind in her work and the rest of us have to make up for it."* The charge nurse could reply, *"Have you addressed your concerns directly with Nancy?"* If the nurse replies, *"No,"* then the charge nurse could state, *"Please talk to Nancy directly with your concerns first."* However, if another nurse shares a similar concern with the charge nurse, then the charge nurse should address this pattern of behavior with Nancy and obtain her perspective.

Victimization

Victimization occurs when a team member feels they are being singled out unfairly or held to higher expectations than their peers. Comments may include, "Why am I getting called out on this when other people are doing this and aren't getting in trouble?" or "I was never told this; why am I always the last to know?" Team members who feel victimized should be reminded by the nurse leader they are held to the same standards as the other members. However, keep in mind that sharing information about other staff members' performance breaches confidentiality, so do not include another employees' performance information in conversations but instead focus on policies and procedures that apply to everyone.[77]

Types of Conflict

There are various sources of conflict that nurses may encounter in their work environment.

Role Conflict: Role conflict arises when individuals have multiple, often conflicting, expectations associated with their roles. In professional settings, an employee may face role conflict when their job responsibilities are unclear or when there are conflicting demands from different supervisors. For example, a project manager might experience tension if their role requires them to enforce strict deadlines while also being expected to accommodate frequent changes in project scope. This type of conflict can lead to stress, decreased job satisfaction, and reduced productivity. Role conflict can be mitigated by clear communication, well-defined job descriptions, and regular feedback to ensure alignment of expectations.[78]

Communication Conflict: Communication conflict occurs when there is a failure in the exchange of information. Misunderstandings, misinterpretations, and lack of effective communication can lead to disputes and frustrations. For instance, in a team setting, if one member interprets a directive differently from others, it can result in duplicated efforts or missed tasks. Communication conflict is often exacerbated by differences in communication styles, cultural backgrounds, or language barriers. Addressing this type of conflict involves fostering an environment of open and clear communication, utilizing active listening techniques, and ensuring that all parties have a mutual understanding of the messages being conveyed.[79]

Goal Conflict: Goal conflict happens when the objectives of individuals or groups are incompatible. In organizations, different departments might pursue goals that are in opposition, such as a sales team aiming for maximum customer satisfaction while a production team focuses on minimizing costs. These conflicting

77. Elizabeth, A. (2019). Managing interpersonal conflict: Steps for success. *Nursing Management, 50*(6), 22-28. https://journals.lww.com/nursingmanagement/Fulltext/2019/06000/Managing_interpersonal_conflict__Steps_for_success.7.aspx
78. Ahmad, M., & Ud din, S. (2023). Effect of role conflict and role ambiguity on employee creativity. *Library Philosophy and Practice (ejournal), 7615*, 1-21. https://digitalcommons.unl.edu/cgi/viewcontent.cgi?article=14720&context=libphilprac
79. Hutagaung, I. (2017). The function of interpersonal communication in conflict management organization. *SHS Web of Conferences, 33*. https://www.researchgate.net/publication/313290661_The_Function_of_Interpersonal_Communication_in_Conflict_Management_Organization

goals can hinder overall progress and lead to tension among team members. To resolve goal conflicts, it is crucial to align individual and departmental goals with the broader objectives of the organization. This can be achieved through strategic planning, crossfunctional collaboration, and regular goal-setting meetings that ensure all efforts are directed towards a common purpose.[80]

Personality Conflict: Personality conflict arises from differences in individual temperaments, attitudes, and behaviors. Such conflicts are common in any setting where diverse personalities interact, such as workplaces, schools, or social groups. For example, a highly extroverted person might clash with a reserved colleague, leading to friction in their interactions. Personality conflicts can negatively impact team cohesion and productivity. Managing these conflicts involves fostering a culture of respect and understanding, providing training in emotional intelligence and conflict resolution, and encouraging individuals to appreciate and leverage the strengths of diverse personalities.[81]

Ethical/Values Conflict: Ethical or values conflict occurs when individuals or groups have fundamentally different beliefs and values. These conflicts are often deeply rooted and can be particularly challenging to resolve. In a corporate environment, an ethical conflict might arise if one employee believes in strict adherence to company policies while another prioritizes flexibility and personal judgment. Values conflicts can also occur over issues such as diversity, environmental responsibility, and corporate social responsibility. Addressing ethical or values conflicts requires creating an environment of mutual respect, where different perspectives are valued. Organizations can benefit from having clear ethical guidelines and fostering an inclusive culture that encourages open dialogue and ethical decision-making.[82]

Conflict Management

Individuals manage conflict differently. During conflict, a person's behavior is typically driven by their commitment to their goals or their commitment to relationships[83]:

- **Commitment to goals:** The extent to which an individual attempts to satisfy their personal concerns or goals.
- **Commitment to relationships:** The extent to which an individual attempts to satisfy the concerns of another party or maintain the relationship with the other party.

Most people use different methods to resolve conflict depending on the situation and what strategy best applies. One approach is not necessarily better than another, and all approaches can be learned and used effectively with practice. However, to effectively manage conflict, it is important to first analyze the situation and then respond accordingly.

80. Gray, J. S., Ozer, D. J., & Rosenthal, R. (2017). Goal conflict and psychological well-being: A meta-analysis. *Journal of Research in Personality, 66*, 27-37. https://doi.org/10.1016/j.jrp.2016.12.003
81. Tehrani, H. D., & Yamini, S. (2020). Personality traits and conflict resolution styles: A meta-analysis. *Personality and Individual Differences, 157*. https://doi.org/10.1016/j.paid.2019.109794
82. Xing, S. (2022). Ethical conflict and knowledge hiding in teams: Moderating role of workplace friendship in education sector. *Front Psychology, 13*. https://doi.org/10.3389/fpsyg.2022.824485.
83. Wagner, J. (2018). *Leadership and Influencing Change in Nursing.* University of Regina Press. https://pressbooks.pub/leadershipandinfluencingchangeinnursing/

A long-standing conflict resolution model created by Thomas and Killmann describes five approaches to dealing with conflict: avoiding, competing, accommodating, compromising, and collaborating. Each of these steps is further described in the following subsections.[84]

Avoidance Approach

An avoidance approach to conflict resolution demonstrates a low commitment to both goals and relationships. This is the most common method of dealing with conflict, especially by people who view conflict negatively. See Table 7.7a for types of avoidance, potential results, and situations when this strategy may be appropriate.[85]

TABLE 7.7A. Avoidance Approach[86]

Types of Avoidance Approaches	Potential Results	Appropriate Use
• Leaving the area • Withdrawing mentally • Changing the subject • Blaming or minimizing • Denying the problem exists • Postponing resolution to a later time (that may never occur) • Displaying emotions (tears, anger, etc.)	• The dispute is not resolved. • Disputes often build up and may eventually explode. • Low team member satisfaction may result from lack of conflict management. • Stress spreads to other parties (e.g., coworkers, family).	• The issue is trivial or unimportant. • Another issue is more urgent. • The potential disadvantages outweigh the potential benefits. • The timing for dealing with the conflict is currently inappropriate (due to overwhelming emotions or lack of information).

Application to Nursing

In a clinical setting, there may be times when it is appropriate to avoid confrontation. For example, on a particularly busy day in the emergency department, a client in a life-threatening condition was recently received. The attending physician shouts orders to the nurse in a disrespectful manner. The nurse avoids addressing the conflict until after the client has been stabilized and then shares their concerns. However, if the physician continues to bark orders to nursing staff in nonemergency situations, avoidance is no longer appropriate, and the conflict must be addressed to establish a positive and respectful working environment.[87]

84. Wagner, J. (2018). *Leadership and Influencing Change in Nursing.* University of Regina Press. https://pressbooks.pub/leadershipandinfluencingchangeinnursing/
85. Wagner, J. (2018). *Leadership and Influencing Change in Nursing.* University of Regina Press. https://pressbooks.pub/leadershipandinfluencingchangeinnursing/
86. Wagner, J. (2018). *Leadership and Influencing Change in Nursing.* University of Regina Press. https://pressbooks.pub/leadershipandinfluencingchangeinnursing/
87. Wagner, J. (2018). *Leadership and Influencing Change in Nursing.* University of Regina Press. https://pressbooks.pub/leadershipandinfluencingchangeinnursing/

Competitive Approach

A competitive approach to conflict management demonstrates a high commitment to goals and a low commitment to relationships. Individuals who use the competitive approach pursue their goals at other individuals' expense and will use whatever power is necessary to win. A competitive approach may be displayed when an individual defends an action, belief, interest, or value they believe to be correct. Competitive approaches may also be supported by infrastructure (agency promotion procedures, courts of law, legislature, etc.).[88] See Table 7.7b for types of competitive approaches, potential results, and appropriate uses.

TABLE 7.7B. Competitive Approach[89]

Types of Competitive Approaches	Potential Results	Appropriate Use
• Using power of authority, position, or majority • Using power of persuasion • Using high-pressure techniques (e.g., threats, force, intimidation) • Disguising the issue • Tying relationship to conflict	• The conflict may escalate or the other party may withdraw. • The quality and durability of agreement may be reduced. • It is assumed the other party will not reciprocate. However, when feeling threatened, people tend to reach for whatever power they have. • The likelihood of future problems between conflicting parties is increased. • Communication and trust decrease.	• Short and quick action is vital. • The competitive strategy may be helpful for certain management decisions (e.g., enforcing unpopular rules, cutting costs, enforcing disciplinary measures).

Application to Nursing

A competitive approach to conflict resolution may be appropriate in a clinical setting if a nurse leader realizes a nurse has made an error while preparing to administer IV medication to a client. The nurse leader may stop the nurse from inaccurately administering the medication and take over completing the procedure. In this case, the goal of client safety outweighs the commitment to the relationship with that nurse. However, after client safety is maintained, it would be inappropriate to continue the competitive approach when debriefing the nurse about a simple human error. Debriefing should focus on educating the nurse about policy and procedures to improve their performance. However, if it is determined the nurse was acting recklessly and disciplinary measures must be instituted by a manager, then the competitive approach may be appro-

88. Wagner, J. (2018). *Leadership and Influencing Change in Nursing.* University of Regina Press. https://pressbooks.pub/leadershipandinfluencingchangeinnursing/
89. Wagner, J. (2018). *Leadership and Influencing Change in Nursing.* University of Regina Press. https://pressbooks.pub/leadershipandinfluencingchangeinnursing/

priate.[90] This approach to responding to errors is often referred to as "Just Culture." Read more about Just Culture in the "Legal Implications" chapter.

Accommodating Approach

An accommodating approach to conflict management demonstrates a low commitment to goals and high commitment to relationships. This approach is the opposite of the competitive approach. It occurs when a person ignores or overrides their own concerns to satisfy the concerns of the other party. An accommodating approach is often used to establish reciprocal adaptations or adjustments, but when the other party does not reciprocate, conflict can result. Accommodators typically do not ask for anything in return but can become resentful when a reciprocal relationship isn't established. If resentment grows, individuals relying on the accommodating approach may shift to a competitive approach from a feeling of "being used" that can lead to conflict.[91] See Table 7.7c for types of the accommodating approach, potential results, and appropriate uses.

TABLE 7.7C. Accommodating Approach[92]

Types of Accommodating Approaches	Potential Results	Appropriate Use
• Playing down the conflict to maintain surface harmony • Self-sacrificing • Yielding to the other point of view	• The accommodating approach builds relationships that encourage more effective future problem-solving. • Accommodation increases the chances that the other party may be more accommodating to your needs in the future. • Communication is not improved.	• The outcome or issue is more important to the other party. • Preserving harmony is more important than the outcome. • It is necessary to build good faith for future problem-solving. • Your position could be damaged by a competitive approach. • Your previous action was incorrect.

Application to Nursing

It may be appropriate to use an accommodating approach when one of the nurses on your team has a challenging client who is taking up a lot of time and effort. By being situationally aware and noticing the nurse has been involved in that client's room for a long period of time, you offer to provide task assistance in an ef-

90. Wagner, J. (2018). *Leadership and Influencing Change in Nursing.* University of Regina Press. https://pressbooks.pub/leadershipandinfluencingchangeinnursing/
91. Wagner, J. (2018). *Leadership and Influencing Change in Nursing.* University of Regina Press. https://pressbooks.pub/leadershipandinfluencingchangeinnursing/
92. Wagner, J. (2018). *Leadership and Influencing Change in Nursing.* University of Regina Press. https://pressbooks.pub/leadershipandinfluencingchangeinnursing/

fort to provide mutual support. You are aware this will increase your workload for a short period of time, but it will assist your colleague and promote a strong team. However, the accommodating approach is no longer appropriate if the nurse continues to expect you to cover their tasks after the situation has been resolved.[93]

Compromising Approach

A compromising approach to conflict resolution strikes a balance between commitment to goals and commitment to relationships. The objective of a compromising approach is a quick solution that will work for both parties. It typically involves both parties giving up something in return for something, thereby "meeting in the middle."[94] See Table 7.7d for types of compromising approaches, potential results, and appropriate uses.

TABLE 7.7D. Compromising Approach

Types of Compromising Approaches	Potential Results	Appropriate Use
• Splitting the difference • Exchanging concessions • Finding middle ground	• Both parties may feel they lost the battle and want to "get even" next time. • A relationship between the two parties is not established, although it does not cause the deterioration of relationships. • There is a danger of stalemate if one or both parties refuse to "give up" anything. • Compromising does not explore the issue in depth.	• Compromising works well when quick solutions are required due to time pressures. • Compromising may be appropriate when collaboration or competition fails. • Short-term solutions are needed until more information can be obtained.

Application to Nursing

Compromise is an appropriate approach to conflict in many clinical settings. For example, you are working with another nurse who rarely assists other team members. The nurse asks you for assistance with a blood draw for a client. You hesitate because you are searching for a lunch tray that has not yet been delivered for a client with diabetes. You ask your colleague to obtain the client's lunch tray while you complete their request for assistance with a blood draw. It would be inappropriate to refuse to assist the nurse based on their reputation because this could impact safe, effective care for the client.[95]

93. Wagner, J. (2018). *Leadership and Influencing Change in Nursing.* University of Regina Press. https://pressbooks.pub/leadershipandinfluencingchangeinnursing/
94. Wagner, J. (2018). *Leadership and Influencing Change in Nursing.* University of Regina Press. https://pressbooks.pub/leadershipandinfluencingchangeinnursing/
95. Wagner, J. (2018). *Leadership and Influencing Change in Nursing.* University of Regina Press. https://pressbooks.pub/leadershipandinfluencingchangeinnursing/

Collaborative Approach

The collaborative approach to conflict resolution demonstrates a high commitment to goals, as well as a high commitment to relationships. The collaborative approach attempts to meet the concerns and priorities of all parties, but trust and willingness for risk are required for this approach to be effective.[96] See Table 7.7e for types of collaborative approaches, potential results, and appropriate uses.

TABLE 7.7E. Collaborative Approach[97]

Type of Collaborative Approaches	Potential Results	Appropriate Use
• Maximizing use of fixed resources • Working to increase resources • Listening and communicating to promote understanding of others' interests and values • Learning from each other's insight	• Collaboration builds relationships and improves potential for future problem-solving. • Collaboration promotes creative solutions.	• Parties are committed to the process and adequate time is available. • The issue is too important to compromise. • New insights can be beneficial in achieving creative solutions. • There are diverse interests and issues at play. • Participants can be future focused.

Application to Nursing

An example of appropriately using the collaborative approach in conflict management in a clinical setting is when discussing vacation time off with team members. During a team meeting, time is available to discuss and focus on what is important and a priority for each member of the team. However, the collaborative approach to conflict management would be inappropriate when discussing the implementation of a new agency policy if the team has little influence in making adjustments.[98]

All approaches to conflict can be appropriate for specific situations, but they can also be inappropriate or overused. When conflict occurs, take time to consider which approach is most beneficial for the situation. Keep in mind that using wrong approaches can escalate conflict, damage relationships, and reduce your ability to effectively meet team goals. Correct conflict management approaches build trust in relationships, accomplish goals, and de-escalate conflict.[99]

96. Wagner, J. (2018). *Leadership and Influencing Change in Nursing.* University of Regina Press. https://pressbooks.pub/leadershipandinfluencingchangeinnursing/
97. Wagner, J. (2018). *Leadership and Influencing Change in Nursing.* University of Regina Press. https://pressbooks.pub/leadershipandinfluencingchangeinnursing/
98. Wagner, J. (2018). *Leadership and Influencing Change in Nursing.* University of Regina Press. https://pressbooks.pub/leadershipandinfluencingchangeinnursing/
99. Wagner, J. (2018). *Leadership and Influencing Change in Nursing.* University of Regina Press. https://pressbooks.pub/leadershipandinfluencingchangeinnursing/

Everyone has the capacity to use any of these approaches for managing conflict and can shift from their natural style as needed. We tend to react with our most dominant natural style when under stress, but other approaches can be learned and applied with practice and self-awareness. When dealing with others who have not developed their capacity to shift from their natural style of conflict management, it is important to consider their underlying needs. By understanding individuals' needs existing beneath the surface of the conflict, you can work with the other person toward achieving a common goal.[100]

Addressing Individual Needs and Approaches

There are times when other individuals take an approach that is not helpful to resolving the conflict. It is important to remember the only person you can control during a conflict is yourself. Be flexible with your approach according to the situation and the team members with whom you are working. If someone is taking an approach that is not beneficial to resolving conflict, it can be helpful to try to understand the needs that underlie their decision to take that approach.[101]

Here are some examples of needs underlying their approaches to conflict and suggested ways to address them[102]:

- People using the **avoidance approach** may need to feel physically and emotionally safe. Take the time to reassure them that their needs will be heard.
- People taking the **competitive approach** often feel the need for something to be accomplished to meet their goals. It may be helpful to say, "We will work out a solution, but it may take some time to get there."
- People using the **accommodating approach** may need to know that no matter what happens during the conversation, your relationship will remain intact. It may be helpful to say, "This decision will not affect our relationship or how we work together."
- People using the **compromising approach** may need to know that they will get something in return. It may be helpful to say, "We will do Action A first, and then we will do Action B for you." However, be sure to be true to your word.
- People using the **collaborative approach** may need to know what you want before they are comfortable sharing their needs. It may be helpful to say, "I need this, this, and this...What do you need?"

Take free online conflict quizzes and assessments to identify your preferred conflict management styles. Access supplementary digital content in the online book using this QR code.

100. Wagner, J. (2018). *Leadership and Influencing Change in Nursing.* University of Regina Press. https://pressbooks.pub/leadershipandinfluencingchangeinnursing/
101. Wagner, J. (2018). *Leadership and Influencing Change in Nursing.* University of Regina Press. https://pressbooks.pub/leadershipandinfluencingchangeinnursing/
102. Wagner, J. (2018). *Leadership and Influencing Change in Nursing.* University of Regina Press. https://pressbooks.pub/leadershipandinfluencingchangeinnursing/

Escalating and De-Escalating Conflict

An approach taken to manage conflict can escalate (increase) or de-escalate (decrease) the conflict. Conflict on a team can take a life of its own and escalate beyond reason if not managed appropriately by nurse leaders. When conflict is not managed appropriately, negative consequences within the team often occur, and client safety can be compromised. Increased rates of absenteeism and turnover may also occur.[103]

Conflict tends to escalate under the following conditions[104]:

- There is an increase in emotions like anger, frustration, etc.
- An individual feels that they are being threatened (i.e., the fight-or-flight response is triggered).
- Other people get involved and choose sides.
- The individuals were not friendly prior to the conflict.
- The individuals desire to engage in conflict.

However, conflict can be de-escalated under the following conditions[105]:

- Attention is focused on solving the problem.
- There is a decrease in emotion and perceived threat.
- The individuals were friendly prior to the conflict.
- The individuals desire to reduce conflict.

Read an example of escalating conflict in the following box.

Example of Escalating Conflict[106]

A conflict begins between two team members who became short-tempered with each other while caring for a client experiencing a medical emergency.

- The parties become aware of the conflict but attempt to deal with it sensibly. Often, they will attribute the problem to "a misunderstanding" and indicate "we can work it out."
- If an appropriate conflict management approach is not used, the parties begin to move from cooperation to competition. ("I'll bend – but only if they bend first.") They begin to view the conflict as resulting from deliberate action on the part of the other. ("Didn't they know this was going to happen?") Positions begin to harden and defensiveness sets in, creating adversarial encounters. Parties begin to strengthen their positions and look to others on the team for support. ("Don't you feel I'm being reasonable?" or "Did you know what that idiot did to me?")

103. Children, Youth, Families & Communities & Michigan State University Extension. (2009). *Module 3 | Part 6 -Managing conflict: Escalating and de-escalating.* Michigan State University Board of Trustees. https://www.canr.msu.edu/uploads/236/64484/MOD_3_MANAGING_CONFLICT_ESCALATING_AND_DE-ESCALATING.pdf

104. Children, Youth, Families & Communities & Michigan State University Extension. (2009). *Module 3 | Part 6 -Managing conflict: Escalating and de-escalating.* Michigan State University Board of Trustees. https://www.canr.msu.edu/uploads/236/64484/MOD_3_MANAGING_CONFLICT_ESCALATING_AND_DE-ESCALATING.pdf

105. Children, Youth, Families & Communities & Michigan State University Extension. (2009). *Module 3 | Part 6 -Managing conflict: Escalating and de-escalating.* Michigan State University Board of Trustees. https://www.canr.msu.edu/uploads/236/64484/MOD_3_MANAGING_CONFLICT_ESCALATING_AND_DE-ESCALATING.pdf

106. The Center for Congregational Health. (2011). *Levels of conflict by Speed Leas.* https://cntr4conghealth.wordpress.com/2011/09/01/levels-of-conflict-by-speed-leas/

- As communication deteriorates, parties rely on assumptions about the other individual and attribute negative motives to them. ("I bet they did that on purpose.") Groupthink can take over the subgroups as each individual seeks others to take on their side. ("We have to appear strong and make a united front.")
- Parties believe that cooperation cannot resolve the problem because of the assumed negative actions of the other. ("I've tried everything to get them to see reason," "It's time to get tough," or "I'm going to put a stop to this.")
- Parties begin to feel righteous and blame the other for the entire problem. Generalizing and stereotyping begin. ("I know what those kinds of people are like. . . We can't let them get away with this.") Parties begin to be judgmental and moralistic and believe they are defending what is "right." ("It's the principle of the matter" or "What will others say if we give in to this?")
- Severe confrontation is anticipated and planned, thus making it inevitable. The parties view this confrontation as acceptable. The objective of the conflict becomes to hurt the other more than being hurt, and the dispute is beyond rational analysis. ("I'm going to make you pay even if we both go down over this," "There is no turning back now," or "They won't make a fool out of me.")

There are positive steps to take to de-escalate conflict with another individual before it gets out of control. See Figure 7.9[107] for steps to de-escalate conflict and implement change.

1 SELF AWARENESS

- Reflect on your own approach and the approach of others.
- Find people you trust to discuss potential solutions.
- Think about who may challenge your perspective rather than who would agree with you.

2 RAISING THE ISSUE

- Decide to raise the issue with the other person(s) when it is important or affects you personally.
- Raise the issue at an appropriate time.
- Commit to a change in your own behaviour(s) that contributes to resolution.
- When raising the issue, use specific examples to limit confusion. Speaking from your perspective will reduce defensiveness. Use "I" language rather than "you."

3 FOLLOW UP

- Follow up with others and assess if a change has been made.
- Determine if the change is continuing to work.
- If the change is not working, decide what adjustments need to be made.

4 WHEN CHANGE IS NOT IMPLEMENTED

- Raise the issue again if necessary.
- Use further problem solving by focusing on what each person needs to create the necessary change and discuss any available options.
- While problem solving, compare the options presented with the necessary outcome (i.e., what is needed).
- If resolution cannot be reached with others, determine what change(s) you can make that would bring some resolution to you personally.

FIGURE 7.9 Steps to De-Escalate Conflict

107. "Dispute Resolution Office, Ministry of Justice (Government of Saskatchewan)" designed by JVDW Designs, is licensed under a CC BY 4.0 International License

Conflict Management Tips

Nurses must develop their own tool kit to manage conflict in a productive, positive way. Due to rapid turnover in the health care environment at this time, new nurses may find themselves in a "charge nurse" position within their first year of practice. See Table 7.7f for tips on managing conflict constructively.[108]

TABLE 7.7F. Conflict Management Tips[109]

Tip	Description
Be Consistent	Convey to the team that expectations are consistent and implemented fairly across the team. Set expectations and make sure the team knows those expectations via department meetings and visual reminders. Follow up to ensure expectations are met. This sets a clear picture of what is required.
Be Team-Focused	Be aware of team members' strengths and weaknesses. Address poor performance and negative attitudes. Teamwork and team dynamics impact client safety and staff retention. Ask team members what they need from you as a leader. Coach team members and staff on a regular basis.
Convey Trust and Integrity	Trustworthiness and integrity are powerful when managing conflict. Team members are more likely to handle difficult situations constructively if they know they are supported by an approachable and supportive team leader. Stay focused on the individual and remind them that you value them and want them to feel heard. It may be helpful to include a statement such as, "As health care members, we are held accountable for positive behaviors with team members."
Lead with Truth	If you need to have a difficult conversation, lead with the tough message and be clear. For example, try saying, "There's something difficult I need to talk with you about. I'm concerned about the feedback I've been receiving from clients." Even in conveying a tough message, you can build trust by showing the employee that you'll be honest with them and share feedback openly. Don't leave the team member guessing about the problem or what they need to do to improve. Clearly state the performance gap, your expectations, the reason it matters, and the timeline for improvement, including a future meeting to review feedback and give a progress update. Provide support and available resources to help them make the needed change.

108. Elizabeth, A. (2019). Managing interpersonal conflict: Steps for success. *Nursing Management, 50*(6), 22-28. https://journals.lww.com/nursingmanagement/Fulltext/2019/06000/Managing_interpersonal_conflict__Steps_for_success.7.aspx
109. Elizabeth, A. (2019). Managing interpersonal conflict: Steps for success. *Nursing Management, 50*(6), 22-28. https://journals.lww.com/nursingmanagement/Fulltext/2019/06000/Managing_interpersonal_conflict__Steps_for_success.7.aspx

TABLE 7.7F. Continued...

Anticipate Reactions	Knowing how a team member will respond when conflicts arise can be a challenge. Common negative reactions to conflicts are defensiveness, deflection, and denial. Defensive comments may include, "No one's ever brought this to me before." You can reply, "I'm invested in you and want to see you succeed. I owe it to you and our department to be transparent with you and share these concerns." Deflection can take the form of an employee asking you why a coworker didn't directly bring up the concern. Often, it's because others are too intimidated by the individual or situation to speak up. Your reply can be, "Accountability between colleagues is always encouraged, but as your leader, I owe it to you to share this feedback. Do you feel your colleagues perceive you as approachable and open to feedback?" Denial may include the employee refuting that the incident of concern ever happened. You can calmly remind the employee that we own others' perceptions of our behaviors and you want to help them understand where some actions may be giving people the wrong impression.
Use Available Resources	Engage in professional development for managing conflicts when they arise. Share knowledge and experiences with other nurse leaders to build networks, partner with other teams within the organization, and use the human resources department when needed.

7.8 NURSING RESPONSIBILITIES IN INTERPROFESSIONAL COLLABORATIVE PRACTICE

Previous sections of this chapter discussed IPEC competencies required for effective interprofessional collaboration and methods for managing conflict. In addition to demonstrating these competencies, nurses also have many other responsibilities related to interprofessional collaborative practice. Nurses plan and participate in interdisciplinary care conferences; assign, delegate, and supervise nursing team members; educate clients and staff; act as client advocates; make client referrals; ensure continuity of care; and contribute to the evaluation of client outcomes. These responsibilities of the nurse are further described in the following subsections.

Planning and Participating in Interdisciplinary Care Conferences

The nurse identifies clients who would benefit from interdisciplinary care conferences. **Interdisciplinary care conferences** are meetings where interprofessional team members professionally collaborate, share their expertise, and plan collaborative interventions to meet client needs. As the interprofessional team member likely to spend the most time at the client's bedside, nurses are key members for advocating for client needs during interdisciplinary care conferences. The nurse utilizes effective communication techniques by expressing and advocating for client needs, listening attentively to suggestions of other team members, formulating a collaborative plan of care, and documenting it in the client's nursing care plan.

Reflective Activity

View the following YouTube video illustrating an interdisciplinary care conference as a client's plan of care is designed and implemented.[110]

Reflective Questions[111]:

- As you watch the video, notice how the professionals from different health disciplines communicate and interact with each other to formulate the plan of care for a client and how the care is continued through multidisciplinary involvement.
- Assess interprofessional collaborative practice of the health care team using the PDF provided.

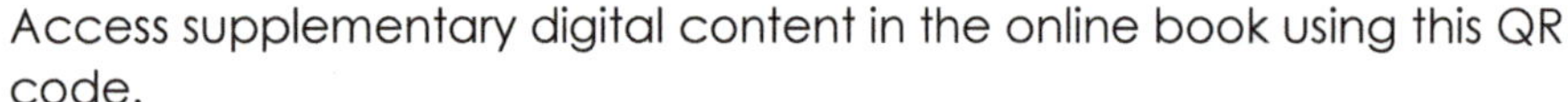

Access supplementary digital content in the online book using this QR code.

Assigning, Delegating, and Supervising

Nurses assign, delegate, and supervise care of other members of the nursing team, such as licensed practical/vocational nurses (LPN/VN) and unlicensed assistive personnel (UAP). Appropriately assigning and delegating care with appropriate supervision are strategies that ensure quality client care is completed efficiently. Read more about assigning and delegating in the "Delegation and Supervision" chapter.

Educating Clients and Staff

Nurses provide client education, train staff, and serve as a staff resource. For example, an RN serves as a resource to unlicensed assistive personnel (UAP) floating to their unit. The RN provides a general orientation of the unit, explains the pertinent needs of the clients as they pertain to the UAP's assigned tasks, and shares how the staff interact and communicate within the unit. The RN ensures the UAP understands the orientation information, is competent in their assigned/delegated tasks, and utilizes the RN as a resource throughout the shift.

---

110. Interprofessional Professionalism Collaborative. (2018, August 15). *IPC case scenario for Mr. Jones part I* [Video]. YouTube. All rights reserved. https://youtu.be/woHaclEtLFw

111. Interprofessional Professionalism Collaborative. (2019). *IPA tool kit.* http://www.interprofessionalprofessionalism.org/toolkit.html

Acting As a Client Advocate

Nurses advocate for client needs with family members, interprofessional team members, health care administrators, and, in some cases, health insurance companies and policy makers. Nurses protect and defend the rights and interests of their clients and ensure their safety, especially if the client is unable to advocate for themselves. For example, clients who are unconscious, developmentally disabled, illiterate, or experiencing confusion often require assertive advocacy with the interprofessional team to effectively meet their needs and preferences.[112] Read more about nurse advocacy in the "Advocacy" chapter.

Making Client Referrals

Nurses assess clients, determine their needs, and make referrals based on potential or actual problem(s). If the assessed needs of the client cannot be met by the collaborative nursing interventions, the nurse seeks out other resources to fulfill the client's needs. For example, nurses often advocate for referrals to community resources such as home health care, support groups, social services, respite care, emergency shelters, transportation, elder day care, and parenting groups. After needed referrals are identified, the nurse obtains necessary provider orders and completes applicable referral forms. This information is shared confidentially with the client and the referral resource.

Ensuring Continuity of Care

Nurses serve a vital role for maintaining **continuity of care** and making any client transition of care smooth and unfragmented. Continuity of care is defined as "the use of information on past events and personal circumstances to make current care appropriate for each individual."[113] Transitions of care include admission to a facility, transfer from one unit to another within the same facility, transfer from one facility to another, or discharge to their home or a long-term care facility. For example, a transfer occurs when a client is moved from a medical unit bed to the intensive care unit.

There is high risk for medical errors during transitions of care. Nurses help make transitions seamless with good handoff reports and documentation while effectively collaborating with the interprofessional team. Read about preventing medication errors during transitions of care in the following box.

112. Gerber, L. (2018). Understanding the nurse's role as a patient advocate. *Nursing, 48(*4), 55-58. https://journals.lww.com/nursing/Fulltext/2018/04000/Understanding_the_nurse_s_role_as_a_patient.15.aspx

113. Kim, S. Y. (2017). Continuity of care. *Korean Journal of Family Medicine, 38*(5), 241. https://doi.org/10.4082/kjfm.2017.38.5.241

PREVENTING MEDICATION ERRORS DURING TRANSITIONS[114]

Key strategies for improving medication safety during transitions of care include the following:

- Implementing formal structured processes for medication reconciliation at all transition points of care. Steps of effective medication reconciliation are to build the best possible medication history by interviewing the client and verifying with at least one reliable information source, reconciling and updating the medication list, and communicating with the client and future health care providers about changes in their medications.
- Partnering with clients, families, caregivers, and health care professionals to agree on treatment plans, ensuring clients are equipped to manage their medications safely, and ensuring clients have an up-to-date medication list.
- Where necessary, prioritize clients at high risk of medication-related harm for enhanced support such as post-discharge contact by a nurse.

SAFELY ADMITTING AND DISCHARGING CLIENTS

Admission refers to an initial visit or contact with a client. **Discharge** refers to the completion of care and services in a health care facility and the client is sent home (or to another health care facility).

Admissions and discharges are more than just the physical movement of an individual. They require a great deal of confidential information sharing to maintain continuity of care. During an admission, nurses use the nursing process to thoroughly assess the client, diagnose nursing problems, establish expected outcomes, and create a nursing care plan. Referrals for other inpatient services, such as a dietician, wound care nurse, chaplain, social worker, or other interprofessional team members, may be initiated. Additionally, the client and their family members are oriented to the setting, and information is provided regarding HIPAA and client rights and responsibilities; medications are reconciled; and other admission tasks are completed based on agency policy.

During discharge, there is also a great deal of information shared with clients regarding follow-up appointments with interprofessional team members, medication reconciliation, and client education.

REPORTING NEW INFORMATION AND CHANGING CONDITIONS

The nurse is often responsible for reporting new information to the interprofessional team regarding inpatients, such as newly reported laboratory or diagnostic results or changes in a client's condition. Here are some examples of a nurse reporting and following up on issues:

- A client receiving BiPAP therapy has worsening oxygen saturation levels and respiratory status. The nurse reports these changes to the respiratory therapist, who reassesses and adjusts the positive pressure settings as needed.
- An inpatient receiving furosemide has new abnormal potassium levels. The nurse reports the newly reported lab results to the provider.

114. Medication Safety in Transitions of Care by World Health Organization is licensed under CC BY-NC-SA 3.0

- A client receiving an antibiotic for the first time develops a rash and shortness of breath. The nurse reports the client's adverse reaction to the prescribing provider and the pharmacist and ensures the allergy is noted in the client's chart.
- A family member shares a recent change in a client's living arrangements that is concerning. The nurse reports updates to the social worker to assist in making alternative living arrangements.

Contributing to the Evaluation of Client Outcomes

In today's complex health care system, data regarding client outcomes is constantly documented and analyzed. This data drives management decisions and is also reported to insurance companies as a component of "pay for performance" reimbursement processes. The nurse is directly involved in this data by establishing expected outcomes customized to the client, evaluating these outcomes, and documenting data supporting outcomes related to collaborative nursing interventions.

7.9 SPOTLIGHT APPLICATION

Allison is a new graduate nurse who is recently transitioned from her orientation period to her scheduled night shift work on a medical telemetry unit. She has a client care assignment of six client. Her client, Mr. Daniels, was admitted from the ER at 2200 shortly before her shift began. He was transferred to the floor with a medical diagnosis of heart failure exacerbation. The client was prescribed IV push furosemide for diuresis. It is now 0500 and the client's morning potassium level is reported from the lab to be 2.9 mmol/L. Allison understands that this level needs to be reported to the admitting physician. Utilizing an ISBARR format, what information should Allison be prepared to phone the physician?

Allison should be prepared to tell the physician her role on the unit and that she is calling to relate information on a critical lab value. She should describe information about the client, including Mr. Daniel's name, position on the unit, and a reminder of when the client was admitted. She should provide a brief synopsis of the stability of the client. If there is relevant information regarding allergies, this should be related at this time as well. The concern related to the lab value and any accompanying symptoms should also be described. Allison should provide insight into the current intake and output status, weight, cardiac rhythm, signs of edema, respiratory status, etc. Allison should outline her request related to orders for potassium replacement. When these orders are received from the provider, she must be sure to repeat back the order to confirm accuracy.

7.10 LEARNING ACTIVITIES

Learning Activities

(Answers to "Learning Activities" can be found in the "Answer Key" at the end of the book. Answers to interactive activities are provided as immediate feedback.)

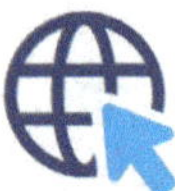

Visit the TeamSTEPPS® Instructor Manual: Specialty Scenarios for multiple AHRQ scenarios requiring application of TeamSTEPPS® to client scenarios. Access supplementary digital content in the online book using this QR code.

Scenario 1

Read this scenario and answer the following questions.

Jill and Neil are both nurses working the same shift. Jill is responsible for clients in Rooms 1–6, and Neil is responsible for clients in Rooms 7–12. Over the course of their shift, both nurses routinely visit their clients' rooms to take vitals and deliver medication.

On one of his rounds, Neil attends to his client in Room 8. He reads the chart and notices Jill's initials signaling that she had already checked on this client. A bit confused, he continues on to his next client. After another hour goes by, Neil returns to Room 8 and again notices Jill's initials on the chart. Neil thinks to himself, "What is she doing? I've got it covered. She's checking my work. She must think I'm incompetent." Neil decides to approach Jill and see what is going on.

Questions:

1. What might have been the initial cause of the conflict?
2. What kind of conflict did it turn into?
3. If Neil provides Jill with a copy of the room assignments, would that resolve the conflict?

Scenario 2

Read this scenario and answer the following questions.

A nursing team is having a routine meeting. One of the nurses, Stephen, is at the end of a 12-hour shift, and another nurse, Tanya, is just beginning hers. Tanya is a senior nurse in the unit with over ten years' experience on this specific unit. Stephen is new to the unit with fewer than three years' experience in nursing. Tanya has been asked to present information to the team about effective time management on the unit. During Tanya's presentation, Stephen is seen rolling his eyes and talking to other members of the team. Tanya breaks from her presentation and asks, "Stephen, do you have anything to add?" Stephen replies, "No, I just don't know why we need to talk about this again." Tanya chooses to avoid engaging with Stephen further and finishes her presentation. Stephen continues to be disruptive throughout the presentation.

After the meeting concludes, Tanya approaches Stephen and asks if he had anything to add from the meeting. Stephen replies, "No, I don't have anything. I just think we all know what the procedure is because we just learned it all during orientation training. Maybe if you don't remember the training, you should take it again." Tanya is shocked by his reply and quickly composes herself. She states, "Stephen, I have worked on this unit for over ten years. I was asked to present that information because there are current issues going on among the staff. Next time please respect my authority and listen to those who come before you."

Questions:

1. What types of conflict are present?
2. What will need to happen to resolve this issue between Tanya and Stephen?
3. Take a moment to think about what your preferred approach to conflict may be. How might you adapt your approach to conflict when working with others?

Scenario 3

Read this scenario and answer the following questions.

Connie, the head nurse on Unit 7, is a respected member of the team. She has been working on this unit for a number of years and is seen by the other nurses as the "go to" person for questions and guidance. Connie is always thorough with clients and demonstrates excellence and quality in her work. Dr. Smith is a well-respected member of the medical profession and an expert in his field of medicine. He has a reputation for excellent bedside manner and is thorough in his approach with clients.

Connie is four hours into her 12-hour shift when she is approached by Dr. Smith. He asks, "Connie, why has the client in Room 2 not received his blood pressure medication over the past few days? I was not notified about this!"

Connie, trying to find a quick solution, replies, "I didn't know that client had been missing medication. I'll go check on it and get back to you."

Dr. Smith is persistent, saying, "You don't need to go check anything. I know this client and should have been informed about the withholding of medication and the reasons why." Connie, again attempting to find a resolution, states, "Well, there must be some communication about this change somewhere . . ."

"There isn't!" Dr. Smith interrupts.

Connie becomes upset and decides to leave the conversation after declaring, "Fine, if you know everything, then you figure it out; you're the one with the medical degree, aren't you?" She storms off.

Connie makes her way to the nurses' station where Dan and Elise are assessing charts and says to them, "You will not believe what Dr. Smith just said to me!"

Dan and Elise look shocked and ask "What?"

Connie explains, "Well, he thinks I don't do my job, when really we nurses are the ones that keep this unit going. Who is he to question my ability to look after clients? I am the most knowledgeable person on this unit!"

Dan and Elise don't know how to reply and decide to avoid the interaction with a simple, "Oh yeah."

Meanwhile, Dr. Smith has made his way to the doctor's lounge and finds his colleague Dr. Lee. Dr. Smith tells him, "That head nurse on Unit 7 is useless. She doesn't know what she is doing and doesn't understand that we must be informed about changes to our clients' medications, does she?" Dr. Lee nods quickly and returns to reviewing his file.

About three hours later, Connie and Dr. Smith have each spoken to several people about the interaction. Connie bumps into another nurse, Jessie, one of her best friends. Connie pulls Jessie aside and says, "You will not believe what I just saw. I was going into the admin office to file my holiday requests and out of the corner of my eye, I saw Dr. Smith lurking around the corner, pretending to look at a chart, spying on me!"

"What? Are you serious? That's not safe," replies Jessie.

Connie is relieved that Jessie is taking her side—it makes her feel as if she is not going crazy. "Yeah, I'm really getting worried about this. First, that creep is accusing me of not doing my job, and then he is wasting his time spying on me. What a loser! Maybe what I should do is file a complaint. That'll show the 'big man' that he isn't that big around here and maybe take him down a notch."

When Jessie gives her an apprehensive look, Connie continues, "Oh Jessie, don't worry. I have a perfect record and this won't affect me. Even if it does, I will have done something good for all the other nurses around here. It is the principle of the matter at this point."

Meanwhile, Dr. Smith has run into an old classmate of his, Dr. Drucker, and says, "Wow! You got hired! So happy to have you in the hospital. I do need to tell you though to be careful of the head nurse on Unit 7 . . ." Dr. Smith describes his troubles with Connie and adds, "She's a real snitch! She makes trouble out of nothing. I was reviewing a chart down the corridor from the admin office, minding my own business and actually getting my work done, when I saw her slip into the admin office to squeal about me to the top bosses! This is something that needs to be watched! We can't have people reporting doctors to administration over nothing. I think I'm going to write her up and get a black mark on that perfect record of hers. I will be fine—everyone knows I'm right. There will be consequences for her."

Questions:

1. Using the scenario above, identify the stages of the conflict escalation.
2. What suggestions might you give to Dan, Elise, Jessie, Dr. Lee, and Dr. Drucker about how to respond to Connie and Dr. Smith?
3. How do you think this conflict will be resolved?

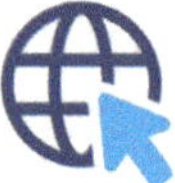

Interactive learning activities have been excluded from the print version of the text. Access free online learning activities in the online book using this QR code.

7.11 GLOSSARY

Admission: Refers to an initial visit or contact with a client.

Brief: A short session to share a plan, discuss team formation, assign roles and responsibilities, establish expectations and climate, and anticipate outcomes and contingencies.

Closed-loop communication: A communication strategy used to ensure that information conveyed by the sender is heard by the receiver and completed.

Communication conflict: Occurs when there is a failure in the exchange of information.

Continuity of care: The use of information on past events and personal circumstances to make current care appropriate for each individual.[115]

Cultural diversity: A term used to describe cultural differences among clients, family members, and health care team members.

Cultural humility: A humble and respectful attitude toward individuals of other cultures that pushes one to challenge their own cultural biases, realize they cannot possibly know everything about other cultures, and approach learning about other cultures as a lifelong goal and process.[116]

CUS statements: Assertive statements that are well-recognized by all staff across a health care agency as implementation of the two-challenge rule. These assertive statements are "I am Concerned – I am Uncomfortable – This is a Safety issue!"[117]

Debrief: An informal information exchange session designed to improve team performance and effectiveness through reinforcement of positive behaviors and reflecting on lessons learned after a significant event occurs.

DESC: A tool used to help resolve conflict. DESC is a mnemonic that stands for Describe the specific situation or behavior and provide concrete data, Express how the situation makes you feel/what your concerns are using "I" messages, Suggest other alternatives and seek agreement, and Consequences are stated in terms of impact on established team goals while striving for consensus.

Discharge: The completion of care and services in a health care facility and the client is sent home (or to another health care facility).

Ethical conflict: Occurs when individuals or groups have fundamentally different beliefs and values.

Feedback: Information is provided to a team member for the purpose of improving team performance. Feedback should be timely, respectful, specific, directed towards improvement, and considerate.[118]

Goal conflict: Happens when the objectives of individuals or groups are incompatible.

Handoff reports: A transfer and acceptance of client care responsibility achieved through effective communication. It is a real-time process of passing client specific information from one caregiver to another, or from one team of caregivers to another, for the purpose of ensuring the continuity and safety of the client's care.[119]

---

115. Kim, S. Y. (2017). Continuity of care. *Korean Journal of Family Medicine, 38*(5), 241. https://doi.org/10.4082/kjfm.2017.38.5.241

116. American Nurses Association. (2021). *Nursing: Scope and standards of practice* (4th ed.). American Nurses Association.

117. AHRQ. (2024). *TeamSTEPPS 3.0.* https://www.ahrq.gov/teamstepps/instructor/index.html

118. AHRQ. (2024). *TeamSTEPPS 3.0.* https://www.ahrq.gov/teamstepps/instructor/index.html

119. Starmer, A. J., Spector, N. D., Srivastava, R., Allen, A. D., Landrigan, C. P., Sectish, T. C., & I-Pass Study Group. (2012). I-PASS, a Mnemonic to Standardize Verbal Handoffs. *Pediatrics, 129*(2), 201-204. https://www.ipassinstitute.com/hubfs/I-PASS-mnemonic.pdf

Horizontal aggression: Hostile behavior among one's peers.

Huddle: A brief meeting during a shift to reestablish situational awareness, reinforce plans already in place, and adjust the teamwork plan as needed.

I'M SAFE: A tool used to assess one's own safety status, as well as that of other team members in their ability to provide safe client care. It is a mnemonic standing for personal safety risks as a result of Illness, Medication, Stress, Alcohol and Drugs, Fatigue, and Eating and Elimination.

Interdisciplinary care conferences: Meetings where interprofessional team members professionally collaborate, share their expertise, and plan collaborative interventions to meet client needs.

Interprofessional collaborative practice: Multiple health workers from different professional backgrounds working together with clients, families, caregivers, and communities to deliver the highest quality of care.

I-PASS: A mnemonic used as a structured communication tool among interprofessional team members. I-PASS stands for Illness severity, Patient summary, Action list, Situation awareness, and Synthesis by the receiver.

ISBARR: A mnemonic for the components of Introduction, Situation, Background, Assessment, Request/Recommendations, and Repeat back.[120,121]

Mutual support: The ability to anticipate and support team members' needs through accurate knowledge about their responsibilities and workload.

Personality conflict: Arises from differences in individual temperaments, attitudes, and behaviors.

Role conflict: Arises when individuals have multiple, often conflicting, expectations associated with their roles.

Shared mental model: The actions of a team leader that ensure all team members have situation awareness and are "on the same page" as situations evolve on the unit.[122]

Situation awareness: The awareness of a team member knowing what is going on around them.[123]

Situation monitoring: The process of continually scanning and assessing the situation to gain and maintain an understanding of what is going on around you.[124]

STEP tool: A situation monitoring tool used to know what is going on with you, your clients, your team, and your environment. STEP stands for Status of the clients, Team members, Environment, and Progress Toward Goal.[125]

TeamSTEPPS®: An evidence-based framework used to optimize team performance across the health care system. It is a mnemonic standing for Team Strategies and Tools to Enhance Performance and Patient Safety.[126]

Two-challenge rule: A strategy for advocating for client safety that includes a team member assertively voicing their concern at least two times to ensure that it has been heard by the decision-maker.

---

120. Institute for Healthcare Improvement (n.d.). *ISBAR trip tick*. http://www.ihi.org/resources/Pages/Tools/ISBARTripTick.aspx
121. Starmer, A. J., Spector, N. D., Srivastava, R., Allen, A. D., Landrigan, C. P., Sectish, T. C., & I-Pass Study Group. (2012). I-PASS, a Mnemonic to Standardize Verbal Handoffs. *Pediatrics, 129*(2), 201-204. https://www.ipassinstitute.com/hubfs/I-PASS-mnemonic.pdf
122. AHRQ. (2024). *TeamSTEPPS: 3.0 Pocket guide*. https://www.ahrq.gov/teamstepps-program/resources/pocket-guide/index.html
123. AHRQ. (2024). *TeamSTEPPS: 3.0 Pocket guide*. https://www.ahrq.gov/teamstepps-program/resources/pocket-guide/index.html
124. AHRQ. (2024). *TeamSTEPPS: 3.0 Pocket guide*. https://www.ahrq.gov/teamstepps-program/resources/pocket-guide/index.html
125. AHRQ. (2024). *TeamSTEPPS: 3.0 Pocket guide*. https://www.ahrq.gov/teamstepps-program/resources/pocket-guide/index.html
126. AHRQ. (2024). *TeamSTEPPS: 3.0 Pocket guide*. https://www.ahrq.gov/teamstepps-program/resources/pocket-guide/index.html

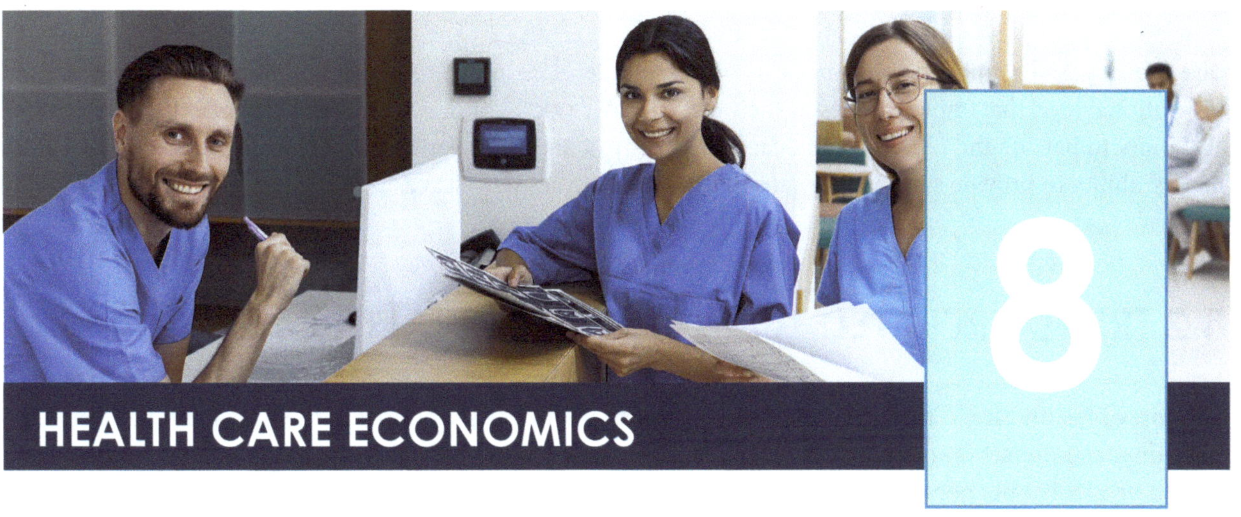

8.1 HEALTH CARE ECONOMICS INTRODUCTION

LEARNING OBJECTIVES

- Summarize the requirements of funding and reimbursement sources for client care services
- Explore how political, social, and demographic trends have affected the client population and delivery of health care
- Analyze the link between economics and quality
- Describe nursing strategies to provide cost-effective care
- Examine economic pressures impacting case management and the management of institutional resources
- Describe the impact of evidence-based practice on health care economics and client care outcomes

Whether health care is a right or a privilege is a historical ethical question debated around the world that ultimately leads to the question, "Who gets what resources?" **Economics** is the study of how individuals and societies make decisions about how to use their limited resources. Health care is considered a limited resource because there isn't enough money or time in the world to purchase and provide care for every individual in every conceivable manner. The ethical question of who pays for that care is referred to as the ethics of rationing health care.

Economics is split into two broad categories called macroeconomics and microeconomics. Macroeconomics looks at decisions that affect the entire society as a whole, whereas microeconomics looks at the financial decisions of businesses and individuals.[1] This chapter will provide an overview of the broad topics of health

1. Khan Academy. (2017, August 8). *Macroeconomics unit: Basic economics concepts.* https://www.khanacademy.org/economics-finance-domain/macroeconomics/macro-basic-economics-concepts

care funding and reimbursement models at a societal level, as well as staffing and budgeting issues at the institutional level that impact nurses in their day-to-day work. Economics in health care affects an individual's ability to pay for and receive health care, the ability of an institution to provide health care services, and nurses' ability to provide safe, quality care to the communities they serve.

8.2 TRENDS RELATED TO INCREASED HEALTH CARE COSTS

The cost of health care in the United States is higher than any other country in the world and has a significant financial impact on our economy.[2] U.S. health care spending grew 4.1 percent in 2022, reaching $4.5 trillion or $13,493 per person. Health care spending accounts for 17.3 percent of our Gross Domestic Product (GDP), the total value of goods produced and services provided annually.[3] See Figure 8.1[4] for a graph of health care cost as a percentage of GDP in the United States compared to other countries around the world.

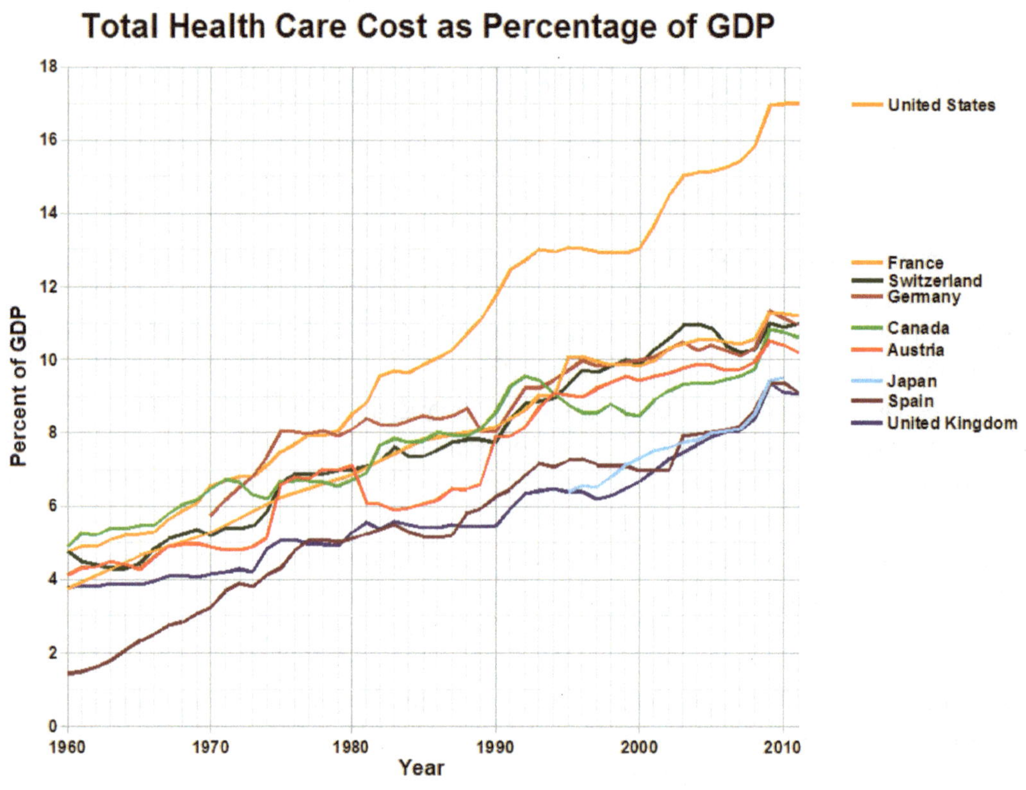

FIGURE 8.1 Comparison of Health Care Costs

2. CMS.gov. (2024). *National health expenditure data - historical.* Centers for Medicare & Medicaid Services. https://www.cms.gov/Research-Statistics-Data-and-Systems/Statistics-Trends-and-Reports/NationalHealthExpendData/NationalHealthAccountsHistorical

3. CMS.gov. (2024). *National health expenditure data - historical.* Centers for Medicare & Medicaid Services. https://www.cms.gov/Research-Statistics-Data-and-Systems/Statistics-Trends-and-Reports/NationalHealthExpendData/NationalHealthAccountsHistorical

4. "Health_Care_Cost_as_Percentage_of_GDP.png" by Delphi234 is licensed under CC0 1.0

Despite spending more money on health care than other high-income countries, the United States has some of the poorest health outcomes, such as the lowest life expectancy, the highest infant mortality rate, and a higher prevalence of chronic diseases.[5] The increasing costs of health care also have several negative impacts on society, employers, and individuals, including the following effects[6]:

- When the government spends more on health care, the national debt increases and funds available for other programs decrease.
- When people spend more on health care, they have less money to spend on other items.
- When health insurance is paid by employers, employees are paid less.
- When employers spend more on health care, the costs of their products and services increase. Jobs may be moved to countries with lower health care costs.
- An increasing number of people cannot afford health care insurance. When people without health care insurance receive health care, they often cannot pay for it. As a result of unpaid bills, this care is indirectly paid for by other people paying increased insurance premiums and taxes.
- People without health care insurance may not seek preventative care and develop a more costly, serious medical disorder that could have been prevented.
- Medical bills that are not covered by health insurance can cause bankruptcy.

There are several national trends affecting the cost of health care and related impacts, including the aging population, increased costs of medical technology, increased prescription medication cost, the Affordable Care Act, social determinants of health, etc. These trends can be further classified as intrinsic or extrinsic factors. **Intrinsic factors** related to increased health care costs are inherent to the characteristics and needs of the population. One significant intrinsic factor is the demographics of the population, such as age, gender, and overall health status. An aging population, for example, typically requires more medical care due to the prevalence of chronic conditions and the natural decline in health associated with aging. Another intrinsic factor is the demand for health care services. As people become more health-conscious, the demand for preventive care, regular check-ups, and advanced treatments rises, leading to increased overall health care spending. Additionally, the extent and nature of health insurance coverage play a crucial role. Comprehensive insurance plans often lead to higher utilization of health care services, as insured individuals are more likely to seek medical care, knowing that a significant portion of the costs will be covered by their insurance.

Extrinsic factors are external elements that impact health care costs. One of the most prominent extrinsic factors is the availability and adoption of medical technology. Advanced diagnostic tools, treatment methods, and surgical techniques can drive up costs due to their high development, implementation, and maintenance expenses. While these technologies can significantly improve client outcomes, they also contribute to rising health care expenditures. Another critical extrinsic factor is the cost of prescription drugs. Pharmaceutical pricing strategies, including research and development costs, marketing, and profit margins, often lead to high prices for medications, especially for new and specialized drugs. Workforce costs are also a significant extrinsic factor. The salaries and benefits of health care professionals, including doctors, nurses, and administrative staff, constitute a substantial portion of health care expenses. These costs are influenced by factors such as education and training requirements, labor market conditions, and regulatory policies. Addressing these extrinsic factors requires strategic planning and policy interventions to balance cost containment with the quality and accessibility of health care services.

---

5. Bush, M. (2018). Addressing the root cause: Rising health care costs and social determinants of health. *North Carolina Medical Journal, 79*(1), 26-29. https://doi.org/10.18043/ncm.79.1.26
6. Schreck, R. I. (2020). *Overview of health care financing.* Merck Manual Consumer Version. https://www.merckmanuals.com/home/fundamentals/financial-issues-in-health-care/overview-of-health-care-financing

Aging Population

According to the Agency for Healthcare Research and Quality (AHRQ), the United States has a growing number of older adults (age 65 years or older) who are living longer than previous generations. It is anticipated that older adults will make up more than 20 percent of the U.S. population by 2030.[7] See Figure 8.2[8] for an illustration of the aging population from the U.S. Census Bureau. This change in demographics will result in increased national health care costs because older adults typically experience more chronic conditions than younger populations, requiring expensive specialty and long-term care.[9]

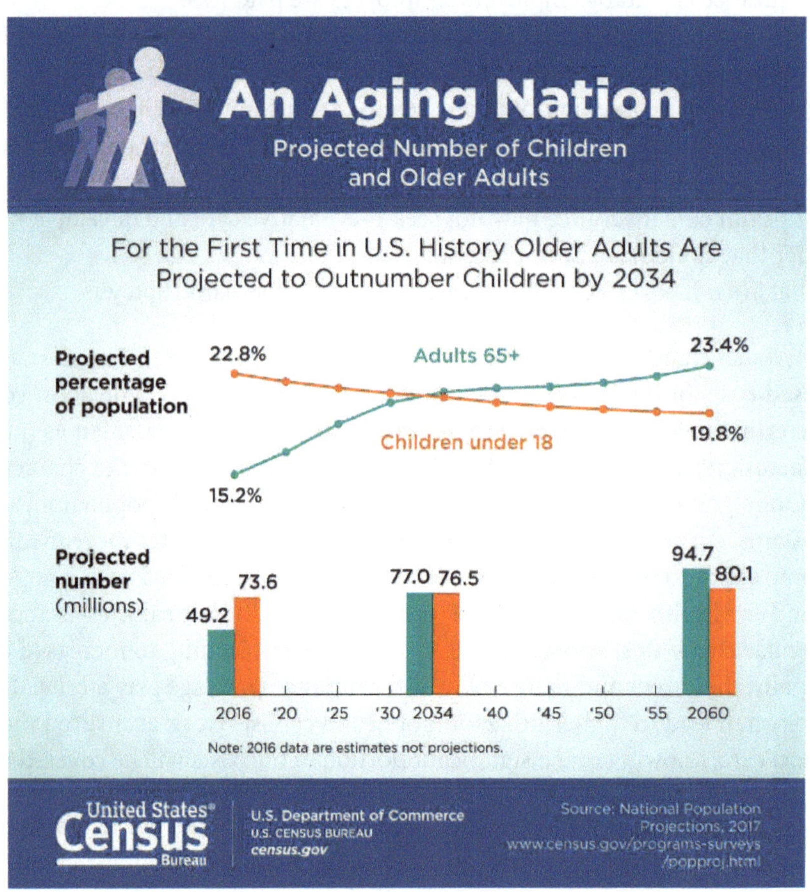

FIGURE 8.2 Aging Population in the United States

Increased Costs of Medical Technology

Highly visible medical technologies, such as organ transplantation, diagnostic imaging systems, and biotechnology products, attract both praise and blame. Evolving medical technologies may save lives and improve a client's health status, but they are also viewed as a dominant cause of continued escalation of medical costs. Research suggests that medical technology accounts for about 10 to 40 percent of the increase in

7. Agency for Healthcare Research and Quality. (n.d.). *Elderly.* https://www.ahrq.gov/topics/elderly.html

8. "graying-america-aging-nation.jpg" by U.S. Census Bureau is in the Public Domain

9. Agency for Healthcare Research and Quality. (n.d.). *Elderly.* https://www.ahrq.gov/topics/elderly.html

health care expenditures over time.[10] These costs also lead to further ethical dilemmas as decisions regarding what scarce resources are provided to which clients are made. See Figure 8.3[11] for an image of common technology used in health care.

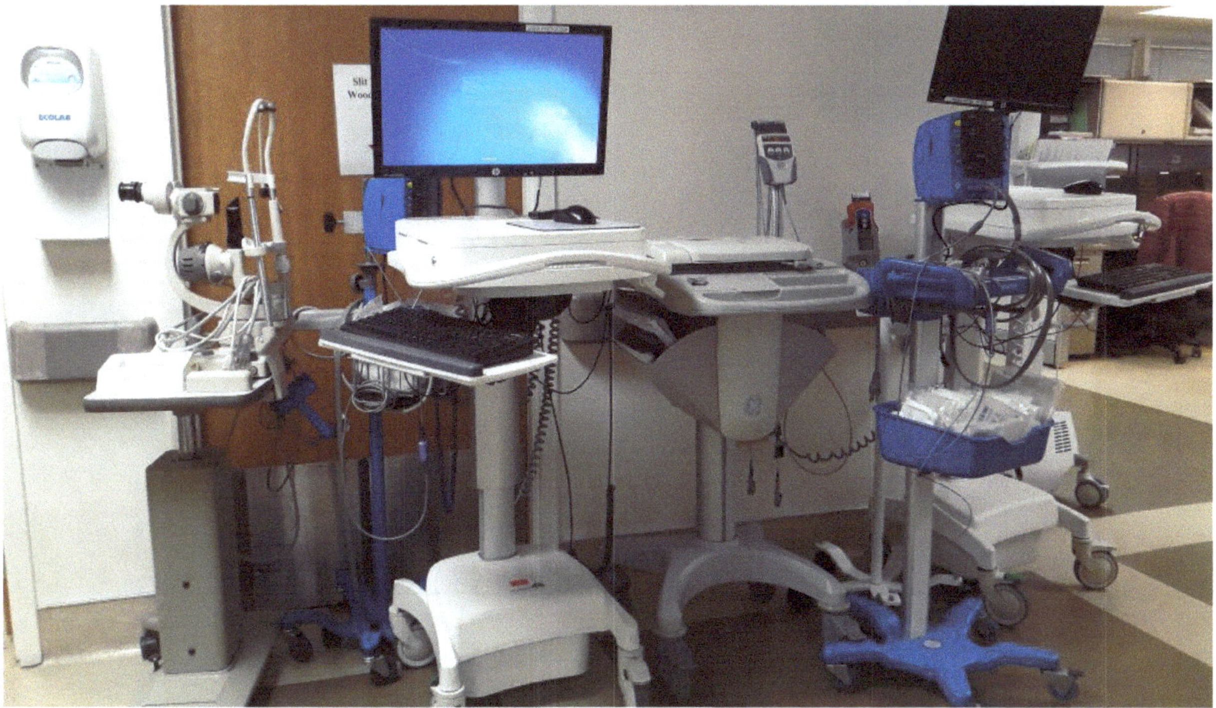

FIGURE 8.3 Health Care Technology

Medical technologies, especially new ones, must justify their costs in a climate of competing claims on limited resources. Resource allocation follows American society's objective of cost effectiveness: if a new technology improves health outcomes at a lower cost than existing technologies, it should be adopted; otherwise, it should not.[12]

Increased Prescription Medication Costs

Retail prices for commonly-used prescription medications continue to increase twice as much as inflation, contributing to increased health care costs and making these life-sustaining medicines potentially unaffordable to many Americans. According to a recent AARP *Rx Price Watch* report, in 2020 prices for 260 commonly used medications increased 2.9 percent while the general rate of inflation was 1.3 percent.[13] For

10. Neumann, P. J., & Weinstein, M. C. (1991). The diffusion of new technology: Costs and benefits to health care. In Institute of Medicine (US) Committee on Technological Innovation in Medicine, Gelijns, A. C., & Halm, E. A. (Eds.). *The changing economics of medical technology.* National Academies Press. https://www.ncbi.nlm.nih.gov/books/NBK234309/
11. "49458105981_fe87fd521c_o.jpg" by Wonderlane is licensed under CC BY 2.0
12. Neumann, P. J., & Weinstein, M. C. (1991). The diffusion of new technology: Costs and benefits to health care. In Institute of Medicine (US) Committee on Technological Innovation in Medicine, Gelijns, A. C., & Halm, E. A. (Eds.). *The changing economics of medical technology.* National Academies Press. https://www.ncbi.nlm.nih.gov/books/NBK234309/
13. Bunis, D. (2021). *Prescription drug price increases continue to outpace inflation.* AARP. https://www.aarp.org/politics-society/advocacy/info-2021/prescription-price-increase-report.html

example, the cost of Symbicort, a medication used to treat asthma and COPD, increased 46 percent, from \$2,940 to \$4,282.[14] See Figure 8.4[15] for an illustration related to prescription medication costs.

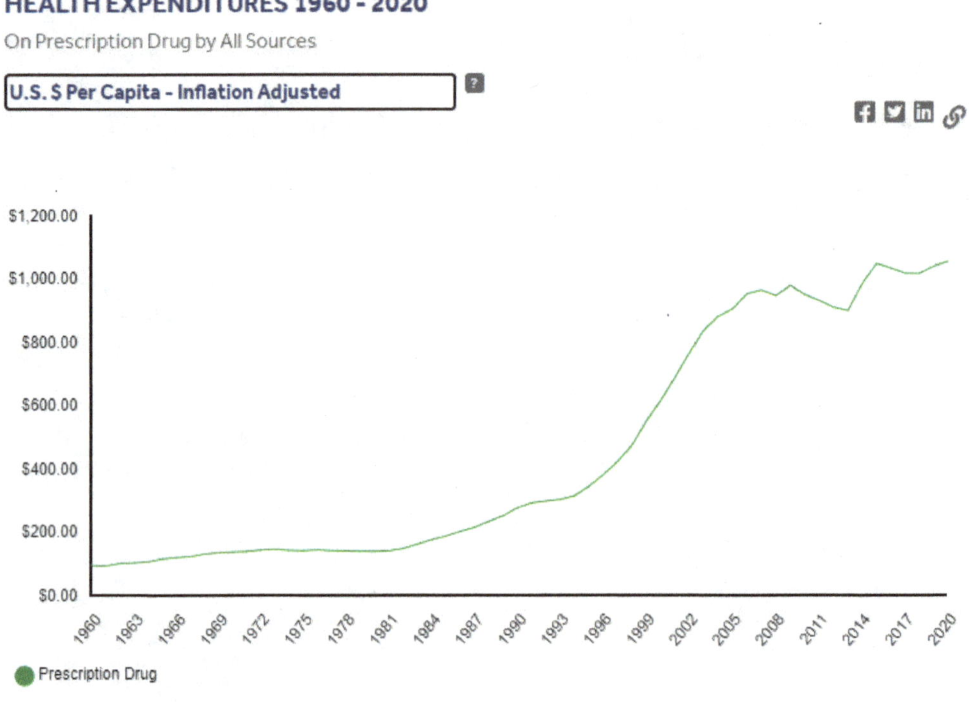

FIGURE 8.4 Prescription Medication Costs

Although the majority of Americans have either public or private insurance that helps them pay for medications, increased medication prices result in higher health insurance premiums and higher taxpayer costs for the Medicare and Medicaid programs. Some insurance companies only cover approved formulary medications. As a result, national organizations like the American Association of Retired Persons (AARP) advocate for national policy changes, such as allowing Medicare to negotiate the prices of prescription medications with drug companies and allowing private insurance plans to have access to those lower prices.[16]

Many consumers find themselves tasked with the difficult decision of purchasing expensive medication or going without prescribed medication and paying for their families' housing and food. Nurses often become involved in case management activities when assisting clients to obtain medications they cannot afford. Nursing case management activities are discussed later in this chapter.

14. Bunis, D. (2021). *Prescription drug price increases continue to outpace inflation.* AARP. https://www.aarp.org/politics-society/advocacy/info-2021/prescription-price-increase-report.html

15. Peterson_KFF Health Systems Tracker. (n.d.). *Health expenditures 1960-2020.* https://www.healthsystemtracker.org/health-spending-explorer/?outputType=%24pop-adjusted&serviceType%5B0%5D=prescriptionDrug&serviceType%5B1%5D=hospitals&serviceType%5B2%5D=allTypes&sourceOfFunds%5B0%5D=allSources&tab=0&yearCompare%5B0%5D=%2A&yearCompare%5B1%5D=%2A&yearRange%5B0%5D=%2A&yearRange%5B1%5D=%2A&yearSingle=%2A&yearType=range

16. Bunis, D. (2021). *Prescription drug price increases continue to outpace inflation.* AARP. https://www.aarp.org/politics-society/advocacy/info-2021/prescription-price-increase-report.html

Affordable Care Act

The Patient Protection and Affordable Care Act (PPACA), also known as the **Affordable Care Act (ACA)** or Obamacare, was signed into law in 2010. The purpose of this legislation was to increase consumers' access to health care coverage and protect them from insurance practices that restricted care or significantly increased the cost of care. The ACA mandated health insurance coverage for employers and individuals. Employers were mandated to provide health care coverage based on the number of their employees, and individuals who were not covered through employer insurance plans were mandated to seek coverage through a newly created Marketplace. The Marketplace provides a central, website that offers three standard health insurance coverage levels to facilitate comparison by consumers. As a result of the ACA and associated Medicaid expansion, 32 million people had health care coverage in 2021.[17]

Read about the Affordable Care Act at HHS.gov. Access supplementary digital content in the online book using this QR code.

Key Provisions of the ACA

The ACA includes the following key provisions[18]:

- Insurers can no longer deny coverage or care for preexisting conditions like diabetes, asthma, and cancer.
- Young adults may remain on their parents' insurance plans until they are 26 (even if they are married, financially independent, or not living with their parents).
- Health insurance plans cannot place annual or lifetime limits on coverage, except for nonessential exceptions, such as cosmetic procedures.
- Many preventive services must be provided, such as:
  - Well-child visits, flu shots, and other common vaccines
  - Screening tests for blood pressure and diabetes
  - Diagnostic screening tests, such mammograms and colonoscopies
  - Counseling services related to mental health and substance use

The ACA also provides an avenue for consumers to appeal insurance companies' denials for care or payment of services and restricts situations in which an insurance carrier may cancel a policy.

17. HealthCare.gov. *Insurance marketplace.* https://www.healthcare.gov/subscribe/?gclid=Cj0KCQjwiqWHBhD2ARIsAPCDzamNRkS3URx_uUvJGdpX15DrZnVbBadXbPmOjBBlLyjtZBn7cLei6WEaAl8GEALw_wcB&gclsrc=aw.ds

18. HHS.gov. *About the Affordable Care Act.* U.S. Department of Health & Human Services. https://www.hhs.gov/healthcare/about-the-aca/index.html

Challenges to the ACA

Although the ACA has significantly increased the number of Americans with health insurance coverage, it continues to be debated. Debates focus on increased taxes, increased insurance premiums, and some people's belief that mandated coverage is governmental intrusion on an individual's rights. The Affordable Care Act has been challenged three times without success. In 2012 the U. S. Supreme Court upheld mandated coverage as a constitutional exercise of Congress' taxing powers because it could be interpreted as an individual's choice to maintain health insurance or pay a tax. However, in 2017 Congress set the penalty for failing to comply with the mandate at zero dollars after multiple attempts to repeal and replace the ACA. In June 2021 the U.S. Supreme Court rejected a third major challenge regarding the constitutionality of the ACA. In a 7-to-2 decision, the U.S. Supreme Court upheld the ACA based on the judgment that the states who brought forth the case did not prove damage to citizens because the fines for not having health coverage had been eliminated since the original legislation was passed.[19]

What to Expect Next

Given the Supreme Court's recent decision regarding the ACA, it is expected the current administration will continue to advocate for the ACA and work towards making ACA tax credits permanent. Congress is also actively debating other legislative proposals to reduce health care costs, such as medication pricing reform and expanding Medicare eligibility age and benefits.[20]

Social Determinants of Health

Social Determinants of Health (SDOH) are the conditions in the environments where people live, learn, work, and play that affect a wide range of outcomes. SDOH include health care access and quality, neighborhood and environment, social and community context, economic stability, and education access and quality. These conditions have a major impact on people's health and well-being, ultimately affecting national health care costs.[21]

SDOH directly impact individuals' health behaviors, their access to routine health care, and development of chronic disease. Yet, the United States spends a significantly lower percentage of its gross domestic product (GDP) on social services as compared to similar countries with better health outcomes.[22]

Healthy People 2030, established by the U.S. Department of Health and Human Services, identifies public health priorities to help individuals, organizations, and communities across the United States improve health and well-being over the next decade by addressing SDOH. One of Healthy People 2030's goals states, "Create social, physical, and economic environments that promote attaining the full potential for health and

19. K&L Gates LLP, Carnevale, A., Hamscho, V., Lawless, T., & Sha Page, K. (2021). *The Affordable Care Act survives Supreme Court challenge: What happens next?* JD Supra. https://www.jdsupra.com/legalnews/the-affordable-care-act-survives-3115372/
20. K&L Gates LLP, Carnevale, A., Hamscho, V., Lawless, T., & Sha Page, K. (2021). *The Affordable Care Act survives Supreme Court challenge: What happens next?* JD Supra. https://www.jdsupra.com/legalnews/the-affordable-care-act-survives-3115372/
21. Healthy People 2030. (n.d.). *Social determinants of health*. U.S. Department of Health and Human Services. https://health.gov/healthypeople/objectives-and-data/social-determinants-health
22. Bush, M. (2018). Addressing the root cause: Rising health care costs and social determinants of health. *North Carolina Medical Journal. 79*(1), 26-29. https://www.ncmedicaljournal.com/content/79/1/26

well-being for all."[23] Nurses act in many ways to address these priorities as they advocate for individuals, families, and communities.

Read more about efforts addressing SDOH for improved economic stability and health care access in Healthy People 2020. Access supplementary digital content in the online book using this QR code.

SDOH Case Study

Maria's Journey Through the Health Care System *(Answers are located in the answer key at the back of the book)*

Maria, a 45-year-old woman, lives in a low-income neighborhood in a large urban area. She works two part-time jobs to support her family of four and has limited access to health care due to financial constraints and transportation issues. Maria has been diagnosed with type 2 diabetes, and her health care outcomes are significantly influenced by various Social Determinants of Health (SDOH).

Maria's low income and unstable employment contribute to her inability to afford healthy food, medications, and regular medical check-ups. This economic instability exacerbates her diabetes, as she often skips doses of her medication to save money and cannot afford nutritious meals that would help manage her condition. The constant stress of making ends meet and providing for her family leads to increased cortisol levels, which can negatively impact her blood sugar control.

1. How can Maria's financial stress impact her ability to manage her diabetes effectively?

2. What programs or policies could be implemented to assist individuals like Maria in managing their health care costs?

Maria has limited knowledge about diabetes management due to a lack of education and access to health information. This impacts her ability to understand and implement lifestyle changes or adhere to treatment plans. With limited education, Maria struggles to find better-paying jobs that could provide health insurance and more financial stability.

3. In what ways can improved health literacy impact Maria's diabetes management?

4. What community resources could be made available to enhance health education for individuals in Maria's situation?

---

23. Healthy People 2030. (n.d.). *Social determinants of health*. U.S. Department of Health and Human Services. https://health.gov/healthypeople/objectives-and-data/social-determinants-health

The availability of health care services in Maria's neighborhood is limited, with long wait times and fewer specialists. This results in delayed diagnoses and treatments for her diabetes-related complications. Maria lacks comprehensive health insurance, making it difficult for her to access primary and specialist care. High out-of-pocket costs deter her from seeking regular medical attention.

5. How does the lack of accessible health care services affect Maria's long-term health outcomes?

6. What are some potential solutions to improve health care access in underserved areas?

Maria lives in a food desert with limited access to fresh fruits and vegetables. She often relies on inexpensive, processed foods that worsen her diabetes. Public transportation in Maria's area is unreliable, making it challenging for her to attend medical appointments. This lack of transportation contributes to missed check-ups and unmanaged diabetes.

7. How does living in a food desert affect Maria's ability to manage her diabetes?

8. What transportation initiatives could help individuals like Maria access healthcare services more easily?

Maria has a limited social network and lacks support from friends and family, which is crucial for managing a chronic condition like diabetes. This isolation can lead to depression and further neglect of her health. Living in a high-crime area, Maria feels unsafe walking outside for exercise, which is essential for diabetes management. This sedentary lifestyle negatively affects her health outcomes.

9. How does a lack of social support contribute to Maria's health challenges?

10. What community programs or interventions could be implemented to enhance social support and safety in high-crime areas?

8.3 HEALTH CARE FUNDING

Health care costs impact both macroeconomics (affecting the entire country and society as a whole) and microeconomics (affecting the financial decisions of businesses and individuals). Health care services are funded by several payment models, including federal government programs (e.g., Medicare and Medicaid), private health insurance (typically provided by employers), and self-pay. Payment models also impact services provided by health care agencies, as well as the services and medications available to consumers. Nurses must be aware of these payment models because of the impact on the allocation of resources they need to provide client care.

Government Funding

Medicare and Medicaid were signed into law in 1965. These programs provide eligible Americans support for their health care needs with taxpayer funding.

Medicare

Medicare is a federal health insurance program used by people aged 65 and older, younger individuals with permanent disabilities, and people with end-stage renal disease requiring dialysis or kidney transplantation. Medicare coverage has four possible components: Part A, Part B, Part C, and Part D.[24] See Figure 8.5[25] for an infographic illustrating Medicare Parts A, B, C, and D.

- **Part A (Hospital Insurance):** Part A covers clients' hospital stays, skilled nursing facility care, hospice care, and some home health care. Part A is free for clients if they or their spouse paid Medicare taxes for a specific amount of time while working. If clients are not eligible for free coverage, they can buy it with premiums based on the number of months they paid Medicare taxes.
- **Part B (Medical Insurance):** Part B covers doctors' services, outpatient care, medical supplies, and preventative care services. Most people pay a standard premium for Part B.
- **Part C (Medicare Advantage Plan):** A Medicare Advantage Plan is a health plan choice offered by private companies approved by Medicare, also referred to as "Part C." These plans provide Part A and Part B coverage, and most also include Part D coverage. Medicare Advantage Plans may offer extra coverage, such as vision, hearing, dental, and/or health and wellness programs.
- **Part D (Prescription Drug Coverage):** Part D helps cover the cost of prescription drugs and vaccinations. To get Medicare drug coverage, clients must enroll in a Medicare-approved plan that offers drug coverage. Different plans vary in cost and what prescription medications they cover, also referred to as a formulary.

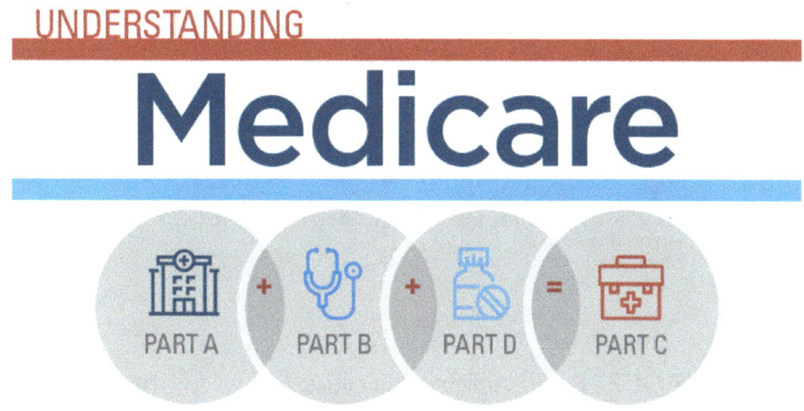

FIGURE 8.5 Medicare

24. Medicare.gov. *What's Medicare?* https://www.medicare.gov/what-medicare-covers/your-medicare-coverage-choices/whats-medicare
25. "Understanding_of_medicare.png" by Samreen Al is licensed under CC BY-SA 4.0

Read more about Medicare at medicare.gov. Access supplementary digital content in the online book using this QR code.

Medicaid

Medicaid is the largest source of health coverage in the United States. It is a joint federal and state program covering eligible individuals with taxpayer funding. To participate in Medicaid, federal law requires states to cover certain groups of individuals, such as low-income families, qualified pregnant women and children, and individuals receiving Supplemental Security Income (SSI). States may choose to cover additional groups, such as individuals receiving home and community-based services and children in foster care who are not otherwise eligible.[26]

In 2014 the Affordable Care Act expanded Medicaid to cover all low-income Americans under the age of 65 years and also expanded coverage for children. Due to the individual states' involvement in Medicaid, coverage of services varies from state to state.[27] See Figure 8.6[28] for an illustration of Medicaid-eligible populations.

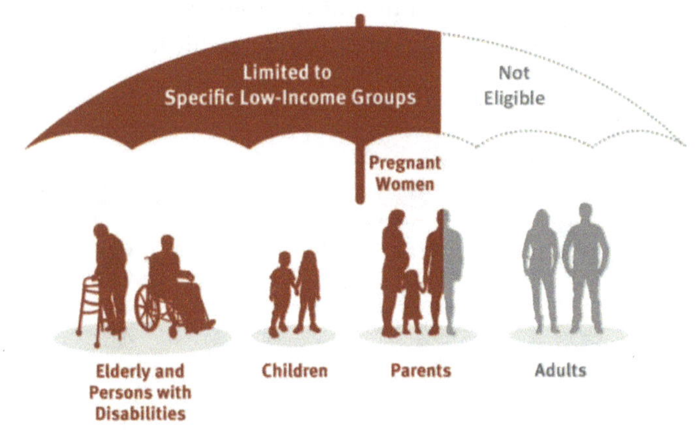

FIGURE 8.6 Medicaid-Eligible Populations

Individuals with Medicaid plans have support in paying for a variety of health services, including hospital care, laboratory and diagnostic testing, skilled nursing care, home health services, preventative care, and regular outpatient provider visits.

26. Medicaid.gov. *Eligibility.* https://www.medicaid.gov/medicaid/eligibility/index.html
27. Healthcare.gov. *Affordable Care Act.* https://www.healthcare.gov/glossary/affordable-care-act/
28. "Medicaid.expansion-1200x846.png" by KFF is licensed under CC BY-NC-ND 4.0

Read more about Medicaid at medicaid.gov. Access supplementary digital content in the online book using this QR code.

Other Government Health Funding

There are several other types of health coverage provided by federal and state programs. Read more about these programs in the following box.

Other Federal and State Health Care Funding Programs[29]

- **State Children's Health Insurance Program (CHIP):** A program designed to help provide coverage for uninsured children whose family income is below average but too high to qualify for Medicaid. The federal government provides matching funds to states for health insurance for these families. Read more details at InsuredKidsNow.gov.
- **Children and Youth With Special Health Care Needs:** This program coordinates funding and resources to provide care to people with special health needs. Read more details at Children With Special Health Care Needs.
- **Tricare:** This program covers about 9 million active duty and retired military personnel and their families. Read more details at TRICARE.
- **Veterans Health Administration (VHA):** This government-operated health care system provides comprehensive health services to eligible military veterans. About 9 million veterans are enrolled. Read more details at Veterans Health Administration.
- **Indian Health Service:** This system of government hospitals and clinics provides health services to about 2 million Native Americans living on or near a reservation. Read more details at Indian Health Service.
- **Federal Employee Health Benefits (FEHB) Program:** This program allows private insurers to offer insurance plans within guidelines set by the government for the benefit of active and retired federal employees and their survivors. Read more details at the Federal Employees Health Benefits (FEHB) Program.
- **Refugee Health Promotion Program:** This program provides short-term health insurance to newly arrived refugees. Read more details at Refugee Health Promotion Program (RHP).

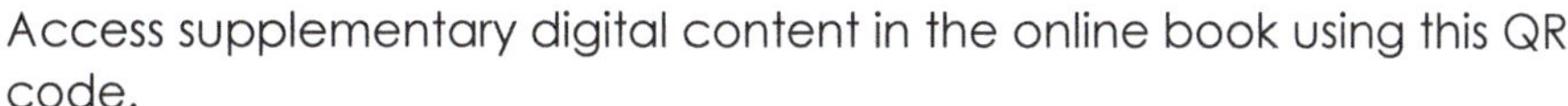

Access supplementary digital content in the online book using this QR code.

29. Schreck, R. I. (2020). *Overview of health care financing.* Merck Manual Consumer Version. https://www.merckmanuals.com/home/fundamentals/financial-issues-in-health-care/overview-of-health-care-financing

Private Insurance

Individuals who are not eligible for government-funded health programs like Medicare or Medicaid can purchase private health insurance. Many individuals with private insurance obtain coverage through their employers' benefit packages, where the costs for coverage are shared between the employer and the employee. If an individual does not receive health insurance through their employer, they may purchase it from the Marketplace established by the Affordable Care Act.

Read more about obtaining health insurance through the ACA Marketplace at healthcare.gov. Access supplementary digital content in the online book using this QR code.

Self-Pay

Some individuals do not have health care coverage provided by their employer, do not qualify for Medicare or Medicaid, and do not elect to purchase health insurance coverage. Instead, these individuals go without coverage and pay health care costs as they arise. See Figure 8.7[30] for a graph illustrating the decreasing numbers of uninsured consumers in the United States over the past several decades. Unfortunately, due to the skyrocketing cost of health care services, significant bills can accrue from a single serious illness or traumatic injury that can put consumers without health care coverage in jeopardy of bankruptcy. Nurses can assist uninsured individuals to better understand coverage options by referring them to a case manager or social worker.

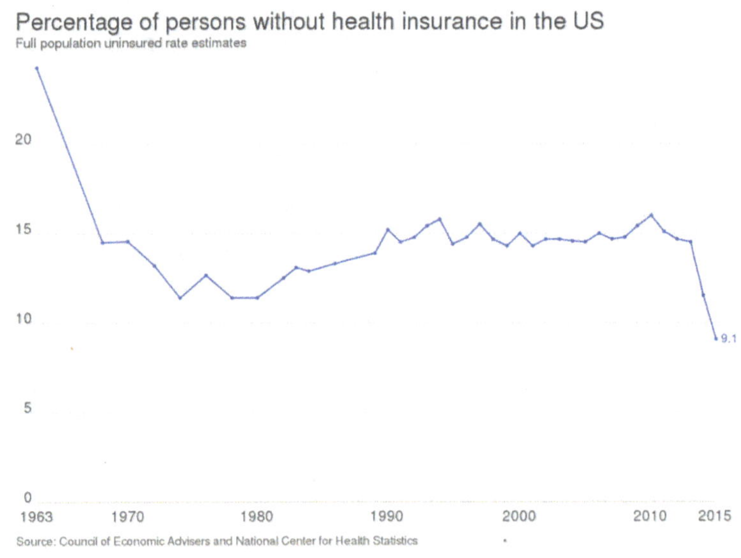

FIGURE 8.7 Uninsured Individuals

30. "Percentage_of_persons_without_health_insurance_in_the_US,_OWID.svg" by Our World In Data is licensed under CC BY 3.0

Types of Insurance Coverage

Health insurance plans have different types of coverage. Common types of health insurance plans are HMO, PPO, POS, HDHP, or HSA.

- **Health Maintenance Organization (HMO):** HMO plans usually have the lowest monthly cost for coverage (i.e., premium) but also have a smaller network of providers and hospitals where the consumer may receive insured care. This means the consumer is restricted to receive care only from specific providers and health facilities. Many HMOs also require the consumer to see their primary care provider to request a referral to see a specialist, which may or may not be approved by the HMO. Additionally, many tests, procedures, surgeries, and medications require "preauthorization" by the HMO, which may or may not be approved. Due to these restrictions, consumers may find they sacrifice flexibility and choice for lower cost of coverage.[31]
- **Preferred Provider Organization (PPO):** PPO plans are typically less restrictive than HMOs. PPOs typically include "in-network" providers and hospitals where costs are lower if care is received in-network, but consumers also have a choice to receive "out-of-network" care at a higher cost. Referrals from a primary care provider are not generally required in a PPO. The monthly premium for a PPO plan is typically higher than an HMO plan, but PPOs allow more consumer flexibility in choosing their health care providers.[32]
- **Point of Service (POS):** POS plans are a combination of HMO and PPO plans, where the insured consumer has a preferred provider network to receive health care services at a lower cost, but also has the flexibility to receive care outside of their network. When consumers venture outside of the network, they often have to pay a significant share of the cost.[33]
- **High Deductible Health Plan (HDHP):** HDHP plans are often popular for younger individuals without chronic health care needs who spend little on health care but require coverage in the event a high-cost injury or illness occurs. HDHPs typically have lower monthly premiums but require the individual to pay more upfront for health care services before the coverage kicks in (referred to as a "deductible"). Individuals with an HDHP often have an associated Health Savings Account (HSA). HDHPs have grown in popularity as more employers offer these plans in an attempt to contain health care costs by shifting more cost-sharing to the consumer.
- **Health Savings Account (HSA):** An HSA is a special account reserved for eligible medical expenses with strict usage rules. Money placed in an HSA can often be deducted from a consumer's pretaxed pay, resulting in tax savings. In addition to purchasing items like glasses, contacts, and over-the-counter medications, HSAs can often be used to pay for deductibles. Some employers deposit a specified amount of money into an employee's HSA every year to help reimburse high deductibles.

Deductible and Copays

Costs paid by an insured individual are commonly referred to as "out-of-pocket expenses." Out-of-pocket expenses include deductibles and co-pays. A **deductible** is the amount of money a consumer pays before the health care plan pays anything. Deductibles generally apply per person per calendar year. Typically, a PPO has higher premiums but lower deductibles than a HDHP.

31. Healthcare.gov (2024). *How to pick a health insurance plan.* https://www.healthcare.gov/choose-a-plan/plan-types/#top
32. Healthcare.gov (2024). *How to pick a health insurance plan.* https://www.healthcare.gov/choose-a-plan/plan-types/#top
33. Healthcare.gov (2024). *How to pick a health insurance plan.* https://www.healthcare.gov/choose-a-plan/plan-types/#top

A **co-pay** is a flat fee the consumer pays at the time of the health care service. For example, when visiting a primary provider, the consumer may pay $20 to the provider at each visit as a co-pay. Some health care plans require co-pays in addition to deductibles.

Nursing Considerations

Understanding a client's health insurance coverage is important because it may impact their choice of health services and their ability to purchase medications and other supplies. Additionally, if a client is self-pay, it is helpful to refer them to resources such as case managers, social workers, or the financial department of the agency. These resources can assist them in obtaining affordable health care coverage through the ACA Marketplace or other government programs.

8.4 HEALTH CARE REIMBURSEMENT MODELS

As discussed in the previous section, hospitals and health care providers are paid for services provided to individuals by government insurance programs (such as Medicare and Medicaid), private insurance companies, or people using their out-of-pocket funds. Traditionally, health care institutions were paid based on a "fee-for-service" model. For example, if a client was admitted to a hospital with pneumonia, the hospital billed that individual's insurance program for the cost of care.

However, as part of a recent national strategy to reduce health care costs, insurance providers have transitioned to "Pay for Performance" reimbursement models that are based on overall agency performance and client outcomes.

Pay for Performance

Pay for Performance, also known as value-based payment, refers to reimbursement models that attach financial incentives to the performance of health care agencies and providers. Pay for Performance models tie higher reimbursement payments to positive client outcomes, best practices, and client satisfaction, thus aligning payment with value and quality.[34] Nurses support higher reimbursement levels to their employers based on their documentation related to nursing care plans and achievement of expected client outcomes.

There are two Pay for Performance models. The first model rewards hospitals and providers with higher reimbursement payments based on how well they perform on process, quality, and efficiency measures. The second model penalizes hospitals and providers for subpar performance by reducing reimbursement amounts.[35] For example, Medicare no longer reimburses hospitals to treat clients who acquire certain preventable conditions during their hospital stay, such as pressure injuries or urinary tract infections associated with use of catheters.[36]

34. Pay for Performance. (2018). *NEJM catalyst*. https://catalyst.nejm.org/doi/full/10.1056/CAT.18.0245
35. Pay for Performance. (2018). *NEJM catalyst*. https://catalyst.nejm.org/doi/full/10.1056/CAT.18.0245
36. James, J. (2012). *Pay-for-performance*. Health Affairs. https://www.healthaffairs.org/do/10.1377/hpb20121011.90233/full/

The Centers for Medicare and Medicaid Services (CMS), spurred by the Affordable Care Act, has led the way in value-based payment with a variety of payment models. CMS is the largest health care funder in the United States with almost 40% of overall health care spending for Medicare and Medicaid. CMS developed three Pay for Performance models that impact hospitals' reimbursement by Medicare. These models are called the Hospital Value-Based Purchasing Program, the Hospital Readmissions Reduction Program, and the Hospital-Acquired Condition Reduction Program. Private insurers are also committed to performance-based payment models. In 2017 *Forbes* reported that almost 50% of insurers' reimbursements were in the form of value-based care models.[37]

HOSPITAL VALUE-BASED PURCHASING PROGRAM

The Hospital Value-Based Purchasing Program (VBP) was designed to improve health care quality and client experience by using financial incentives that encourage hospitals to follow established best clinical practices and improve client satisfaction scores via client satisfaction surveys. Reimbursement is based on hospital performance on measures divided into four quality domains: safety, clinical care, efficiency and cost reduction, and client and caregiver-centered experience.[38] The VBP program rewards hospitals based on the quality of care provided to Medicare clients and not just the quantity of services that are provided. Hospitals may have their Medicaid payments reduced by up to 2% if not meeting the quality metrics.

Read more about client satisfaction surveys. Access supplementary digital content in the online book using this QR code.

HOSPITAL READMISSIONS REDUCTION PROGRAM

The Hospital Readmissions Reduction Program (HRRP) penalizes hospitals with higher rates of client readmissions compared to other hospitals. HRRP was established by the Affordable Care Act and applies to clients with specific conditions, such as heart attacks, heart failure, pneumonia, chronic obstructive pulmonary disease (COPD), hip or knee replacements, and coronary bypass surgery. Hospitals with poor performance receive a 3% reduction of their Medicare payments. However, it was discovered that hospitals with higher proportions of low-income clients were penalized the most, so Congress passed legislation in 2019 that divided hospitals into groups for comparison based on the socioeconomic status of their client populations.[39]

HOSPITAL-ACQUIRED CONDITION REDUCTION PROGRAM

The Hospital-Acquired Condition Reduction Program (HACRP) was established by the Affordable Care Act. This Pay for Performance model reduces payments to hospitals based on poor performance regarding client safety and hospital-acquired conditions, such as surgical site infections, hip fractures resulting from falls, and pressure injuries. This model has saved Medicare approximately $350 million per year.[40]

37. Pay for Performance. (2018). *NEJM catalyst*. https://catalyst.nejm.org/doi/full/10.1056/CAT.18.0245
38. Pay for Performance. (2018). *NEJM catalyst*. https://catalyst.nejm.org/doi/full/10.1056/CAT.18.0245
39. Pay for Performance. (2018). *NEJM catalyst*. https://catalyst.nejm.org/doi/full/10.1056/CAT.18.0245
40. Pay for Performance. (2018). *NEJM catalyst*. https://catalyst.nejm.org/doi/full/10.1056/CAT.18.0245

The HACRP model measures the incidence of hospital-acquired conditions, including central line-associated bloodstream infections (CLABSI), catheter-associated urinary tract infections (CAUTI), surgical site infections (SSI), *Methicillin-Resistant Staphylococcus Aureus* (MRSA), and *Clostridium Difficile* (C. diff).[41] As a result, nurses have seen changes in daily practices based on evidence-based practices related to these conditions. For example, stringent documentation is now required for clients with Foley catheters that indicates continued need and associated infection control measures.

OTHER CMS PAY FOR PERFORMANCE MODELS

CMS has created other value-based payment programs for agencies other than hospitals, including the End-Stage Renal Disease (ESRD) Quality Initiative Program, the Skilled Nursing Facility Value-Based Program (SNFVBP), the Home Health Value-Based Program (HHVBP), and the Value Modifier (VM) Program. The VM program is aimed at Medicare Part B providers who receive high, average, or low ratings based on quality and cost measurements as compared to peer agencies.

Impacts of Value-Based Payment

Pay for Performance (i.e., value-based payment) stresses quality over quantity of care and allows health care payers to use reimbursement to encourage best clinical practices and promote positive health outcomes. It focuses on transparency by using metrics that are publicly reported, thus incentivizing organizations to protect and strengthen their reputations. In this manner, Pay for Performance models encourage accountability and consumer-informed choice.[42] See Figure 8.8[43] for an illustration of Pay for Performance.

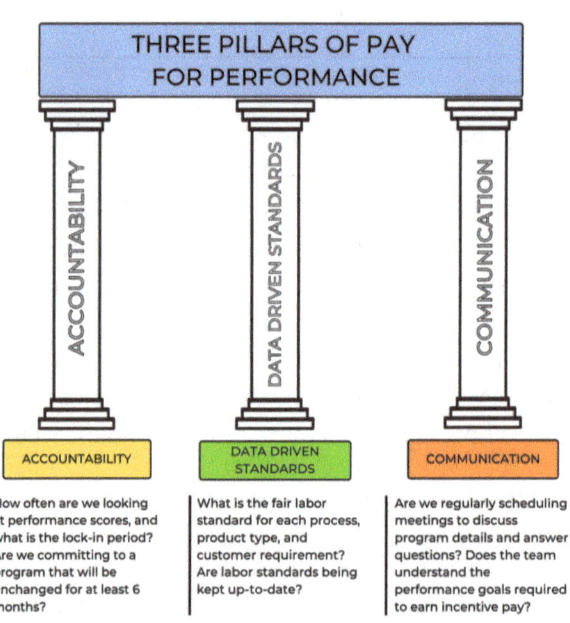

FIGURE 8.8 Pay for Performance

41. Pay for Performance. (2018). *NEJM catalyst.* https://catalyst.nejm.org/doi/full/10.1056/CAT.18.0245
42. Pay for Performance. (2018). *NEJM catalyst.* https://catalyst.nejm.org/doi/full/10.1056/CAT.18.0245
43. "Pillars of Pay Performance.png" by Meredith Pomietlo for Chippewa Valley Technical College is licensed under CC BY 4.0

Pay for Performance models have reduced health care costs and decreased the incidence of poor client outcomes. For example, 30-day hospital readmission rates have been falling since 2012, indicating HRRP and HACRP are having an impact.[44]

However, there are also disadvantages to value-based payment. As previously discussed, initial research indicated hospitals with higher proportions of low-income clients were being penalized the most, resulting in additional legislation to compare hospital performance in groups based on their clients' socioeconomic status. Nursing leaders continue to emphasize strategies that further address social determinants of health and promote health equity.[45] Read more about equity and social determinants of health in the following subsection.

Nursing Considerations

Nurses have a direct impact on activities related to quality care and reimbursement rates received by their employer. There are several categories of actions nurses can take to improve quality client care, reduce costs, and improve reimbursement. By incorporating these actions into their daily care, nurses can help ensure the funding they need to provide quality client care is received by their employer and resources are allocated appropriately to their clients.

The following categories of actions to improve quality of care are based on the Institute of Medicine (IOM) report *To Err Is Human: Building a Safer Health Care System and Crossing the Quality Chasm*[46]:

- **Effectiveness and Efficiency:** Nurses support their institution's effectiveness and efficiency with individualized nursing care planning, good documentation, and care coordination. With accurate and timely documentation and care coordination, there is reduced care duplication and waste. Coordinating care also helps to reduce the risk of hospital readmissions.
- **Timeliness:** Nurses positively impact timeliness by prioritizing and delegating care. This helps reduce client wait times and delays in care. Read more about these concepts in the "Delegation and Supervision" and "Prioritization" chapters in this book.
- **Safety:** Nurses pay attention to their clients' changing conditions and effectively communicate these changes with appropriate health care team members. They take any concerns about client care up the chain of command until their concerns are resolved.
- **Client-Centered Care:** Nurses support this quality measure by ensuring nursing care plans are individualized for each client. Effective care plans can improve client compliance, resulting in improved client outcomes.
- **Evidence-Based Practice:** Nurses provide care based on evidence-based practice. **Evidence-Based Practice (EBP)** is defined by the American Nurses Association as, "A lifelong problem-solving approach that integrates the best evidence from well-designed research studies and evidence-based theories; clinical expertise and evidence from assessment of the health care consumer's history and condition, as well

44. Pay for Performance. (2018). *NEJM catalyst.* https://catalyst.nejm.org/doi/full/10.1056/CAT.18.0245
45. Pay for Performance. (2018). *NEJM catalyst.* https://catalyst.nejm.org/doi/full/10.1056/CAT.18.0245
46. Avalere Health LLC. (2015). *Optimal nurse staffing to improve quality of care and patient outcomes: Executive summary* [White paper]. https://cdn2.hubspot.net/hubfs/4850206/ANA/NurseStaffingWhitePaper_Final.pdf?__hstc=53609399.b25284991e95c5d4f1c55a49e826489f.1612299494138.1628353446072.1628356381954.16&__hssc=53609399.3.1628356381954&__hsfp=1865500357

as health care resources; and client, family, group, community, and population preferences and values."[47] EBP is a component of *Scholarly Inquiry*, one of the ANA's Standards of Professional Practice. Nurses' implementation of EBP ensures proper resources are allocated to the appropriate clients. EBP promotes safe, efficient, and effective health care.[48,49] Read more information about EBP in the "Quality and Evidence-Based Practice" chapter of this book.

- **Equity:** Health care institutions care for all members of their community regardless of client demographics and their associated **social determinants of health (SDOH)**. SDOH are conditions in the places where people live, learn, work, and play that affect a wide range of health risks and outcomes. Health disparities in communities with poor SDOH have been consistently documented in reports by the Agency for Healthcare Research and Quality (AHRQ).[50]

Nurses address negative determinants of health by advocating for interventions that reduce health disparities and promote the delivery of equitable health care resources. The term **health disparities** describes the differences in health outcomes that result from SDOH. Advocating for resources that enhance quality of life can significantly influence a community's health outcomes. Examples of resources that promote health include safe and affordable housing, access to education, public safety, availability of healthy foods, local emergency/health services, and environments free of life-threatening toxins.

A related term is **health care disparity** that refers to differences in access to health care and insurance coverage. Health disparities and health care disparities can lead to decreased quality of life, increased personal costs, and lower life expectancy. More broadly, these disparities also translate to greater societal costs, such as the financial burden of uncontrolled chronic illnesses. An example of nurses addressing health care disparities are nurse practitioners providing health care according to their scope of practice to underserved populations in rural communities.

The ANA promotes nurse advocacy in workplaces and local communities. There are many ways nurses can promote health and wellness within their communities through a variety of advocacy programs at the federal, state, and community level.[51] Read more information in the "Advocacy" chapter of this book. Read more about advocacy and reducing health disparities in the following boxes.

Read more about ANA Policy and Advocacy. Access supplementary digital content in the online book using this QR code.

47. American Nurses Association. (2021). *Nursing: Scope and standards of practice* (4th ed.). American Nurses Association.
48. American Nurses Association. (2021). *Nursing: Scope and standards of practice* (4th ed.). American Nurses Association.
49. Stevens, K. (2013). The impact of evidence-based practice in nursing and the next big ideas. *OJIN: The Online Journal of Issues in Nursing, 18*(2). https://ojin.nursingworld.org/MainMenuCategories/ANAMarketplace/ANAPeriodicals/OJIN/TableofContents/Vol-18-2013/No2-May-2013/Impact-of-Evidence-Based-Practice.html
50. Centers for Disease Control and Prevention. (2020, May 6). *Social determinants of health: Know what affects health.* https://www.cdc.gov/socialdeterminants/index.htm
51. Agency for Healthcare Research and Quality. (2021). *2019 national healthcare quality and disparities report.* https://www.ahrq.gov/research/findings/nhqrdr/nhqdr19/index.html

Read more about addressing health disparities in the "Diverse Patients" chapter in Open RN *Nursing Fundamentals, 2e*. Access supplementary digital content in the online book using this QR code.

8.5 BUDGETS AND STAFFING

Economics and health care reimbursement models impact health care institutional budgets that ultimately impact nurse staffing. A **budget** is an estimate of revenue and expenses over a specified period of time, usually over a year. There are two basic types of health care budgets that affect nursing: capital and operating budgets. **Capital budgets** are used to plan investments and upgrades to tangible assets that lose or gain value over time. Capital is something that can be touched, such as buildings or computers. **Operating budgets** include personnel costs and annual facility operating costs.[52] Typically 40% of the operating budgets of health care agencies are dedicated to nursing staffing. As a result, nursing is often targeted for reduced hours and other cutbacks.[53]

What is the value of a nurse? Nurses are priceless to the clients, families, and communities they serve, but health care organizations are tasked with calculating the cost of delivering safe, high-quality nursing care using affordable staffing models. All members of the health care team must understand the relationship between economics, resources, budgeting, and staffing, and how these issues affect their ability to provide safe, quality care to their clients.

As health care agencies continue to adapt to meet "Pay for Performance" reimbursement models and deliver cost-effective care to an aging population with complex health needs, many nurses are experiencing changes in staffing models.[54] Strategies implemented by agencies to facilitate cost-effective nurse staffing include acuity-based staffing, team nursing, mandatory overtime, floating, on call, and off with benefits. Agencies may also use agency nurses when nurse shortages occur.

Acuity-Based Staffing

Historically, inpatient staffing patterns focused on "nurse-to-client ratios" where a specific number of clients were assigned to each registered nurse during a shift. **Acuity-based staffing** is a client assignment model that takes into account the level of client care required based on the severity of a client's illness or condition. As a result of acuity-based staffing, the number of clients a nurse cares for often varies from shift to shift as the needs of the clients change. Acuity-based staffing promotes efficient use of resources by ensuring nurses have adequate time to care for complex clients. Read more information about acuity-based staffing in the "Prioritization" chapter.

52. American Nurses Association. (n.d.). *Nurse staffing*. https://www.nursingworld.org/practice-policy/nurse-staffing/#staffinfo
53. Kenton, W. (2024). *Capital budgeting*. Investopedia. https://www.investopedia.com/terms/c/capitalbudgeting.asp
54. American Nurses Association. (n.d.). *Nurse staffing*. https://www.nursingworld.org/practice-policy/nurse-staffing/#staffinfo

Team Nursing

Team nursing is a common staffing pattern that uses a combination of Registered Nurses (RNs), Licensed Practical/Vocational Nurses (LPN/VNs), and Unlicensed Assistive Personnel (UAP) to care for a group of clients. The RN is the leader of a nursing team, making assignments and delegating nursing care to other members of the team with appropriate supervision. Team nursing is an example of allocating human resources wisely to provide quality and cost-effective care. In order for team nursing to be successful, team members must use effective communication and organize their shift as a team. Read more about team nursing in the "Delegation and Supervision" chapter of this book.

Mandatory Overtime

When client numbers and acuity levels exceed the number of staff scheduled for a shift, nurses may experience mandatory overtime as an agency staffing tool. **Mandatory overtime** requires a nurse to stay and care for clients beyond their scheduled shift when there is a lack of nursing staff (often referred to as short staffing). The American Nurses Association recognizes mandatory overtime as a dangerous staffing practice because of client safety concerns related to overtired staff. Depending on state laws, nurses can be held liable for client abandonment or neglect charges for refusing to stay when mandated. Nurses should be aware of state and organizational policies related to mandatory overtime.[55]

Read more about ANA's advocacy for adequate nurse staffing. Access supplementary digital content in the online book using this QR code.

Floating

Floating is a common agency staffing strategy that asks nurses to temporarily work on a different unit to help cover a short-staffed shift. Floating can reduce personnel costs by reducing overtime payments for staff. It can also reduce nurse burnout occurring from working in an environment without enough personnel.

Nurses must be aware of their rights and responsibilities when asked to float because they are still held accountable for providing safe client care according to their state's Nurse Practice Act and professional standards of care. Before accepting a floating assignment, nurses should ensure the assignment is aligned with their skill set and they receive orientation to the new environment before caring for clients. If an error occurs and the nurse is held liable, the fact they received a floating assignment does not justify the error. As the ANA states, nurses don't just have the right to refuse a floating client assignment; they have the obligation to do so if it is unsafe.[56] The ANA has developed several questions to guide nurses through the decision process of accepting client assignments. Review these questions in the following box.

55. American Nurses Association. (n.d.). *Nurse staffing*. https://www.nursingworld.org/practice-policy/nurse-staffing/#staffinfo
56. American Nurses Association. (n.d.) *Top issues for staff nurses*. https://www.nursingworld.org/practice-policy/nurse-staffing/

ANA's Suggested Questions When Deciding on Accepting a Client Assignment[57]

- What is the assignment? Clarify what is expected; do not assume. Be certain about the details.
- What are the characteristics of the clients being assigned? Don't just respond to the number of clients assigned. Make a critical assessment of the needs of each client and their complexity and stability. Be aware of the resources available to meet those needs.
- Do you have the expertise to care for the clients? Always ask yourself if you are familiar with caring for the types of clients assigned? If this is a "float assignment," are you cross-trained to care for these clients? Is there a "buddy system" in place with staff who are familiar with the unit? If there is no cross-training or "buddy system," has the client load been modified accordingly?
- Do you have the experience and knowledge to manage the clients for whom you are being assigned care? If the answer to the question is "No," you have an obligation to articulate your limitations. Limitations in experience and knowledge may not require refusal of the assignment, but rather an agreement regarding supervision or a modification of the assignment to ensure client safety. If no accommodation for limitations is considered, the nurse has an obligation to refuse an assignment for which they lack education or experience.
- What is the geography of the assignment? Are you being asked to care for clients who are in close proximity for efficient management, or are the clients at opposite ends of the hall or in different units? If there are geographic difficulties, what resources are available to manage the situation? If the clients are in more than one unit and you must go to another unit to provide care, who will monitor clients out of your immediate attention?
- Is this a temporary assignment? When other staff are located for assistance, will you be relieved? If the assignment is temporary, it may be possible to accept a difficult assignment knowing that there will soon be reinforcements. Is there a pattern of short staffing at this agency, or is this truly an emergency?
- Is this a crisis or an ongoing staffing pattern? If the assignment is being made because of an immediate need or crisis in the unit, the decision to accept the assignment may be based on that immediate need. However, if the staffing pattern is an ongoing problem, you have the obligation to identify unmet standards of care that are occurring as a result of ongoing staffing inadequacies. This may result in a formal request for peer review using the appropriate channels.
- Can you take the assignment in good faith? If not, you will need to have the assignment modified or refuse the assignment. Consult your state's Nurse Practice Act regarding clarification of accepting an assignment in good faith.

On Call and Off With Benefits

When staffing projected for a shift exceeds the number of clients admitted and their acuity, agencies often decrease staffing due to operating budget limitations. Two common approaches that agencies use to reduce staffing on a shift-to-shift basis are placing nurses "on call" or "off with benefits."

57. American Nurses Association. (n.d). *Nurse staffing.* https://www.nursingworld.org/practice-policy/nurse-staffing/

On Call

On call is an agency staffing strategy when a nurse is not immediately needed for their scheduled shift. The nurse may have the options to report to work and do work-related education or stay home. When a nurse is on call, they typically receive a reduced hourly wage and have a required response time. A required response time means if a nurse who is on call is needed later in the shift, they need to be able to report and assume client care in a designated amount of time.

Off With Benefits

A nurse may be placed "**off with benefits**" when not needed for their scheduled shift. When a nurse is placed off with benefits, they typically do not receive an hourly wage and are not expected to report to work or be on call, but still accrue benefits such as insurance and paid time off.

Agency Nursing

Agency nursing is an industry in health care that provides nurses to hospitals and health care facilities in need of staff. Nurse agencies employ nurses to work on an as-needed basis and place them in facilities that have staffing shortages.

Advocacy by the ANA for Appropriate Nurse Staffing

According to the ANA, there is significant evidence showing appropriate nurse staffing contributes to improved client outcomes and greater satisfaction for both clients and staff. Appropriate staffing levels have multiple client benefits, including the following[58]:

- Reduced mortality rates
- Reduced length of client stays
- Reduced number of preventable events, such as falls and infections

Nurses also benefit from appropriate staffing. Appropriate workload allows nurses to utilize their full expertise, without the pressure of fatigue. A recent report suggested that staff levels should depend on the following factors[59]:

- Client complexity, acuity, or stability
- Number of admissions, discharges, and transfers
- Professional nurses' and other staff members' skill level and expertise
- Physical space and layout of the nursing unit
- Availability of technical support and other resources

Read more information about client acuity tools in the "Prioritization" chapter.

58. American Nurses Association. (n.d). *Nurse staffing.* https://www.nursingworld.org/practice-policy/nurse-staffing/
59. American Nurses Association. (n.d.). *Questions to ask in making the decision to accept a staffing assignment for nursing.* https://www.nursingworld.org/practice-policy/nurse-staffing/questions-to-ask-in-making-the-decision-to-accept-a-staffing-assignment-for-nurses/

Visit ANA's interactive Principles of Nurse Staffing infographic. Access supplementary digital content in the online book using this QR code.

Cost-Effective Nursing Care

One of ANA's Standards of Professional Performance is *Resource Stewardship*. The *Resource Stewardship* standard states, "The registered nurse utilizes appropriate resources to plan, provide, and sustain evidence-based nursing services that are safe, effective, financially responsible, and used judiciously."[60] Nurses have a fiscal responsibility to demonstrate resource stewardship to the employing organization and payer of care. This responsibility extends beyond direct client care and encompasses a broader role in health care sustainability. By effectively managing resources, nurses help reduce unnecessary expenditures and ensure that funds are allocated where they are most needed. This can include everything from minimizing waste in the use of medical supplies to optimizing staffing levels to avoid both overworking and underutilizing nursing staff.

Nurses can help contain health care costs by advocating for clients and ensuring their care is received on time, the plan of care is appropriate and individualized to them, and clear documentation has been completed. These steps reduce waste, avoid repeated tests, and ensure timely treatments that promote positive client outcomes and reduce unnecessary spending. Nurses routinely incorporate these practices to provide cost-effective nursing care in their daily practice:

- Keeping supplies near the client's room
- Preventing waste by only bringing needed supplies into a client's room
- Avoiding prepackaged kits with unnecessary supplies
- Avoiding "Admission Bags" with unnecessary supplies
- Using financially-sound thinking
  - Understanding health care costs and reimbursement models
  - Charging out supplies and equipment according to agency policy
- Being productive
  - Organizing and prioritizing
  - Using effective time management
  - Grouping tasks when entering client rooms (i.e., clustering cares)
  - Assigning and delegating nursing care to the nursing team according to the state Nurse Practice Act and agency policy
  - Using effective team communication to avoid duplication of tasks and request assistance when needed
  - Updating and individualizing clients' nursing care plans according to their current needs
  - Documenting for continuity of client care that avoids duplication and focuses on effective interventions based on identified outcomes and goals

60. American Nurses Association. (2021). *Nursing: Scope and standards of practice* (4th ed.). American Nurses Association.

8.6 RESOURCE STEWARDSHIP AND CASE MANAGEMENT

Resource Stewardship

Resource Stewardship is one of the Standards of Professional Performance established by the American Nursing Association (ANA). **Resource stewardship** is defined as using appropriate resources to plan, provide, and sustain evidence-based nursing services that are safe, effective, financially responsible, and used judiciously. See the following box for competencies associated with the ANA's *Resource Stewardship* Standard of Professional Performance.[61]

Competencies of ANA's Resource Stewardship Standard of Professional Performance[62]

- Partners with the health care consumer and other stakeholders to identify care needs and necessary resources to achieve desired outcomes.
- Collaborates with the health care consumer and other stakeholders to assess costs, availability, risks, and benefits in decisions about care.
- Secures appropriate resources to address needs across the health care continuum.
- Advocates for equitable resources that support and enhance nursing practice and health outcomes.
- Integrates connected health technologies into practice to promote positive interactions between health care consumers and care providers.
- Uses organizational and community resources to implement interprofessional plans.
- Addresses discriminatory health care practices and the adverse impact on allocation of resources.

Case Management

Nurses are tasked with daily case management activities and allocating appropriate resources to their clients. Two common types of case management that staff nurses provide are educating clients about using appropriate levels of care and encouraging the use of cost-effective health care team members.

Several levels of care are available to clients for their health care services:

- **Emergency department care** has specialized providers and high-level diagnostics and should be reserved for immediate and potentially life-threatening needs.
- **Urgent care** is an elevated level of care above an outpatient visit, yet below the needs of an emergency visit. Nurses should refer clients to this setting if they have a health need that needs attention within the next 24 hours but is not life-threatening.

61. American Nurses Association. (2021). *Nursing: Scope and standards of practice* (4th ed.). American Nurses Association.
62. American Nurses Association. (2021). *Nursing: Scope and standards of practice* (4th ed.). American Nurses Association.

- **Outpatient health settings** provide health maintenance for chronic disease or treatment of nonurgent acute conditions. They also provide preventative services like well-baby checks and immunizations. In the outpatient setting, the nurse recognizes the client's time with a provider is limited, so the majority of a nurse's time is often spent providing client education, answering questions, and coordinating care.
- **Inpatient and acute care** typically occurs in a hospital setting where skilled nursing, diagnostic tests, and medical treatments are required. Nursing goals in these settings are to address immediate health concerns, stabilize the client, and prepare them for discharge. Most inpatient stays are 72 hours or less, so nurses must provide efficient care that includes adequate client education regarding follow-up care after discharge.
- **Assisted living** refers to licensed facilities that provide safe living accommodations and three meals daily. Residents receive assistance with medications and ADLs and may receive general nursing care.[63]
- **Skilled nursing facilities**, commonly referred to as "nursing homes" or "long-term care facilities," are licensed facilities that provide 24-hour licensed nursing services. Residents may require total assistance with ADLs.[64]
- **Home health** refers to services provided in a client's home that may include nursing, home health aide, physical therapy (PT), occupational therapy (OT), and speech therapy.[65]
- **Hospice** offers palliative and supportive services providing physical, psychological, social, and spiritual care for dying clients and their families. Services may be provided in the client's home or an inpatient setting. Hospice may include nursing, home health aide, social worker, chaplain, PT, OT, ST, nutritional therapy, and volunteer services.[66]
- **Telehealth** is a fairly new and expanding health delivery model. Telehealth is a form of an outpatient health service where the client and member of the health care team are able to connect remotely using telephone calls or video conferencing on a computer with an Internet connection. Devices may be provided to monitor vital signs and other health indicators. Telehealth enhances client access to multiple providers without the burden of travel. Telehealth has become an important resource in rural communities, especially due to social distancing required by the COVID-19 pandemic.[67]

Nurses can also address the economic pressures within the health care system by utilizing and advocating for cost-effective care by providers on the health care team. In this manner, limited health care resources are allocated wisely, and consumers receive the health care they need. For example, many nurse practitioners (NPs) and physician assistants (PAs) function as primary providers in outpatient settings and provide preventative services, treat self-limited acute medical conditions, and manage chronic disease. NPs and PAs are trained to refer clients for specialized care when indicated. Some NPs and PAs work in specialized inpatient areas and serve as the primary point of contact during a client's hospital stay. Nurses recognize the time of specialty physicians is limited and unnecessary referrals can be costly to the client. By using and advocating for the wise use of these health care human resources, nurses can help reduce the overall cost of health care.

63. Utah Department of Health. (n.d.). *Levels of care.* https://health.utah.gov/hflcra/facinfo/HFLevelsOfCare.PDF
64. Utah Department of Health. (n.d.). *Levels of care.* https://health.utah.gov/hflcra/facinfo/HFLevelsOfCare.PDF
65. Utah Department of Health. (n.d.). *Levels of care.* https://health.utah.gov/hflcra/facinfo/HFLevelsOfCare.PDF
66. Utah Department of Health. (n.d.). *Levels of care.* https://health.utah.gov/hflcra/facinfo/HFLevelsOfCare.PDF
67. Health Resources & Services Administration. (2024). *What is telehealth?* https://telehealth.hhs.gov/patients/understanding-telehealth/

8.7 SPOTLIGHT APPLICATION

Emma is assigned to care for a 64-year-old client readmitted with heart failure (HF). Emma recognizes the client's name during shift report as the reporting nurse comments how this client was a "frequent flyer," and he was just discharged last week. The reporting nurse spends little time describing the client's actual condition and focuses comments on how the client "might as well put his name plaque on the door" because he is here so frequently. Emma does agree that the client has been readmitted very frequently with HF exacerbations but is concerned by the dismissive comments by her peer. She is determined to spend time with this client on this admission and find out more about his home environment, support system, and self-care.

Reflective Questions

- How do the frequent readmissions affect the client's health care costs and the hospital's reimbursement levels by Medicare and private insurance companies?
- What additional nursing interventions might help prevent future frequent readmissions and reduce costs?

Emma engages in a conversation with the client about his dietary habits at home. He reports that his wife passed away one year ago from breast cancer, and he has been preparing his own meals since that time by using easy-to-prepare and cheap foods. Canned soups, boxed meals, and chips are common staples in his diet. Through Emma's conversation with the client, she can see that the client needs dietary instruction and further education about monitoring his fluid retention with daily weights. He seems engaged in exploring different food preparations and was unaware that foods could exacerbate his heart failure. When Emma asked if he had been taught about this on previous admissions, he stated that no one took the time to talk with him about his home situation. He reports that he received pamphlets but never really took the time to read them because the print was so small. Emma reflects on how preventative education opportunities were missed and increased costs were incurred by the client and the health care organization as a result.

8.8 LEARNING ACTIVITIES

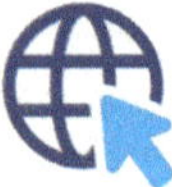

Interactive learning activities have been excluded from the print version of the text. Access free online learning activities in the online book using this QR code.

8.9 GLOSSARY

Acuity-based staffing: A client assignment model that takes into account the level of client care required based on the severity of a client's illness or condition.

Affordable Care Act (ACA): Legislation enacted in 2010 to increase consumers' access to health care coverage and protect them from insurance practices that restrict care or significantly increase the cost of care.

Budget: An estimate of revenue and expenses over a specified period of time, usually over a year.

Capital budgets: Budgets used to plan investments and upgrades to tangible assets that lose or gain value over time. Capital is something that can be touched, such as buildings or computers.

Co-pay: A flat fee the consumer pays at the time of receiving a health care service as a part of their health care plan.

Deductible: The amount of money a consumer pays for health care before their insurance plan pays anything. These amounts generally apply per person per calendar year.

Economics: The study of how society makes decisions about its limited resources.

Evidence Based Practice (EBP): A lifelong problem-solving approach that integrates the best evidence from well-designed research studies and evidence-based theories; clinical expertise and evidence from assessment of the health care consumer's history and condition, as well as health care resources; and client, family, group, community, and population preferences and values.

Extrinsic factors: External elements that impact health care costs.

Floating: An agency strategy that asks nurses to temporarily work on a different unit to help cover a short-staffed shift.

Health care disparity: Differences in access to health care and insurance coverage.

Health disparities: Differences in health outcomes that result from social determinants of health (SDOH).

Intrinsic factors: Factors that are inherent to the characteristics and needs of the population.

Mandatory overtime: A requirement by agencies for nurses to stay and care for clients beyond their scheduled shift when short staffing occurs.

Medicaid: A joint federal and state program covering groups of eligible individuals, such as low-income families, qualified pregnant women and children, and individuals receiving Supplemental Security Income (SSI). States may choose to cover additional groups, such as individuals receiving home and community-based services and children in foster care who are not otherwise eligible.

Medicare: A federal health insurance program used by people aged 65 and older, younger individuals with permanent disabilities, and people with end-stage renal disease requiring dialysis or a kidney transplant.

Off with benefits: An agency staffing strategy when a nurse is not needed for their scheduled shift. The nurse does not typically receive an hourly wage and is not expected to report to work, but they still accrue benefits such as insurance and paid time off.

On call: An agency staffing strategy when a nurse is not immediately needed for their scheduled shift. They may have options to stay at work and complete work-related education or stay home.

Operating budgets: Budgets including personnel costs and annual facility operating costs.

Pay for Performance: A reimbursement model, also known as value-based payment, that attaches financial incentives based on the performance of health care agencies and providers.

Resource stewardship: Using appropriate resources to plan, provide, and sustain evidence-based nursing services that are safe, effective, financially responsible, and used judiciously.

Social Determinants of Health (SDOH): Conditions in the places where people live, learn, work, and play, such as unstable housing, low income areas, unsafe neighborhoods, or substandard education that affect a wide range of health risks and outcomes.

Team nursing: A common staffing pattern that uses a combination of Registered Nurses (RNs), Licensed Practical/Vocational Nurses (LPN/VNs), and Unlicensed Assistive Personnel (UAP) to care for a group of clients.

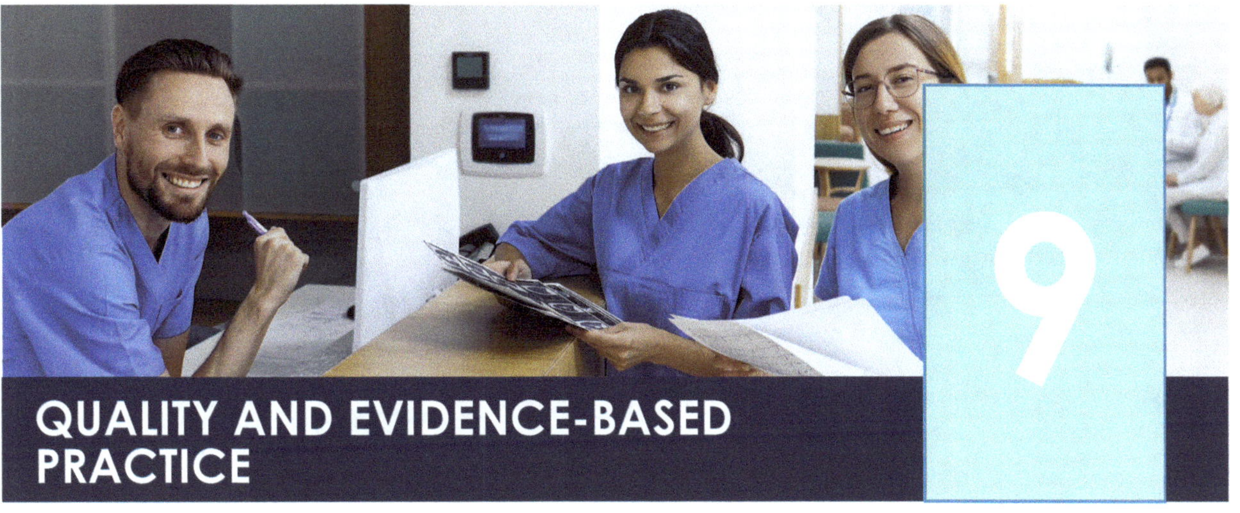

9.1 QUALITY AND EVIDENCE-BASED PRACTICE INTRODUCTION

LEARNING OBJECTIVES

- Examine the role of utilization review and continuous quality improvement
- Describe the role of research in providing evidence-based, quality client care
- Identify the accreditation process for agencies
- Explain quality client care based on standards of nursing practice
- Examine the role of government, nursing, and other organizations in developing standards for quality nursing practice
- Explain how informatics systems promote quality and safety in health care delivery
- Examine the role of the nurse in workplace quality improvement processes

Florence Nightingale was a pioneer in the evaluation of quality nursing care. She identified the role of a nurse within the health care team and measured client outcomes to support the value of a nurse. See an example of one of Florence Nightingale's diagrams comparing the causes of mortality in the Army in Figure 9.1.[1] Over the years nursing theorists and governing agencies have continued the evaluation work of Florence Nightingale by collecting data, using statistics, and creating reports to ensure the best quality care is being delivered to all clients.

1. "Nightingale-mortality.jpg" by Florence Nightingale is licensed under Public Domain

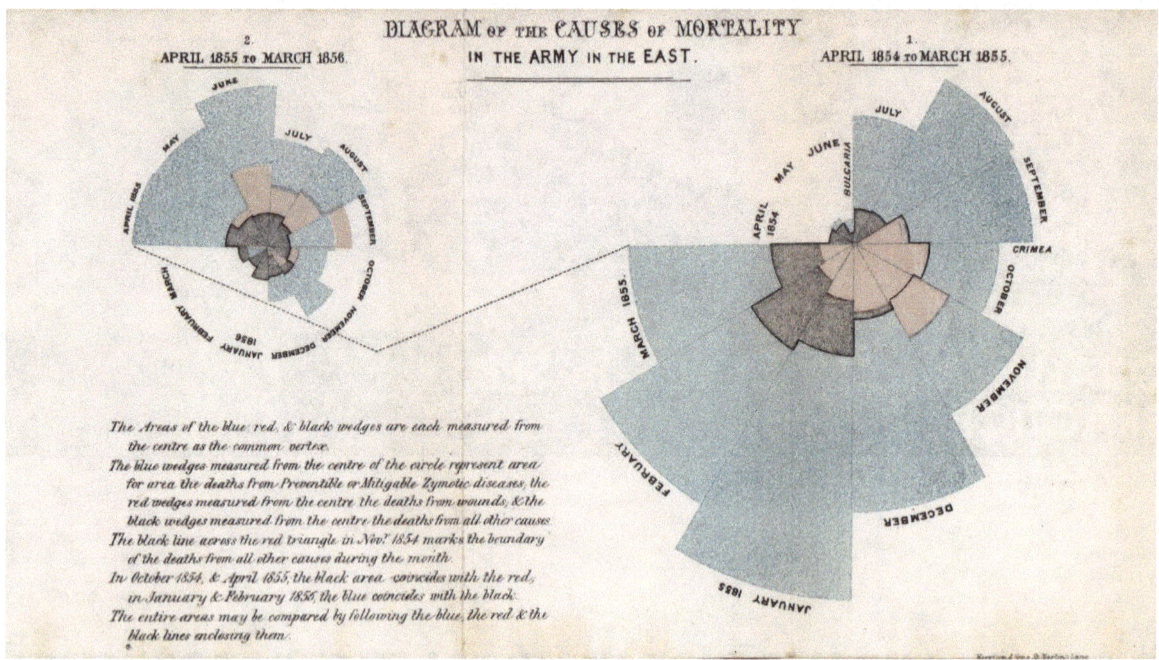

FIGURE 9.1 Florence Nightingale's Diagram of the Causes of Mortality

In previous chapters we discussed how delegation, prioritization, and working as part of an interdisciplinary team all contribute to the delivery of effective and high-quality care. However, a common question by nurses and other health care stakeholders is, "What is the definition of quality health care?" A second question is, "How is quality measured and evaluated in health care to determine if standards are met?" A third related question is, "How do nurses incorporate research and evidence-based practices into their nursing practice?" This chapter will review how quality nursing care is defined, measured, and evaluated and how nurses implement evidence-based practices into their daily nursing practice.

9.2 QUALITY CARE

Quality is defined in a variety of ways that impact nursing practice.

ANA Definition of Quality

The American Nurses Association (ANA) defines **quality** as, "The degree to which nursing services for health care consumers, families, groups, communities, and populations increase the likelihood of desirable outcomes and are consistent with evolving nursing knowledge."[2] The phrases in this definition focus on three aspects of quality: services (nursing interventions), desirable outcomes, and consistency with evolving nursing knowledge (evidence-based practice). Alignment of nursing interventions with current

2. American Nurses Association. (2021). *Nursing: Scope and standards of practice* (4th ed.). American Nurses Association.

evidence-based practice is a key component for quality care.[3] Evidence-based practice (EBP) will be further discussed later in this chapter.

Quality of Practice is one of the ANA's Standards of Professional Performance. **ANA Standards of Professional Performance** are "authoritative statements of the actions and behaviors that all registered nurses, regardless of role, population, specialty, and setting are expected to perform competently." See the competencies for the ANA's *Quality of Practice* Standard of Professional Performance in the following box.[4]

Competencies of ANA's Quality of Practice Standard of Professional Performance[5]

- Ensures that nursing practice is safe, effective, efficient, equitable, timely, and person-centered.
- Incorporates evidence into nursing practice to improve outcomes.
- Uses creativity and innovation to enhance nursing care.
- Recommends strategies to improve nursing care quality.
- Collects data to monitor the quality of nursing practice.
- Contributes to efforts to improve health care efficiency.
- Provides critical review and evaluation of policies, procedures, and guidelines to improve the quality of health care.
- Engages in formal and informal peer review processes of the interprofessional team.
- Participates in quality improvement initiatives.
- Collaborates with the interprofessional team to implement quality improvement plans and interventions.
- Documents nursing practice in a manner that supports quality and performance improvement initiatives.
- Recognizes the value of professional and specialty certification.

Reflective Questions

1. What *Quality of Practice* competencies have you already demonstrated during your nursing education?
2. What *Quality of Practice* competencies are you most interested in mastering?
3. What questions do you have about the ANA's *Quality of Practice* competencies? Where could you find answers to those questions (e.g., instructors, preceptors, health care team members, guidelines, or core measures)?

This chapter will review content related to the competencies of the ANA's *Quality of Practice* Standard of Professional Performance. Additional information about peer review is discussed in the "Leadership and Management" chapter, and specialty certification is discussed in the "Preparation for the RN Role" chapter.

3. Stevens, K. R. (2013). The impact of evidence-based practice in nursing and the next big ideas. *OJIN: The Online Journal of Issues in Nursing, 18*(2), manuscript 4. https://ojin.nursingworld.org/MainMenuCategories/ANAMarketplace/ANAPeriodicals/OJIN/TableofContents/Vol-18-2013/No2-May-2013/Impact-of-Evidence-Based-Practice.html
4. American Nurses Association. (2021). *Nursing: Scope and standards of practice* (4th ed.). American Nurses Association.
5. American Nurses Association. (2021). *Nursing: Scope and standards of practice* (4th ed.). American Nurses Association.

Quality and Safety Education for Nurses

The Quality and Safety Education for Nurses (QSEN) project advocates for safe, quality client care by defining six competencies for prelicensure nursing students: Patient-Centered Care, Teamwork and Collaboration, Evidence-Based Practice, Quality Improvement, Safety, and Informatics. These competencies are further discussed in the "Advocacy" chapter.

Framework of Quality Health Care

A definition of quality that has historically guided the measurement of quality initiatives in health care systems is based on the framework for improvement originally created by the Institute of Medicine (IOM). The IOM name changed to the National Academy of Medicine in 2015. The IOM framework includes the following six criteria for defining quality health care[6,7]:

- **Safe:** Avoiding harm to clients from the care that is intended to help them.
- **Effective:** Providing services based on scientific knowledge to all who could benefit and refraining from providing services to those not likely to benefit (i.e., avoiding underuse and misuse).
- **Client-centered:** Providing care that is respectful of and responsive to individual client preferences, needs, and values and ensuring that client values guide all clinical decisions.
- **Timely:** Reducing waits and sometimes harmful delays for both those who receive and those who provide care.
- **Efficient:** Avoiding waste, including waste of equipment, supplies, ideas, and energy.
- **Equitable:** Providing care that does not vary in quality because of personal characteristics such as gender, ethnicity, geographic location, and socioeconomic status.

This framework continues to guide quality improvement initiatives across America's health care system. The evidence-based practice (EBP) movement began with the public acknowledgement of unacceptable client outcomes resulting from a gap between research findings and actual health care practices. For EBP to be successfully adopted and sustained, it must be adopted by nurses and other health care team members, system leaders, and policy makers. Regulations and recognitions are also necessary to promote the adoption of EBP. For example, the Magnet Recognition Program promotes nursing as a leader in catalyzing adoption of EBP and using it as a marker of excellence.[8]

Magnet Recognition Program

The Magnet Recognition Program is an award from the American Nurses Credentialing Center (ANCC) that recognizes organizational commitment to nursing excellence. The award recognizes organizations worldwide where nursing leaders have successfully aligned their nursing strategic goals to improve the

6. Agency for Healthcare Research & Quality. (2022). *Six domains of health care quality.* https://www.ahrq.gov/talkingquality/measures/six-domains.html
7. Institute of Medicine (US) Committee on Quality of Health Care in America. (2001). *Crossing the quality chasm: A new health system for the 21st century.* National Academies Press. https://pubmed.ncbi.nlm.nih.gov/25057539/
8. Stevens, K. R. (2013). The impact of evidence-based practice in nursing and the next big ideas. *OJIN: The Online Journal of Issues in Nursing, 18*(2), manuscript 4. https://ojin.nursingworld.org/MainMenuCategories/ANAMarketplace/ANAPeriodicals/OJIN/TableofContents/Vol-18-2013/No2-May-2013/Impact-of-Evidence-Based-Practice.html

organization's client outcomes. To nurses, Magnet Recognition means education and development are available through every stage of their career. To clients, it means quality care is delivered by nurses who are supported to be the best that they can be.[9] See Figure 9.2[10] for an image related to the Magnet Recognition Program.

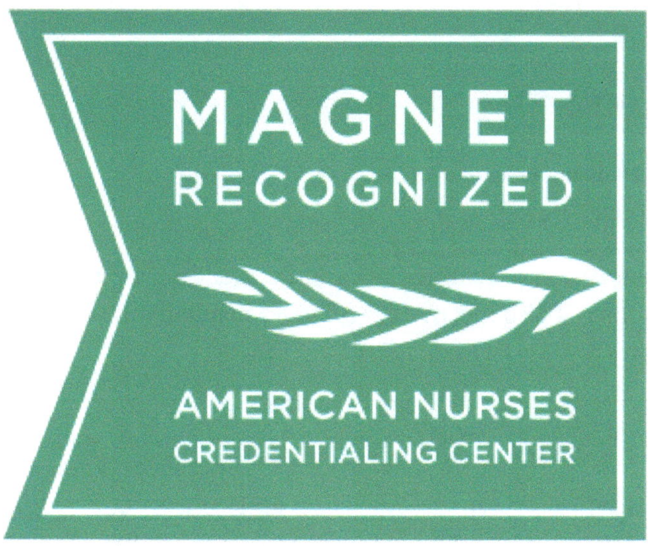

FIGURE 9.2 Magnet Recognition

Reimbursement Models

Quality health care is also defined by value-based reimbursement models used by Medicare, Medicaid, and private insurance companies paying for health services. As discussed in the "Health Care Reimbursement Models" section of the "Health Care Economics" chapter, value-based payment reimbursement models use financial incentives to reward quality health care and positive client outcomes. For example, Medicare no longer reimburses hospitals to treat clients who acquire certain preventable conditions during their hospital stay, such as pressure injuries or urinary tract infections associated with use of catheters.[11] These reimbursement models directly impact the evidence-based care nurses provide at the bedside and the associated documentation of assessments, interventions, and nursing care plans to ensure quality performance criteria are met.

CMS Quality Initiatives

The Centers for Medicare & Medicaid Services (CMS) establishes quality initiatives that focus on several key quality measures of health care. These quality measures provide a comprehensive understanding and

9. American Nurses Credentialing Center. (2024). *ANCC magnet recognition program.* https://www.nursingworld.org/organizational-programs/magnet/
10. "Magnet_Recognition_Logo_CMYK_-png-.png" by Mattmitchell37 is licensed under CC BY-SA 4.0
11. James, J. (2012). *Pay-for-performance.* Health Affairs. https://www.healthaffairs.org/do/10.1377/hpb20121011.90233/full/

evaluation of the care an organization delivers, as well as clients' responses to the care provided. These quality measures evaluate many areas of health care, including the following[12]:

- Health outcomes
- Clinical processes
- Client safety
- Efficient use of health care resources
- Care coordination
- Client engagement in their own care
- Client perceptions of their care

These measures of quality focus on providing the care the client needs when the client needs it, in an affordable, safe, effective manner. It also means engaging and involving the client, so they take ownership in managing their care at home.

Visit the CMS *What is a Quality Measure* web page. Access supplementary digital content in the online book using this QR code.

Accreditation

Accreditation is a review process that determines if an agency is meeting the defined standards of quality determined by the accrediting body. The main accrediting organizations for health care are as follows:

- The Joint Commission
- National Committee for Quality Assurance
- American Medical Accreditation Program
- American Accreditation Healthcare Commission

The standards of quality vary depending on the accrediting organization, but they all share common goals to improve efficiency, equity, and delivery of high-quality care. Two terms commonly associated with accreditation that are directly related to quality nursing care are core measures and client safety goals. Please see Table 9.2 for more information on accrediting organizations.

12. CMS.gov. (2024). *Quality measures.* https://www.cms.gov/Medicare/Quality-Initiatives-Patient-Assessment-Instruments/QualityMeasures

TABLE 9.2. Accrediting Organizations[13,14,15,16]

Organization	Overview	History	Accreditation Process	Standards	Impact
The Joint Commission	Non-profit organization accrediting and certifying health care organizations and programs in the U.S.	Founded in 1951, aims to improve public health care quality and safety	Conducts rigorous on-site surveys to assess compliance with standards covering client care, medication safety, infection control, and overall performance	Developed with input from health care professionals, providers, and consumers and designed to help measure, assess, and improve performance	Recognized as a symbol of quality, reflecting commitment to high performance standards
National Committee for Quality Assurance (NCQA)	Private, non-profit organization improving health care quality through evidence-based standards, measures, programs, and accreditation	Established in 1990, provides quality information for health care decision-making	Comprehensive review of policies and procedures, including quality management, utilization management, credentialing, and member rights	Widely regarded standards used by CMS and state governments for quality oversight	Demonstrates commitment to improving health care quality and adhering to high performance standards
American Medical Accreditation Program (AMAP)	Program by AMA aimed at improving medical care quality by setting high standards for physicians	Launched in the late 1990s, assesses physicians' qualifications and ethical standards	Detailed review process, including verification of credentials, practice history assessment, and compliance with CME requirements	Ensures physicians provide high-quality care, maintain competency, and adhere to ethical practices	Recognizes physicians' commitment to high-quality care and medical practice standards

13. Joint Commission International. (2024). *Who we are.* https://www.jointcommission.org/?utm_campaign=tjc_brand__1_core&utm_source=google&utm_medium=cpc&gad_source=1&gclid=CjwKCAjwnK60BhA9EiwAmpHZw55yd91qdT0f3Q6nauq82Oo3uHe5nPJKBwT81CxvmdtkGrjdc26GchoCvz8QAvD_BwE
14. NCQA. (2024). *About NCQA.* https://www.ncqa.org/about-ncqa/
15. AMA Ed Hub. (2024). *About the AMA's CME accreditation.* https://edhub.ama-assn.org/pages/ama-cme
16. ACHC. (2024). *About accreditation.* https://www.achc.org/

TABLE 9.2. Continued...

American Accred-itation Healthcare Commission (AAHC) / URAC	Independent, non-profit organization promot-ing health care quali-ty through accreditation, certification, and measurement	Founded in 1990, expanded from utiliza-tion review to a wide range of health care services	Thorough re-view of policies, procedures, and performance, including on-site visits and compliance assessment	Developed by a broad array of stakehold-ers to pro-mote evidence-based prac-tices, client safety, and continuous improvement	Recognized as a mark of excellence, demonstrates commitment to quality and accountability

Core Measures

Core measures are national standards of care and treatment processes for common conditions. These processes are proven to reduce complications and lead to better client outcomes. Core measure compliance reports show how often a hospital successfully provides recommended treatment for certain medical conditions. In the United States, hospitals must report their compliance with core measures to The Joint Commission, CMS, and other agencies.[17]

In November 2003, The Joint Commission and CMS began work to align common core measures, so they are identical. This work resulted in the creation of one common set of measures known as the *Specifications Manual for National Hospital Inpatient Quality Measures.* These core measures are used by both organizations to improve the health care delivery process. Examples of core measures include guidelines regarding immunizations, tobacco treatment, substance use, hip and knee replacements, cardiac care, strokes, treatment of high blood pressure, and the use of high-risk medications in the elderly. Nurses must be aware of core measures and ensure the care they provide aligns with these recommendations.[18]

Read more about the National Hospital Inpatient Quality Measures. Access supplementary digital content in the online book using this QR code.

National Patient Safety Goals

Patient safety goals are guidelines specific to organizations accredited by The Joint Commission that focus on health care safety problems and ways to solve them. The National Patient Safety Goals (NPSG) were first established in 2003 and are updated annually to address areas of national concern related to client

17. John Hopkins Medicine. (n.d.). *Core measures.* https://www.hopkinsmedicine.org/patient_safety/core_measures.html
18. The Joint Commission. (n.d.). *Measures.* https://www.hopkinsmedicine.org/patient_safety/core_measures.html

safety, as well as to promote high-quality care. The NPSG provide guidance for specific health care settings, including hospitals, ambulatory clinics, behavioral health, critical access hospitals, home care, laboratory, skilled nursing care, and surgery.

The following goals are some examples of NPSG for hospitals[19]:

- Identify patients correctly
- Improve staff communication
- Use medicines safely
- Use alarms safely
- Prevent infection
- Identify patient safety risks
- Prevent mistakes in surgery

Nurses must be aware of the current NPSG for their health care setting, implement appropriate interventions, and document their assessments and interventions. Documentation in the electronic medical record is primarily used as evidence that an organization is meeting these goals.

Read the current agency-specific National Patient Safety Goals. Access supplementary digital content in the online book using this QR code.

9.3 MEASURING AND IMPROVING QUALITY

Now that we have discussed the various ways that quality health care is defined, let's discuss how quality care is measured, evaluated, and improved.

Utilization Review

Thinking back to value-based reimbursement models discussed in the "Health Care Economics" chapter, recall how health care agencies are reimbursed from Medicare, Medicaid, and private insurance based on their quality performance measures. A **utilization review** is an investigation of health care services performed by doctors, nurses, and other health care team members to ensure money is not wasted covering unnecessary or inefficient expenditures for proper treatment. Utilization review also allows organizations to objectively measure how their health care services and resources are being used to best meet their clients' needs. Information from clients' medical records is analyzed, along with client demographics, to evaluate resource

19. The Joint Commission. (2025). *2025 national patient safety goals.* https://www.jointcommission.org/standards/national-patient-safety-goals/

allocation, efficiency, and quality of health promotion initiatives.[20] See Figure 9.3[21] for an illustration of utilization review related to costs.

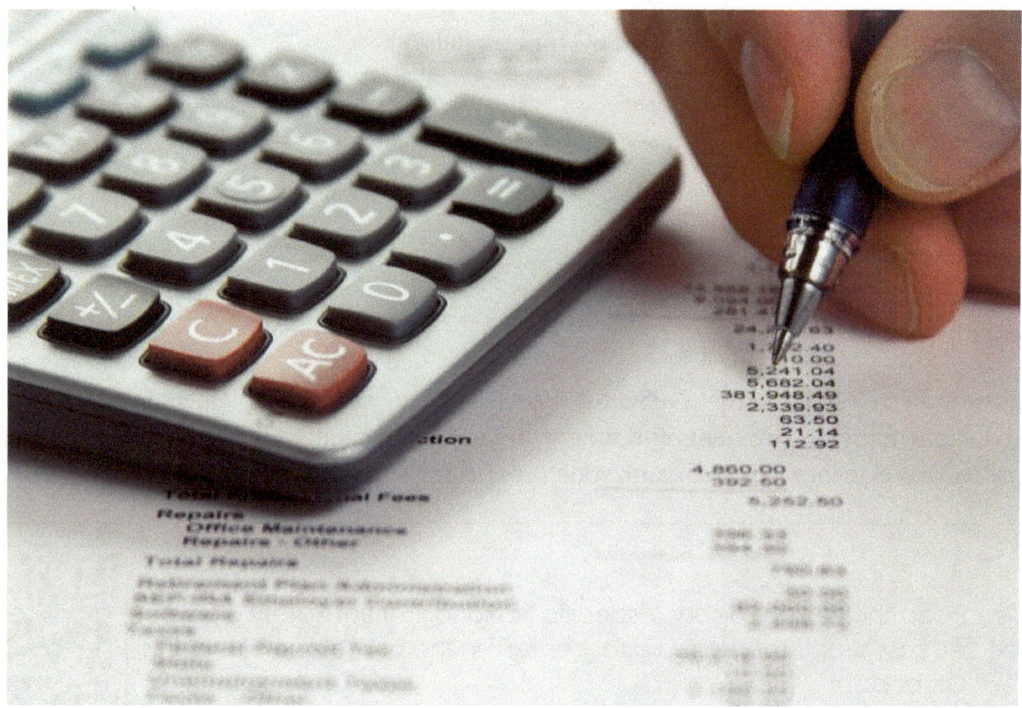

FIGURE 9.3 Utilization Review

Using Informatics to Promote Quality

Utilization review relies on the collection of meaningful data from health records to determine if quality metrics are being met. **Informatics** refers to using information and technology to communicate, manage knowledge, mitigate error, and support decision-making.[22] Informatics allows members of the health care team to share, store, and analyze health-related information. Nurses have an important role in informatics. **Nursing informatics** is the science and practice of integrating nursing knowledge with information and communication technologies to promote the health of people, families, and communities worldwide.[23] It is a nursing specialty with certification available from the ANCC. See Figure 9.4[24] for an artistic rendition of informatics.

---

20. Institute of Medicine (US) Committee on Utilization Management by Third Parties, Gray, B. H., & Field, M. J., (Eds.). (1989). *Controlling costs and changing patient care? The role of utilization management.* National Academies Press. https://www.ncbi.nlm.nih.gov/books/NBK235000
21. "Analyzing_Financial_Data_(5099605109).jpg" by Dave Dugdale is licensed under CC BY-SA 2.0
22. QSEN Institute. (n.d.). *QSEN competencies: Quality improvement (QI).* https://qsen.org/competencies/pre-licensure-ksas/#quality_improvement
23. AMIA. (n.d.). *Informatics: Research and practice.* https://amia.org/about-amia/why-informatics/informatics-research-and-practice
24. "informatics-1322241_1920.jpg" by mariojsantos at Pixabay.com is licensed under CC0

These are several benefits of using informatics in health care[25]:

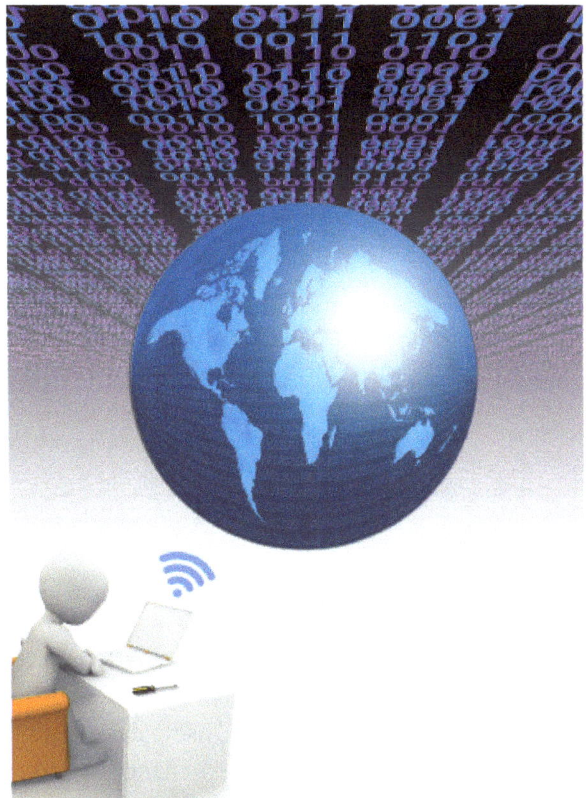

FIGURE 9.4 Informatics

- **Improvement of Client Safety:** Informatics allows for up-to-date information sharing by both the client and members of the health care team. Using informatics can help to reduce the occurrence of medication errors, as well as monitor client side effects and overall health status. For example, barcode scanning has reduced medication errors by ensuring the correct dose is administered to the correct client at the correct time.
- **Reduction of Delays in Care:** Some health care informatics systems allow for direct communication between health care team members and clients. The ability to ask and answer questions without needing to schedule an office appointment promotes the ability for care to be delivered efficiently in a cost-effective manner.
- **Reduction of Waste:** The use of informatics to share information between care team members reduces waste associated with duplication of tests or exams when more than one provider is on the care team. Additionally, clients can request their records be shared with health providers from other health organizations, which reduces duplication and unnecessary spending across the nation.
- **Promotion of Client-Centered Care:** Many informatics systems have "portal" options where the client and/or designated personnel are able to be active participants in the care planning and health promotion processes. Informatics offers an inclusive environment for clients to communicate and share directly with their care team regardless of physical location and timing.
- **Support of Quality Improvement:** The continuous process of quality improvement requires the ability to collect and analyze data in a systematic and reliable manner. Using informatics provides members of the health care team a secure place to store data, as well as the ability to review in a timely manner.

Quality Indicators

The National Database of Nursing Quality Indicators (NDNQI) was developed as a national nursing database used to evaluate quality in nursing care. This database was purchased by Press Ganey in 2014. In collaboration with the American Nursing Association (ANA), the original NDNQI database established nurse-sensitive quality indicators such as these[26]:

25. Otokiti, A. (2019). Using informatics to improve healthcare quality. *International Journal of Health Care Qual Assurance, 32*(2), 425-430. https://doi.org/10.1108/ijhcqa-03-2018-0062
26. Montalvo, I. (2007). The National Database of Nursing Quality Indicators (NDNQI). *The Online Journal of Issues in Nursing, 12*(3). https://ojin.nursingworld.org/MainMenuCategories/ANAMarketplace/ANAPeriodicals/OJIN/TableofContents/Volume122007/No3Sept07/NursingQualityIndicators.html

- Nursing Care Hours Per Patient Day
- Hospital-Acquired Pressure Injuries
- RN Job Satisfaction

Nurses use quality indicators to support practice changes with evidence directly related to improved client outcomes.

Read about current quality measures promoting clinical excellence at the Press Ganey website. Access supplementary digital content in the online book using this QR code.

Quality Improvement

Quality Improvement (QI) is a systematic process using measurable data to improve health care services and the overall health status of clients.[27] QI is one of the competencies of the Quality and Safety Education (QSEN) project and defined as, "using data to monitor the outcomes of care processes and using improvement methods to design and test changes to continuously improve the quality and safety of health care systems."[28]

The overall goal of the QI process is to improve the quality and safety of health care. The process of quality improvement is very similar to the nursing process, but its purpose is to answer these three main questions:

- What are we trying to accomplish?
- How will we know if a change is an improvement?
- What changes can we make that will result in an improvement?

See Figure 9.5[29] for an illustration of the quality improvement process.

27. Study.com. (n.d.). *What is economics? - Definition, history, timeline & importance* [Video]. https://study.com/academy/lesson/what-is-economics-definition-history-timeline-importance.html
28. QSEN Institute. (n.d.). *QSEN competencies: Quality improvement (QI)*. https://qsen.org/competencies/pre-licensure-ksas/#quality_improvement
29. "Model_for_Improvement.jpg" by Cliffnorman is licensed under CC BY-SA 4.0

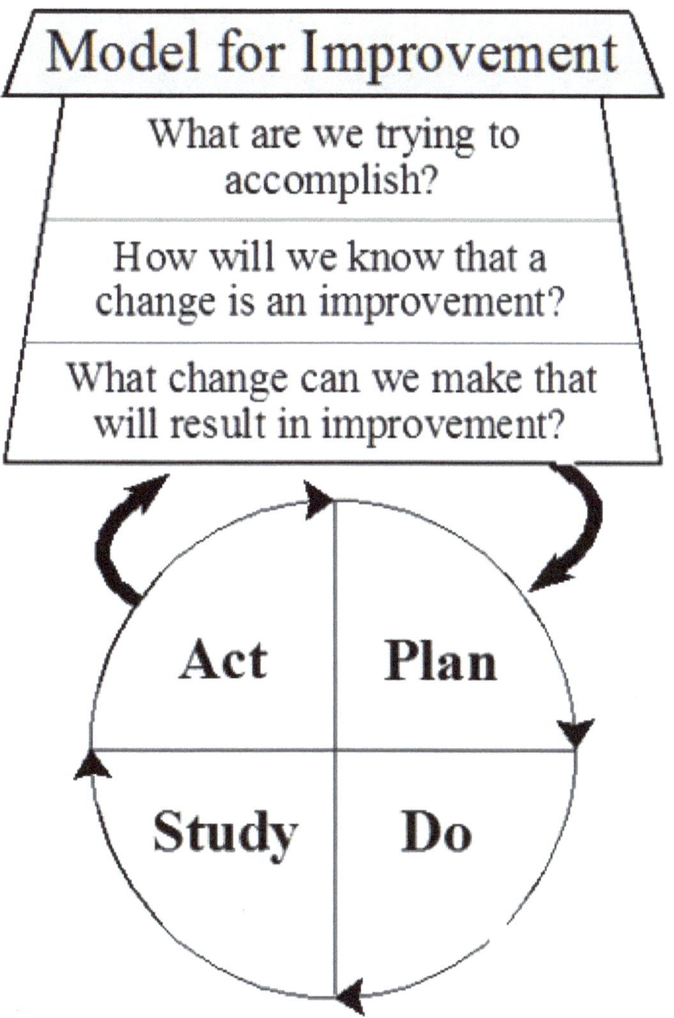

FIGURE 9.5 Quality Improvement Process

To answer these questions, QI is a continuous process in which a project is planned, interventions are implemented, data is collected, results are studied, and outcomes are evaluated. The process is repeated after additional planning. During the QI process, four key steps are used to evaluate current client care and determine if changes are needed. These components are referred to as Plan, Do, Study, and Act:

- **Plan:** The first step in the QI process is to identify what you will be testing or focusing on and what will be measured. Similar to the nursing process where subjective and objective data are collected, the nurse determines what data will be needed during the QI process. The nurse also determines a timeline for the QI project, such as one year, including a specific framework for when data is collected and when it will be reviewed. For example, fall rates will decrease 10% in one year.
- **Do:** After the plan is determined, the nurse works with a health care team to implement the project and ensure data collection occurs.
- **Study:** During this phase, the nurse works with the health care team to review and analyze the data that was collected and determine if the outcomes were achieved or not.

- **Act:** In the fourth step of the QI process, the team discusses the outcomes. In this step the team identifies barriers, strengths, and weaknesses and then decides if additional changes are needed in nursing practice. The QI process is continuous, so the QI team uses outcome findings to continue the process of Plan, Do, Study, and Act to ensure safe, quality client care.

PDSA Fall Rates Example

Reducing Client Fall Rates

Objective: Decrease the client fall rate in the hospital by 10% within one year.

Plan

1. **Identify the Focus:** The QI project will focus on reducing client falls in the hospital.
2. **Determine What to Measure:** The primary metric will be the fall rate, calculated as the number of falls per 1,000 client days.
3. **Collect Data:** Baseline fall rates will be collected for the past year to understand current performance.
4. **Set Goals:** Aim to reduce the fall rate by 10% within one year.
5. **Develop a Timeline:**
    - **Initial Planning and Baseline Data Collection:** Month 1
    - **Intervention Implementation:** Months 2-4
    - **Data Collection and Monitoring:** Months 2-12
    - **Initial Data Analysis:** Month 6
    - **Final Data Analysis and Review:** Month 12

Do

1. **Implement Interventions:** Conduct fall prevention training sessions for all nursing staff. Ensure that client rooms are free from clutter and that non-slip mats are in place. Install bed alarms and provide non-slip socks for clients. Implement a protocol for frequent rounding, especially for high-risk clients.
2. **Data Collection:** Continuously collect data on fall incidents, including the circumstances of each fall.

Study

1. **Data Analysis:** Review the fall rates monthly and compare them to the baseline data. Analyze trends and identify any patterns in the fall incidents. Determine if the interventions are associated with a reduction in fall rates.
2. **Outcome Evaluation:** Assess whether the goal of a 10% reduction in fall rates is being met. Identify any unexpected outcomes.

Act

1. **Discuss Outcomes:** Hold meetings with the health care team to discuss the results. Identify barriers to successful implementation (e.g., lack of compliance with protocols, insufficient training). Recognize strengths (e.g., effective use of bed alarms, positive feedback from staff).

2. **Make Adjustments:** If the fall rate has not decreased as expected, identify additional changes that might be needed (e.g., more frequent training, adjusting the rounding protocol). If successful, consider ways to further enhance the fall prevention program.
3. **Continuous Improvement:** Use the findings to plan the next cycle of improvements. Set new goals based on the outcomes and continue the PDSA cycle to maintain and further improve client safety

See Figure 9.6[30] for an illustration comparing the QI process to the nursing process.

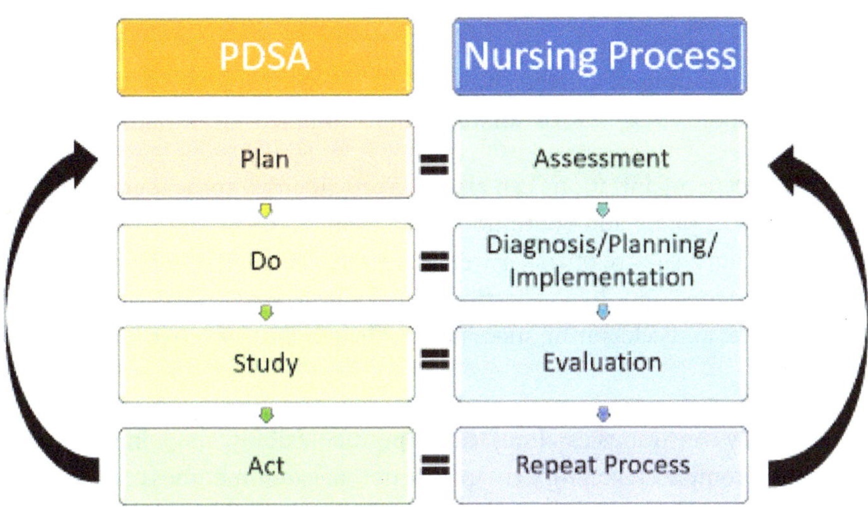

FIGURE 9.6 Comparison of the QI Process and the Nursing Process (Source: Amy Tyznik, MPTC)

It is important to note that quality improvement is different from nursing research. QI evaluates processes in place and determines if changes are needed, whereas the goal of research is to identify new innovations in nursing practice.[31]

Barriers to Quality Improvement

Barriers to quality improvement (QI) in health care organizations can be multifaceted, arising from a range of systemic, cultural, and practical challenges. One of the primary barriers is resistance to change among health care professionals. This resistance can stem from a lack of understanding of QI principles, fear of additional workload, or skepticism about the effectiveness of new practices. Overcoming this barrier requires

30. "Comparison_QI Process_Nursing Process.jpg" by Amy Tyznik, MPTC for Open RN is licensed under CC BY 4.0
31. Agency for Healthcare Research and Quality. (2013). *Module 4. Approaches to quality improvement*. Practice facilitation handbook. https://www.ahrq.gov/ncepcr/tools/pf-handbook/mod4.html

robust education and training programs that highlight the benefits of QI initiatives and provide staff with the skills and knowledge needed to implement changes effectively. Also, having transparent conversations, discussing the process steps, and engaging staff questions are paramount.[32]

Another significant barrier is inadequate data management systems. Quality improvement relies heavily on accurate and timely data to identify areas for improvement, track progress, and measure outcomes. However, many health care organizations struggle with fragmented or outdated information systems that hinder data collection and analysis. Investing in modern, integrated health information technologies can facilitate better data management and support QI efforts. It also saves significant manpower and staff resources, allowing for more rapid identification of issues and trends.[33]

Resource constraints also pose a substantial challenge to quality improvement in health care. Financial limitations, staffing shortages, and limited time can impede the ability to implement and sustain QI initiatives. Organizations may find it difficult to allocate the necessary resources for training, process redesign, and continuous monitoring. Addressing this barrier often requires strategic planning, prioritization of QI projects, and seeking external funding or partnerships to support initiatives. Many organizations may have quality departments while others may utilize nursing staff to complete QI initiatives.[34]

Cultural factors in health care organizations can also impede quality improvement. Organizational culture that does not prioritize client safety and continuous improvement can undermine QI efforts. This barrier can be addressed by fostering a culture of transparency, accountability, and collaboration. Leadership plays a crucial role in setting the tone and demonstrating a commitment to quality improvement. Engaging all levels of staff in QI processes and celebrating successes can help build a positive culture that supports ongoing improvement.[35]

Lastly, regulatory and policy constraints can limit the scope and flexibility of QI initiatives. Health care organizations operate within a complex regulatory environment that can sometimes create barriers to innovative practices. Navigating these regulations while attempting to implement QI can be challenging. Advocacy for policy changes that support QI, along with a thorough understanding of existing regulations, can help organizations find ways to work within or adapt to these constraints.[36]

---

32. Giannitrapani, K., Satija. A., Ganesh, A., Gamboa, R., Fereydooni, S., Hennings, T., Chandrashekaran, S., Mickelsen, J., DeNatale, M., Spruijt, O., Bhatnagar, S., & Lorenz, K. A. (2021). Barriers and facilitators of using quality improvement to foster locally initiated innovation in palliative care services in India. *Journal of General Internal Medicine, 36*(2), 366-373. https://doi.org/10.1007/s11606-020-06152-y.
33. Giannitrapani, K., Satija. A., Ganesh, A., Gamboa, R., Fereydooni, S., Hennings, T., Chandrashekaran, S., Mickelsen, J., DeNatale, M., Spruijt, O., Bhatnagar, S., Lorenz, K. A. (2021). Barriers and facilitators of using quality improvement to foster locally initiated innovation in palliative care services in India. *Journal of General Internal Medicine, 36*(2), 366-373. https://doi.org/10.1007/s11606-020-06152-y.
34. Alexander, C., Tschannen, D., Argetsinger, D., Hakim, H., & Milner, K. A. (2022). A qualitative study on barriers and facilitators of quality improvement engagement by frontline nurses and leaders. *Journal of Nursing Management, 30*(3), 694-701. https://doi.org/10.1111/jonm.13537.
35. Alexander, C., Tschannen, D., Argetsinger, D., Hakim, H., & Milner, K. A. (2022). A qualitative study on barriers and facilitators of quality improvement engagement by frontline nurses and leaders. *Journal of Nursing Management, 30*(3), 694-701. https://doi.org/10.1111/jonm.13537.
36. Alexander, C., Tschannen, D., Argetsinger, D., Hakim, H., & Milner, K. A. (2022). A qualitative study on barriers and facilitators of quality improvement engagement by frontline nurses and leaders. *Journal of Nursing Management, 30*(3), 694-701. htttps://doi.org/10.1111/jonm.13537.

9.4 EVIDENCE-BASED PRACTICE AND RESEARCH

There are many ties between safe, quality client-centered care; evidence-based practice; research; and quality improvement. These concepts fall under the umbrella term "scholarly inquiry." All nurses should be involved in scholarly inquiry related to their nursing practice, no matter what agency they work. The American Nursing Association (ANA) Standard of Professional Performance called *Scholarly Inquiry* lists competencies related to incorporating evidence-based practice and research for all nurses. See the following box for a list of these competencies.[37]

Competencies of ANA's Scholarly Inquiry Standard of Professional Performance[38]

- Identifies questions in the health care or practice setting that can be answered by scholarly inquiry.
- Uses current evidence-based knowledge, combined with clinical expertise and health care consumer values and preferences, to guide practice in all settings.
- Participates in the formulation of evidence-based practice.
- Uses evidence to expand knowledge, skills, abilities, and judgement; to enhance role performance; and to increase knowledge of professional issues for themselves and others.
- Shares peer-reviewed, evidence-based findings with colleagues to integrate knowledge into nursing practice.
- Incorporates evidence and nursing research when initiating changes and improving quality in nursing practice.
- Articulates the value of research and scholarly inquiry and their application to one's practice and health care setting.
- Promotes ethical principles of research in practice and the health care setting.
- Reviews nursing research for application in practice and the health care setting.

Reflective Questions

1. What *Scholarly Inquiry* competencies have you already demonstrated during your nursing education?
2. What *Scholarly Inquiry* competencies are you most interested in mastering?
3. What questions do you have about the ANA's *Scholarly Inquiry* competencies?

Nursing practice should be based on solid evidence that guides care and ensures quality. Evidence-based practice (EBP) is the foundation for providing effective and efficient health care that promotes improved client outcomes. **Evidence-based practice** is defined by the American Nurses Association as, "A lifelong problem-solving approach that integrates the best evidence from well-designed research studies and evidence-based theories; clinical expertise and evidence from assessment of the health care consumer's history and condition, as well as health care resources; and client, family, group, community, and population preferences and values."[39] See Figure 9.7[40] for an illustration of evidence-based practice.

37. American Nurses Association. (2021). *Nursing: Scope and standards of practice* (4th ed.). American Nurses Association.
38. American Nurses Association. (2021). *Nursing: Scope and standards of practice* (4th ed.). American Nurses Association.
39. American Nurses Association. (2021). *Nursing: Scope and standards of practice* (4th ed.). American Nurses Association.
40. "Flowchart-sm.png" by Bates98 is licensed under CC BY_SA 4.0

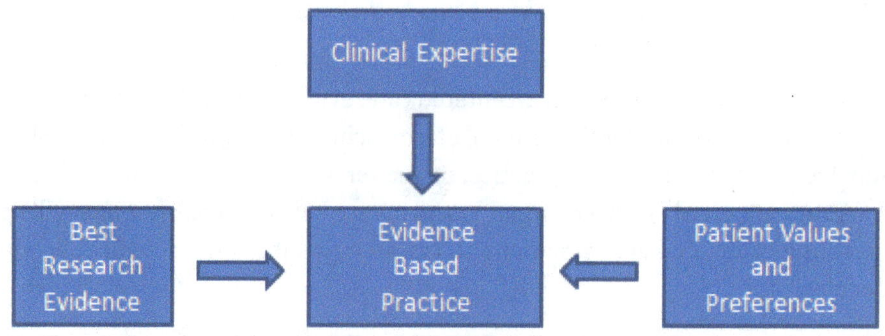

FIGURE 9.7 Evidence-based Practice

Evidence-based practice is the foundation nurses rely on to ensure their interventions, policies, and procedures are based on data supporting positive client outcomes. EBP relies on scholarly research that generates new nursing knowledge, as well as quality improvement processes that review client outcomes resulting from current nursing practice, to continually improve quality care. EBP encourages health care team members to incorporate new research findings into their practice, referred to as translating evidence into practice. Nurses must recognize the partnership between EBP and research; EBP cannot exist without continual scholarly research, and research requires nurses to evaluate research findings and incorporate them into their practice.[41]

Read examples of nursing evidence-based projects from Johns Hopkins. Access supplementary digital content in the online book using this QR code.

Newly graduated nurses may become immediately involved with evidence-based practice and quality improvement processes. The Quality and Safety Education (QSEN) project further elaborates on evidence-based practice for entry-level nurses with the definition of EBP as, "integrating best current evidence with clinical expertise and client/family preferences and values for delivery of optimal health care." See Table 9.4 for the knowledge, skills, and attitudes associated with the QSEN competency of evidence-based practice for entry-level nurses.

41. Chien, L. Y. (2019). Evidence-based practice and nursing research. *The Journal of Nursing Research: JNR, 27*(4), e29. https://doi.org/10.1097/jnr.0000000000000346

TABLE 9.4. QSEN: Knowledge, Skills, and Attitudes Associated With Evidence-Based Practice

Knowledge	Skills	Attitudes
Demonstrate knowledge of basic scientific methods and processes. Describe EBP to include the components of research evidence, clinical expertise, and client/family values.	Participate effectively in appropriate data collection and other research activities. Adhere to Institutional Review Board (IRB) guidelines. Base individualized care plan on client values, clinical expertise, and evidence.	Appreciate strengths and weaknesses of scientific bases for practice. Value the need for ethical conduct of research and quality improvement. Value the concept of EBP as integral to determining best clinical practice.
Differentiate clinical opinion from research and evidence summaries. Describe reliable sources for locating evidence reports and clinical practice guidelines.	Read original research and evidence reports related to area of practice. Locate evidence reports related to clinical practice topics and guidelines.	Appreciate the importance of regularly reading relevant professional journals.
Explain the role of evidence in determining best clinical practice. Describe how the strength and relevance of available evidence influences the choice of interventions in provision of client-centered care.	Participate in structuring the work environment to facilitate integration of new evidence into standards of practice. Question rationale for routine approaches to care that result in less-than-desired outcomes or adverse events.	Value the need for continuous improvement in clinical practice based on new knowledge.
Discriminate between valid and invalid reasons for modifying evidence-based clinical practice based on clinical expertise or client/family preferences.	Consult with clinical experts before deciding to deviate from evidence-based protocols.	Acknowledge own limitations in knowledge and clinical expertise before determining when to deviate from evidence-based best practices.

Reflective Questions: Read through the knowledge, skills, and attitudes in Table 9.4.

1. How are you currently integrating evidence-based practice when providing client care?
2. Where do you find information on current evidence-based practice?
3. Have you witnessed any routine approaches to care that resulted in less-than-desired outcomes or adverse events?
4. What else would you like to learn about evidence-based nursing practice?

Keeping Current on Evidence-Based Practices

Health care is constantly evolving with new technologies and new evidence-based practices. Nurses must dedicate themselves to being lifelong learners. After graduating from nursing school, it is important to remain current on evidence-based practices. Many employers subscribe to electronic evidence-based clinical tools that nurses and other health care team members can access at the bedside. Nurses also independently stay up-to-date on current evidence-based practice by reading nursing journals; attending national, state, and local nursing conferences; and completing continuing education courses. See the box below for examples of ways to remain current on evidence-based practices.

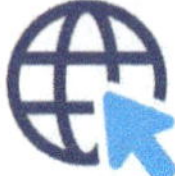

Examples of Evidence-Based Clinical Supports, Nursing Journals, and Conferences

- *American Nurse* (published by the American Nurses Association)
- *American Journal of Nursing*
- Cochrane Library
- ECRI Guidelines Trust
- Agency for Healthcare Research and Quality – EPC Evidence-Based Reports
- *Journal of Clinical Nursing*
- Lippincott Advisor
- Turning Research Into Practice (TRIP) Database
- UpToDate
- American Nursing Association – Events and Continuing Education

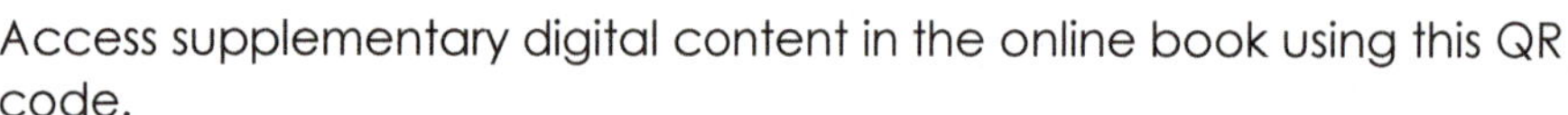

Access supplementary digital content in the online book using this QR code.

Research

Earlier in this chapter we discussed the process of quality improvement and the manner in which it is used to evaluate current nursing practice by determining where gaps exist and what improvements can be made. **Nursing research** is a different process than QI. The American Nurses Association (ANA) defines nursing research as, "Systematic inquiry designed to develop knowledge about issues of importance to the nursing professions."[42] The purpose of nursing research is to advance nursing practice through the discovery of new information. It is also used to provide scholarly evidence regarding improved client outcomes resulting from evidence-based nursing interventions.

42. American Nurses Association. (2021). *Nursing: Scope and standards of practice* (4th ed.). American Nurses Association.

Nursing research is guided by a systematic, scientific approach. Research consists of reviewing current literature for recurring themes and evidence, defining terms and current concepts, defining the population of interest for the research study, developing or identifying tools for collecting data, collecting and analyzing the data, and making recommendations for nursing practice. As you can see, the scholarly process of nursing research is more complex than the Plan, Do, Study, Act process of QI and typically requires more time and resources to complete.[43]

Nurse researchers often use the PICOT format to organize the overall goals of the research project. The PICOT mnemonic assists nurses in answering the clinical question to be studied.[44] See Figure 9.8[45] for an image of PICOT. PICOT terms are further defined in the following box.

PICOT
P - Population/Problem: Who are the patients and what will be studied?
I - Intervention: What specific intervention will be implemented?
C - Comparison: What alternative(s) will be used to compare results to the treatment intervention?
O - Outcome: What will be measured and how? What is the identified goal?
T - Timeframe: How long will the interventions be implemented and data collected?

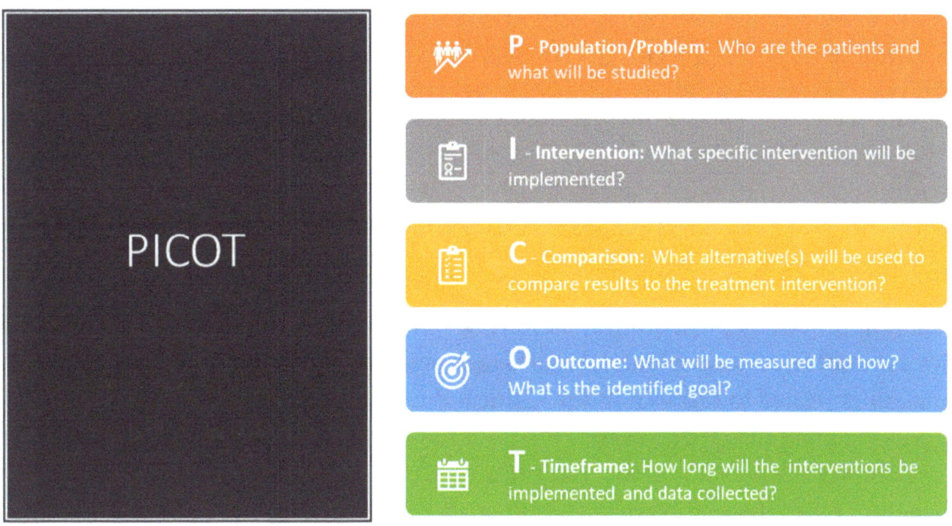

FIGURE 9.8 PICOT

43. American Association of Colleges of Nursing. (2006). *Nursing research.* https://www.aacnnursing.org/News-Information/Position-Statements-White-Papers/Nursing-Research

44. Lansing Community College Library. (2025). *Nursing: PICOT.* https://libguides.lcc.edu/c.php?g=167860&p=6198388

45. "PICOT.png" by Kim Ernstmeyer for Chippewa Valley Technical College is licensed under CC BY 4.0

PICOT

P: Population/Problem: Who are the clients who will be studied (e.g., age, race, gender, disease, or health status, etc.) and what problem is being addressed (e.g., mortality, morbidity, compliance, satisfaction, etc.)?

I: Intervention: What is the specific intervention to be implemented with the research population (e.g., therapy, education, medication, etc.)?

C: Comparison: What is the alternative intervention that will be used to compare to the treatment intervention (e.g., placebo, no intervention, different medication, etc.)?

O: Outcome: What will be measured and how will it be measured and with what identified goal (e.g., fewer symptoms, increased satisfaction, reduced mortality, etc.)?

T: Time Frame: How long will the interventions be implemented and data collected for this research?

After the researcher has completed the PICOT question, these additional questions should also be considered to protect clients' rights and reduce the potential for ethical conflicts:

- Was the study approved by the Institutional Review Board (IRB)? The IRB, also known as an independent ethics committee, reviews research studies to protect the rights and welfare of participants.[46] Read more about ethics related to research in the "Ethical Practice" chapter.
- Were the participants protected? Researchers have the responsibility to protect human rights, uphold HIPAA, and respect the personal values of the participants.
- Did the benefits of the intervention outweigh the risk(s)? Researchers have the responsibility to identify if there is a possibility for increased harm to the clients because of the research project.
- Were informed consents obtained? All research participants must provide written informed consent before a study can begin. Researchers must ensure the participants were fully informed of the study, provided risks and benefits, and allowed to exit the study at any time.
- Were vulnerable populations protected? Populations of study that include infants, minorities, children, elderly, socioeconomically disadvantaged, prisoners, etc., are considered vulnerable populations, and researchers must ensure their rights and safety are accounted for.

After the nurse researcher confirms participants' rights are protected and has established a PICOT question, the next step is to design the research study and review existing research. Research designs are categorized by the type of data that is collected and reviewed. See Figure 9.9[47] for an illustration of different types of research. The three basic types of nursing research are quantitative studies, qualitative studies, and meta-analyses. See definitions and examples of these types in the following box.

---

46. U. S. Food & Drug Administration. (2025). *Institutional review boards frequently asked questions: Guidance for institutional review boards and clinical investigators.* https://www.fda.gov/regulatory-information/search-fda-guidance-documents/institutional-review-boards-frequently-asked-questions

47. "Quantitative_methods.png" by Remydiligent1 is licensed under CC BY-SA 4.0

Types of Research

- **Quantitative Studies:** These studies provide objective data by using number values to explain outcomes. Researchers can use statistical analysis to determine the strength of the findings, as well as identify correlations.

View an example of an quantitative research study. Access supplementary digital content in the online book using this QR code.

- **Qualitative Studies:** These studies provide subjective data, often focusing on the perception or experience of the participants. Data is collected through observations and open-ended questions and is often referred to as experimental data. Data is interpreted by recurring themes in participants' views and observations.

View an example of a qualitative research study. Access supplementary digital content in the online book using this QR code.

- **Meta-Analyses:** A meta-analysis, also referred to as a "systematic review," compares the results of independent research studies asking similar research questions. A meta-analysis often collects both quantitative and qualitative data to provide a well-rounded evaluation by providing both objective and subjective outcomes. This research design often requires more time and resources, but it also promotes consistency and reliability through the identification of common themes.

View an example of a meta-analysis/systematic review. Access supplementary digital content in the online book using this QR code.

Experimental Research
- Uses a control group and experimental group
- Experimental Research is needed to suggest a cause and effect relationship

Content Analysis
- Analysis of texts and media
- Counting the number of occurrences of a particular phenomena

Survey Research
- Questionnaires, Interviews, and Sample Polls
- Represents response using statistically using graphs, charts, tables, or percentages

Meta-Analysis
- Analyze patterns in existing research
- Combining the results from a collection of existing research

FIGURE 9.9 Research

Nurses must understand the types of research designs to accurately understand and apply the research findings. Additionally, only research from peer-reviewed scholarly journals should be used. Scholarly journals use a process called "peer review" to ensure high quality. An article that is **peer reviewed** has been reviewed independently by at least two other academic experts in the same field as the author(s) to ensure accuracy.

Nurses must also be aware of the difference between primary and secondary sources of scholarly evidence. A **primary source** is the original study or report of an experiment or clinical problem. The evidence is typically written and published by the individual(s) conducting the research and includes a literature review, description of the research design, statistical analysis of the data, and discussion regarding the implications of the results.

A **secondary source** is written by an author who gathers existing data provided from research completed by another individual. A secondary source analyzes and reports on findings from other research projects and may interpret findings or draw conclusions. In nursing research secondary sources of evidence are typically published as a systematic review and meta-analysis.

View QUT Library's primary vs. secondary sources YouTube video. Access supplementary digital content in the online book using this QR code.[48]

By understanding these basic research concepts, nurses can accurately implement current evidence-based practice based on continually evolving nursing research.

48. QUT Library. (2020, November 22). *Primary vs. secondary sources* [Video]. YouTube. All rights reserved. https://youtu.be/FZRxYfWYEBI

9.5 SPOTLIGHT APPLICATION

Joanne is a newly graduated nurse working on a general medical floor in a large urban teaching hospital. She is typically assigned between four and six clients during her shift depending on the acuity mix. Many of her clients are direct admit clients or are transferred from the emergency department. Joanne has recently noticed a significant delay on weekend shifts with room turnover and new client admittance.

Joanne voiced her concerns regarding the delays to her unit manager. Her manager agreed that room turnover delays on the weekend have significantly increased in recent months. She reported that she will investigate the delays further. A few weeks pass and Joanne's manager reports back that there have been staff reductions in the organization's environmental services staff on the weekend shifts. As a result, room cleaning has been delayed significantly. Joanne's manager has voiced her concerns regarding the delays, but administration has been reluctant to hire additional staff. Joanne and her manager both feel strongly that investment in staff is needed.

Reflective Questions

1. What strategies might Joanne and her manager utilize to reflect the significance of these staff shortages?
2. How might they gather and present information to demonstrate the need for additional environmental services personnel?
3. What stakeholders would be important to engage in this discussion?
4. Create a PICOT question for this scenario.

When considering the impact of care delays in a health care organization, it is important to gather data to substantiate the significance of delayed care. Joanne and her manager might begin to look at organizational throughput or transfer data to determine how long clients are being held in emergency rooms or other settings during the weekend shifts compared to weekday shifts. Additionally, it would be important for the organization to determine if these delayed admits impeded the ability of the emergency department to accept clients and if the organization was subsequently placed on client divert due to an inability to care for clients in the emergency room setting. Engaging house supervisors, charge nurses, informatics specialists, etc., may be helpful in determining the significance of the delay and potential quality implications. An example PICOT question to help examine this scenario may be structured as: What is the impact of one additional environmental services FTE compared to existing staffing patterns on organizational throughput times over a three-month period?

9.6 LEARNING ACTIVITIES

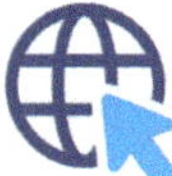

Interactive learning activities have been excluded from the print version of the text. Access free online learning activities in the online book using this QR code.

9.7 GLOSSARY

Accreditation: A review process to determine if an agency meets the defined standards of quality determined by the accrediting body.

ANA Standards of Professional Performance: Authoritative statements of the actions and behaviors that all registered nurses, regardless of role, population, specialty, and setting are expected to perform competently.

Core measures: National standards of care and treatment processes for common conditions. These processes are proven to reduce complications and lead to better client outcomes.

Evidence-Based Practice (EBP): A lifelong problem-solving approach that integrates the best evidence from well-designed research studies and evidence-based theories; clinical expertise and evidence from assessment of the health care consumer's history and condition, as well as health care resources; and client, family, group, community, and population preferences and values.[49]

Informatics: Using information and technology to communicate, manage knowledge, mitigate error, and support decision-making.[50] This allows members of the health care team to share, store, and analyze health-related information.

Meta-analysis: A type of nursing research (also referred to as a "systematic review") that compares the results of independent research studies asking similar research questions. This research often collects both quantitative and qualitative data to provide a well-rounded evaluation by providing both objective and subjective outcomes.

Nursing informatics: The science and practice integrating nursing, its information and knowledge, with information and communication technologies to promote the health of people, families, and communities worldwide.

Nursing research: The systematic inquiry designed to develop knowledge about issues of importance to the nursing profession.[51] The purpose of nursing research is to advance nursing practice through the discovery of new information. It is also used to provide scholarly evidence regarding improved client outcomes resulting from nursing interventions.

National Patient Safety Goals: Guidelines specific to organizations accredited by The Joint Commission that focus on problems in health care safety and ways to solve them.

Peer-reviewed: Scholarly journal articles that have been reviewed independently by at least two other academic experts in the same field as the author(s) to ensure accuracy and quality.

Primary source: An original study or report of an experiment or clinical problem. The evidence is typically written and published by the individual(s) conducting the research and includes a literature review, description of the research design, statistical analysis of the data, and discussion regarding the implications of the results.

---

49. American Nurses Association. (2021). *Nursing: Scope and standards of practice* (4th ed.). American Nurses Association.
50. QSEN Institute. (n.d.). *QSEN competencies: Quality improvement (QI).* https://qsen.org/competencies/pre-licensure-ksas/#quality_improvement
51. American Nurses Association. (2021). *Nursing: Scope and standards of practice* (4th ed.). American Nurses Association.

Qualitative studies: A type of study that provides subjective data, often focusing on the perception or experience of the participants. Data is collected through observations and open-ended questions and often referred to as experimental data. Data is interpreted by developing themes in participants' views and observations.

Quality: The degree to which nursing services for health care consumers, families, groups, communities, and populations increase the likelihood of desirable outcomes and are consistent with evolving nursing knowledge.

Quality Improvement (QI): A systematic process using measurable data to improve health care services and the overall health status of clients. The QI process includes the steps of Plan, Do, Study, and Act.

Quantitative studies: A type of study that provides objective data by using number values to explain outcomes. Researchers can use statistical analysis to determine strength of the findings, as well as identify correlations.

Secondary source: Evidence is written by an author who gathers existing data provided from research completed by another individual. This type of source analyzes and reports on findings from other research projects and may interpret findings or draw conclusions. In nursing research these sources are typically published as a systematic review and meta-analysis.

Utilization review: An investigation by insurance agencies and other health care funders on services performed by doctors, nurses, and other health care team members to ensure money is not wasted covering things that are unnecessary for proper treatment or are inefficient. This review also allows organizations to objectively measure how effectively health care services and resources are being used to best meet their clients' needs.

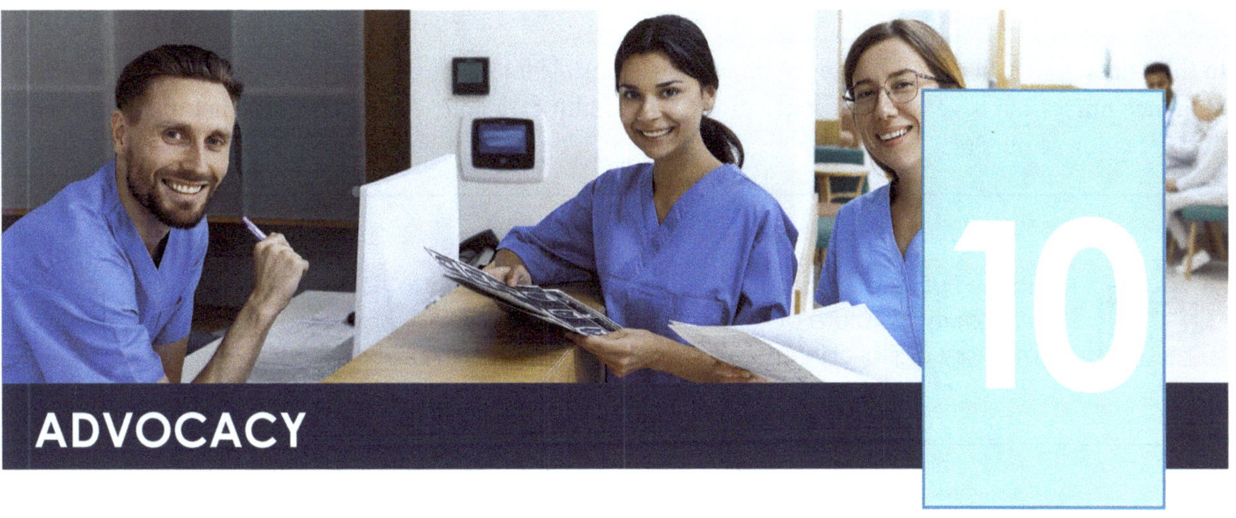

10.1 ADVOCACY INTRODUCTION

LEARNING OBJECTIVES

- Assess the effects of current health care policies on health care consumers and nursing practice
- Explore the role of professional organizations in nursing practice
- Discuss legislative policy-making activities that influence nursing practice and health care
- Examine various positions on unions and collective bargaining
- Compare various workplace advocacy models

What do you think of when you hear the word "advocacy"? Nurses act as advocates for their clients (e.g., individuals, families, communities, or populations) by protecting their "client rights" and voicing their needs. Nurses have a long history of acting as client advocates. Early nurses advocated for professional nurses' value and knowledge and fought for implementation of best practices, safety measures, and other quality improvements. Florence Nightingale advocated for practice changes that improved environmental conditions in health care and reduced life-threatening infections by using data to support her recommendations. Lillian Wald worked to establish public health nursing and improve the lives of immigrant communities.

More recently, nurses led the establishment of Nurse Practice Acts in each state and pushed for multistate licensing via the Nurse Licensure Compact (NLC). The American Nurses Association (ANA) declared 2018 as the "Year of Advocacy" to highlight the importance of advocacy in the nurse's role. Nurses continue to advocate for building healthier communities as demonstrated in the *Future of Nursing 2020-2030: Charting a Path to Achieve Health Equity* report.[1]

1. National Academies of Sciences, Engineering, and Medicine. (2021). *The Future of nursing 2020-2030: Charting a path to achieve health equity.* The National Academies Press. https://doi.org/10.17226/25982

In this chapter, we will review how every nurse is responsible for client advocacy and examine the powerful influence nurses can have on local, state, and federal health care policies that affect the nation's health and the profession of nursing.

Read the *Future of Nursing 2020-2030: Charting a Path to Achieve Health Equity* at Future of Nursing: Campaign for Action. Access supplementary digital content in the online book using this QR code.

10.2 BASIC ADVOCACY CONCEPTS

Advocacy

The American Nurses Association (ANA) emphasizes that advocacy is fundamental to nursing practice in every setting. See Figure 10.1[2] for an illustration of advocacy. **Advocacy** is defined as the act or process of pleading for, supporting, or recommending a cause or course of action. Advocacy may be for individuals, groups, organizations, communities, society, or policy issues[3]:

- **Individual:** The nurse educates health care consumers so they can consider actions, interventions, or choices related to their own personal beliefs, attitudes, and knowledge to achieve the desired outcome. In this way, the health care consumer learns self-management and decision-making.[4]
- **Interpersonal:** The nurse empowers health care consumers by providing emotional support, assistance in obtaining resources, and necessary help through interactions with families and significant others in their social support network.[5]
- **Organization and Community:** The nurse supports cultural and social transformation of organizations, communities, or populations. Registered nurses understand their obligation to help improve environmental and societal conditions related to health, wellness, and care of the health care consumer.[6]
- **Policy:** The nurse promotes inclusion of the health care consumers' voices into policy, legislation, and regulation about issues such as health care access, reduction of health care costs and financial burden, protection of the health care consumer, and environmental health, such as safe housing and clear water.[7]

Advocacy at each of these levels will be further discussed in later sections of this chapter.

2. "Advocacy_-_The_Noun_Project.svg" by OCHA Visual Information Unit is licensed under CC0
3. American Nurses Association. (2021). *Nursing: Scope and standards of practice* (4th ed.). American Nurses Association.
4. American Nurses Association. (2021). *Nursing: Scope and standards of practice* (4th ed.). American Nurses Association.
5. American Nurses Association. (2021). *Nursing: Scope and standards of practice* (4th ed.). American Nurses Association.
6. American Nurses Association. (2021). *Nursing: Scope and standards of practice* (4th ed.). American Nurses Association.
7. American Nurses Association. (2021). *Nursing: Scope and standards of practice* (4th ed.). American Nurses Association.

FIGURE 10.1 Advocacy

Advocacy is one of the ANA's Standards of Professional Performance. The Standards of Professional Performance are "authoritative statements of the actions and behaviors that all registered nurses, regardless of role, population, specialty, and setting, are expected to perform competently."[8] See the following box to read the competencies associated with the ANA's *Advocacy* Standard of Professional Performance.[9]

Competencies of ANA's Advocacy Standard of Professional Performance[10]

- Champions the voice of the health care consumer.
- Recommends appropriate levels of care, timely and appropriate transitions, and allocation of resources to optimize outcomes.
- Promotes safe care of health care consumers, safe work environments, and sufficient resources.
- Participates in health care initiatives on behalf of the health care consumer and the system(s) where nursing happens.
- Demonstrates a willingness to address persistent, pervasive systemic issues.
- Informs the political arena about the role of nurses and the vital components necessary for nurses and nursing to provide optimal care delivery.
- Empowers all members of the health care team to include the health care consumer in care decisions, including limitation of treatment and end-of-life care.

8. American Nurses Association. (2021). *Nursing: Scope and standards of practice* (4th ed.). American Nurses Association.
9. American Nurses Association. (2021). *Nursing: Scope and standards of practice* (4th ed.). American Nurses Association.
10. American Nurses Association. (2021). *Nursing: Scope and standards of practice* (4th ed.). American Nurses Association.

- Embraces diversity, equity, inclusivity, health promotion, and health care for individuals of diverse geographic, cultural, ethnic, racial, gender, and spiritual backgrounds across the life span.
- Develops policies that improve care delivery and access for underserved and vulnerable populations.
- Promotes policies, regulations, and legislation at the local, state, and national levels to improve health care access and delivery of health care.
- Considers societal, political, economic, and cultural factors to address social determinants of health.
- Role models advocacy behavior.
- Addresses the urgent need for a diverse and inclusive workforce as a strategy to improve outcomes related to the social determinants of health and inequities in the health care system.
- Advances policies, programs, and practices within the health care environment that maintain, sustain, and restore the environment and natural world.
- Contributes to professional organizations.

Reflective Questions

1. What *Advocacy* competencies have you already demonstrated during your nursing education?
2. What *Advocacy* competencies are you most interested in performing next?
3. What questions do you have about ANA's *Advocacy* competencies?

10.3 INDIVIDUAL AND INTERPERSONAL ADVOCACY

As discussed previously, the American Nurses Association (ANA) defines advocacy at the individual level as educating health care consumers so they can consider actions, interventions, or choices related to their own personal beliefs, attitudes, and knowledge to achieve the desired outcome. In this way, the health care consumer learns self-management and decision-making.[11] Advocacy at the interpersonal level is defined as empowering health care consumers by providing emotional support, assistance in obtaining resources, and necessary help through interactions with families and significant others in their social support network.[12]

What does advocacy look like in a nurse's daily practice? The following are some examples provided by an oncology nurse[13]:

- **Ensure Safety.** Ensure the client is safe when being treated in a health care facility and when they are discharged by communicating with case managers or social workers about the client's need for home health or assistance after discharge so it is arranged before they go home.

11. American Nurses Association. (2021). *Nursing: Scope and standards of practice* (4th ed.). American Nurses Association.
12. American Nurses Association. (2021). *Nursing: Scope and standards of practice* (4th ed.). American Nurses Association.
13. Nitzky, A. (2018). *Six ways nurses can advocate for patients.* Oncology Nursing News. https://www.oncnursingnews.com/view/six-ways-nurses-can-advocate-for-patients

- **Give Clients a Voice.** Give clients a voice when they are vulnerable by staying in the room with them while the doctor explains their diagnosis and treatment options to help them ask questions, get answers, and translate information from medical jargon.
- **Educate.** Educate clients on how to manage their current or chronic conditions to improve the quality of their everyday life. For example, clients undergoing chemotherapy can benefit from the nurse teaching them how to take their anti-nausea medication in a way that will be most effective for them and will allow them to feel better between treatments.
- **Protect Client Rights.** Know clients' wishes for their care. Advocacy may include therapeutically communicating a client's wishes to an upset family member who disagrees with their choices. In this manner, the client's rights are protected and a healing environment is established.
- **Double-Check for Errors.** Know that everyone makes mistakes. Nurses often identify, stop, and fix errors made by interprofessional team members. They flag conflicting orders from multiple providers and notice oversights. Nurses should read provider orders and carefully compare new orders to previous documentation. If an order is unclear or raises concerns, a nurse should discuss their concerns with another nurse, a charge nurse, a pharmacist, or the provider before implementing it to ensure client safety.
- **Connect Clients to Resources.** Help clients find resources inside and outside the hospital to support their well-being. Know resources in your agency, such as case managers or social workers who can assist with financial concerns, advance directives, health insurance, or transportation concerns. Request assistance from agency chaplains to support spiritual concerns. Promote community resources, such as client or caregiver support networks, Meals on Wheels, or other resources to meet their needs.

Nurses must recognize their unique position in client advocacy to empower individuals to provide them with the support and resources to make their best judgment. The intimate and continuous nature of the nurse-client relationship places nurses in a prime position to identify and address the needs and concerns of their clients. This relationship is built on trust, empathy, and consistent interaction, which allows nurses to gain a deep understanding of their clients' values, preferences, and personal circumstances. By leveraging this close proximity and strong rapport, nurses can effectively advocate for their clients, ensuring that their voices are heard, and their wishes are respected in all aspects of care.[14]

The power of the nurse-client relationship extends beyond the immediate clinical environment. Nurses often act as liaisons between clients and the broader health care team, facilitating communication and ensuring that client preferences are integrated into care plans. This advocacy role is crucial in navigating complex health care systems where clients may feel overwhelmed or marginalized. Nurses can help demystify medical jargon, explain treatment options, and support clients in making informed decisions that align with their values and goals. Through education and emotional support, nurses empower clients to take an active role in their own care, enhancing client autonomy and satisfaction.[15]

In addition to direct client care, nurses play a pivotal role in identifying systemic issues that affect client outcomes. Their frontline perspective provides valuable insights into the barriers clients face in accessing quality care, such as socioeconomic challenges, cultural barriers, and institutional policies. By advocating for policy changes and improvements in health care delivery, nurses contribute to creating a more equitable and client-centered health care system. Their advocacy efforts can lead to the implementation of practices

14. Nsiah, C., Siakwa, M., & Ninnoni, J. P. K. (2019). Registered nurses' description of patient advocacy in the clinical setting. *Nursing Open, 6*(3), 1124-1132. https://doi.org/10.1002/nop2.307.
15. Nsiah, C., Siakwa, M., & Ninnoni, J. P. K. (2019). Registered nurses' description of patient advocacy in the clinical setting. *Nursing Open, 6*(3), 1124-1132. https;//doi.org/10.1002/nop2.307.

and policies that better address the needs of diverse client populations, ultimately improving health outcomes on a broader scale.[16]

Nurses' advocacy is also essential in situations where clients are unable to speak for themselves, such as in cases of severe illness, disability, or end-of-life care. In these instances, nurses must be vigilant in recognizing and addressing the needs of vulnerable clients, ensuring that their rights and dignity are upheld. This may involve working closely with families and caregivers, coordinating with interdisciplinary teams, and navigating ethical dilemmas to provide the best possible care for the client.

10.4 COMMUNITY AND ORGANIZATION ADVOCACY

Nurses advocate for issues in their communities and their organizations.

Addressing Social Determinants of Health

Advocacy is commonly perceived as acting on behalf of a client, but it can be a much broader action than affecting a single client and their family members. Nurses advocate for building healthier communities by addressing **social determinants of health (SDOH)**. SDOH are the conditions in the environments where people live, learn, work, and play that affect a wide range of outcomes. SDOH include health care access and quality, neighborhood and environment, social and community context, economic stability, and education access and quality. Social determinants of health (SDOH) have a major impact on people's health, well-being, and quality of life. See Figure 10.2[17] for an illustration of SDOH.[18]

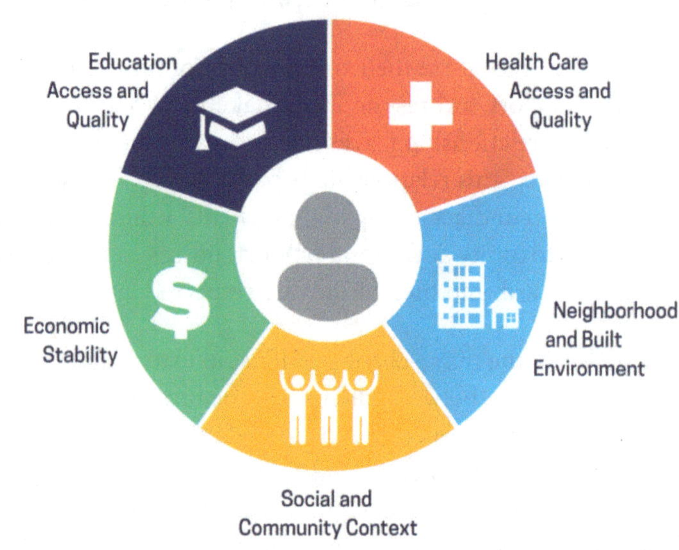

FIGURE 10.2 Social Determinants of Health

16. Nsiah, C., Siakwa, M., & Ninnoni, J. P. K. (2019). Registered nurses' description of patient advocacy in the clinical setting. *Nursing Open, 6*(3), 1124-1132. https://doi.org/10.1002/nop2.307.

17. "Healthy People 2030 SDOH Graphic.png" by U.S. Department of Health and Human Services, Office of Disease Prevention and Health Promotion is in the Public Domain. Access for free at https://health.gov/healthypeople/objectives-and-data/social-determinants-health

18. Healthy People 2030. (n.d.). *Social determinants of health.* U.S. Department of Health and Human Services. https://health.gov/healthypeople/objectives-and-data/social-determinants-health

Specific examples of addressing SDOH include the following goals:

- Improving safe housing and public transportation
- Decreasing discrimination and violence
- Expanding quality education and job opportunities
- Increasing access to nutritious foods and physical activity opportunities
- Promoting clean air and clean water
- Enhancing language and literacy skills[19]

SDOH contribute to health disparities and inequities among different socioeconomic groups. For example, individuals who don't have access to grocery stores with healthy foods are less likely to have good nutrition, increasing their risk for health conditions like heart disease, diabetes, and obesity, and potentially lowering their life expectancy relative to people who do have access to healthy foods.[20]

One of Healthy People 2030's goals specifically relates to advocacy regarding SDOH. The goal states, "Create social, physical, and economic environments that promote attaining the full potential for health and well-being for all." Across the United States, people and organizations at the local, state, territorial, tribal, and national levels are working hard to improve health and reduce health disparities by addressing SDOH.[21] Read more information about these advocacy efforts in the following box.

Read more about efforts addressing SDOH at Healthy People 2030. Access supplementary digital content in the online book using this QR code.

Understanding and addressing SDOH is crucial for effective health care advocacy, as it provides a comprehensive view of the various elements that impact clients' well-being. These determinants include economic stability, education, social and community context, health and health care access, and the neighborhood and built environment.

- **Economic stability:** Factors such as income, employment, and financial security directly affect individuals' ability to access health care services, afford medications, and maintain healthy lifestyles. Advocates can use this understanding to push for policies that address income inequality, create job opportunities, and provide financial support for those in need. By advocating for economic policies that reduce poverty and enhance financial stability, health care advocates can help mitigate one of the most significant barriers to health.
- **Education:** Higher levels of education are associated with better health outcomes, as education enhances health literacy, empowers individuals to make informed health decisions, and provides opportunities for better employment. Advocacy efforts can focus on improving access to quality education, promoting

19. Healthy People 2030. (n.d.). *Social determinants of health.* U.S. Department of Health and Human Services. https://health.gov/healthypeople/objectives-and-data/social-determinants-health
20. Healthy People 2030. (n.d.). *Social determinants of health.* U.S. Department of Health and Human Services. https://health.gov/healthypeople/objectives-and-data/social-determinants-health
21. Healthy People 2030. (n.d.). *Social determinants of health.* U.S. Department of Health and Human Services. https://health.gov/healthypeople/objectives-and-data/social-determinants-health

health education programs, and supporting lifelong learning initiatives. By addressing educational disparities, advocates can contribute to long-term improvements in health and well-being.

- **Social and community context:** Strong social support and community connections can improve mental health, reduce stress, and foster a sense of belonging, all of which are essential for overall well-being. Health care advocates can work to strengthen community resources, promote social cohesion, and address issues such as discrimination and violence. Efforts to build safer, more supportive communities can lead to healthier and more resilient populations.
- **Access to health and health care:** Barriers such as lack of insurance, geographic limitations, and inadequate health care infrastructure can prevent individuals from receiving necessary care. Advocacy in this area can focus on expanding health care coverage, improving health care delivery systems, and ensuring that marginalized populations have access to quality care. By promoting equitable access to health care services, advocates can help reduce health disparities and improve outcomes for underserved communities.
- **Neighborhood and environment:** Poor housing conditions, lack of safe recreational spaces, and limited access to nutritious food can lead to adverse health outcomes. Advocates can work to improve urban planning, support affordable housing initiatives, and promote policies that ensure access to healthy food options. Creating healthier environments can have a substantial impact on public health.[22] Nursing union goals are typically to advocate for the improvement of benefits, wages, client safety, and workplace conditions. Advocacy is accomplished by collective bargaining. **Collective bargaining** refers to the negotiation of wages and other conditions of employment by an organized body of employees. See Figure 10.3[23] for an image of a union worker.

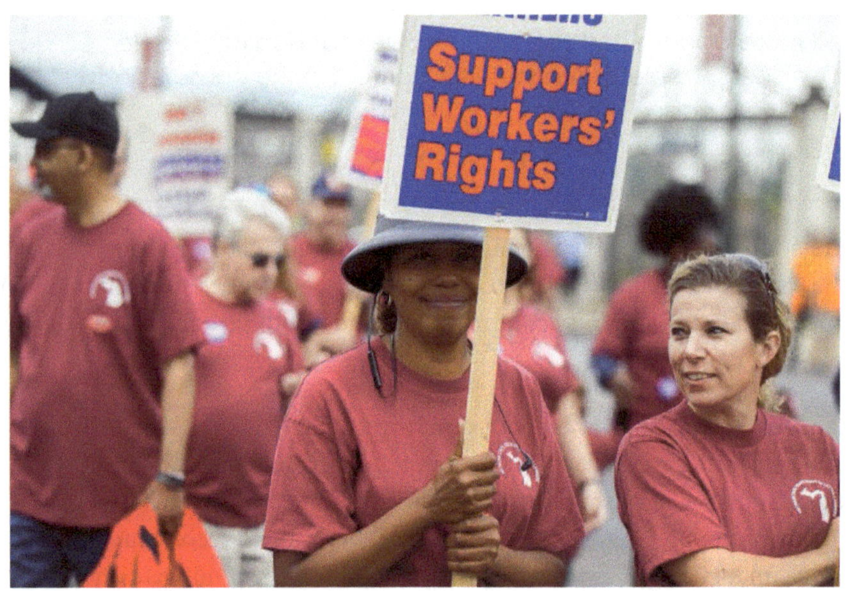

FIGURE 10.3 Union Worker

22. Healthy People 2030. (n.d.). *Social determinants of health.* U.S. Department of Health and Human Services. https://health.gov/healthypeople/objectives-and-data/social-determinants-health[/footnote Analysis of individuals' social determinants of health provides a holistic understanding of the factors that influence health. By addressing economic stability, education, social and community context, health and healthcare access, and the neighborhood and built environment, advocates can develop comprehensive strategies to improve health outcomes and reduce disparities. Recognizing and addressing SDOH enables healthcare advocates to promote policies and initiatives that create healthier, more equitable communities, ultimately leading to better health for all.

23. "Debbie_Stabenow_marches_on_Labor_Day_2017_21318919_10155403813215528_8762450224354658172_o.jpg" by Office of Debbie Stabenow is in the Public Domain

Although there is no single union that represents all nurses across the country, there are several nursing unions such as the National Nurses United, SEIU United Healthcare, and The United Food and Commercial Workers International Union. The National Nurses United union is the largest nursing union in the United States and has joined with other unions across the country to address unsafe staffing. Read more about these unions in the following box.

Read more about nursing unions:

- National Nurses United
- SEIU United Healthcare
- The United Food and Commercial Workers International Union

Access supplementary digital content in the online book using this QR code.

Nursing unions can provide several potential benefits to the nursing profession. They may improve job security, improve working conditions, negotiate for better pay and benefits, protect seniority, establish staffing ratios, address workplace violence and incivility, and provide a well-defined grievance process. Unionized nurses earn an average of $200-$400 more per week than nonunionized nurses. Unions assist with grievance processes for resolving disagreements between employees and management. Examples of grievances include the promotion of one employee over another who has more seniority, disputes over holiday pay, and problems related to employee discipline.[24]

However, there are also potential disadvantages of unions, such as the cost of dues (up to $90/month per nurse), difficulty in removal of incompetent nurses, mandatory strikes with no pay, the issue of seniority taking precedence over good performance, and creation of working environments that can be adversarial between management and nursing. Additionally, many nursing unions are not organized or led by nurses, causing the belief that some unions are more interested in collecting dues than in improving the work environment for nurses. Although there has been research to determine if unions are good for nurses and good for clients, the findings are not conclusive. Some studies have shown that unionized hospitals have lower mortality rates, but higher failure-to-rescue and pressure injury rates. Another study found that unionized hospitals had higher levels of job dissatisfaction but higher levels of nurse retention.[25,26]

Workplace Advocacy Models

Nurses can advocate for improvements in the workplace via various mechanisms, such as shared governance and the ANCC Magnet Recognition Program, and by participation in professional organizations. Nurses can also seek legislative solutions for workplace problems by advocating for legislation such as whistleblower protection.[27] Whistleblower protection is further discussed in the "Policy Advocacy" section of this chapter.

---

24. Rowland, T. (2020). *The pros and cons of nursing unions* [Blog]. Soliant. https://blog.soliant.com/nursing/the-pros-and-cons-of-nursing-unions/
25. Dube, A. Kaplan, E., & Thompson, O. (2016). Nurse unions and patient outcomes. *ILR Review, 69*(4), 803-833. https://doi.org/10.1177%2F0019793916644251
26. Seago, J. A., Spetz, J., Ash, M., Herrera, C., & Keane, D. (2011). Hospital RN job satisfaction and nurse unions. *Journal of Nursing Administration, 41*(3), 109-114. https://doi.org/10.1097/nna.0b013e31820c726f
27. American Nurses Association. (n.d.). *Five opportunities and challenges for workforce advocacy program.* https://www.nursingworld.org/practice-policy/advocacy/

SHARED GOVERNANCE

Shared governance refers to a shared leadership model between management and employees working together to achieve common goals. Shared governance models are believed to promote nurses' empowerment, engagement, autonomy, accountability, and collaboration while also striving to improve client safety, quality care, and positive outcomes. This style of management encourages and empowers nurses to be part of making decisions that impact their daily work environments. When organizations utilize a shared governance model, employees feel valued and invested in the organization's success. Nurse engagement also improves both staff and client outcomes, such as increased job satisfaction and client satisfaction.[28] Implementation of a shared governance model has led to organizational cost savings, decrease in meeting times, fewer sick days used by employees, and a decrease in staff turnover.[29] See the following box for an example of effective shared governance.

Example of Effective Shared Governance[30]

A busy telemetry unit wants to address issues with low client satisfaction scores and an increase in both central line and indwelling catheter days. A quality improvement project is instituted by a multidisciplinary team that works to communicate the project's goals and objectives, respecting each team member's expertise and input. The team initiates daily multidisciplinary rounding on the unit. Six months after the implementation of multidisciplinary rounding, client satisfaction scores improve, and a decrease in both central line and indwelling catheter days is noted. Multidisciplinary rounding provides a collaborative team approach, acknowledging the expertise and leadership role of each discipline with the same end goal of improving client outcomes.

MAGNET RECOGNITION PROGRAM

Nurses can advocate for their excellence in the workplace by participating in activities required for Magnet Recognition. As previously discussed in this book, the **Magnet Recognition Program** is an organizational credential from the American Nurses Credentialing Center (ANCC) recognizing quality client outcomes, nursing excellence, and innovations in professional nursing practice. The Magnet Recognition Program requires nursing advocacy in the areas of technology, education, policies, and process development. This advocacy is accomplished by creating unit-based practice councils who meet regularly to discuss unit policies, practices, and outcomes. Additionally, an organization-wide practice council includes a representative from each unit council and reviews organizational-wide policies and practices. Read more about the Magnet Recognition Program in the following box.

28. Kroning, M., & Hopkins, K. (2019). Healthcare organizations thrive with shared governance. *Nursing Management, 50*(5), 13-15. https://doi.org/10.1097/01.numa.0000557781.40049.2d
29. Anthony, M. (2004). Shared governance models: The theory, practice, and evidence. *Online Journal of Issues in Nursing, 9*(1), 7. https://pubmed.ncbi.nlm.nih.gov/14998357/
30. Kroning, M., & Hopkins, K. (2019). Healthcare organizations thrive with shared governance. *Nursing Management, 50*(5), 13-15. https://doi.org/10.1097/01.numa.0000557781.40049.2d

Read more about the Magnet Recognition Program. Access supplementary digital content in the online book using this QR code.

Professional Nursing Organizations

Professional organizations provide easy access to nursing advocacy work being done across the nation and the world. There are over 100 local, state, and national organizations that advocate for the nursing profession. Professional nursing organizations may advocate for specific nursing issues in certain areas of practice, such as critical-care nursing (American Association of Critical-Care Nurses, AACN) or broader national nursing issues, such as the American Nurses Association (ANA). Professional organizations also provide opportunities for continuing education, advanced certification, and participation in political action committees. Membership in state and national organizations helps nurses stay up-to-date on current evidence-based practices and research findings.

Review a list of national, state, and international nursing organizations. Access supplementary digital content in the online book using this QR code.

Organization Advocacy

Nurses advocate for organizational issues in the nursing profession and the workplace through participation in unions, collective bargaining, workplace advocacy models, and professional organizations.

Unions and Collective Bargaining

A nursing union is a type of labor union that advocates for the interest of its nurse members. According to the Bureau of Labor Statistics, 20 percent of RNs and 10 percent of LPNs/VNs in the United States are union members.[31]

10.5 POLICY ADVOCACY

National, state, and local policies impact nurses at all levels of care, from nurse administrators to bedside nurses, making it essential for nurses to take an active role in advocating for their clients, their profession,

31. Rowland, T. (2020). *The pros and cons of nursing unions* [Blog]. Soliant. https://blog.soliant.com/nursing/the-pros-and-cons-of-nursing-unions/

and their community. Nurses advocate for improved access to basic health care, enhanced funding of health care services, and safe practice environments by participating in policy discussions. Nurses also participate in state and national policy discussions affecting nursing practice. For example, nurses advocate for the removal of practice barriers so nurses can practice according to the full extent of their education, certification, and licensure; address reimbursement based on the value of nursing care; and expand funding for nursing education.[32]

When advocating, nurses must view themselves as knowledgeable professionals who have the power to influence policy and decision-makers. A nurse can advocate for improved policies through a variety of pathways. Each method provides a unique opportunity for the nurse to impact the health of individuals and communities, the profession of nursing, and the overall health care provided to clients. These are few easy ways for nurses to get involved:

- Becoming involved in professional nursing organizations
- Engaging in conversations with local, state, and federal policymakers on health care related issues
- Participating in shared governance committees regarding workplace policies

Health Care Legislative Policies

Legislative policies are external rules and regulations that impact health care practice and policy at the national, state, and local levels. These regulations seek to protect clients and nurses by defining safe practices, quality standards, and requirements for health care organizations and insurance companies. Nurses have been involved in the adoption of these rules and regulations and continue to advocate for new and updated legislation affecting health care.

Examples of federal legislation addressing health care include advocating for the Patient's Bill of Rights, client privacy and confidentiality, improved access to health care, and protections for individuals who report unethical or illegal activities in the health care environment (i.e., whistleblower legislation). Examples of legislation at the state level include topics such as right-to-die and physician-assisted suicide, medicinal marijuana use, and nurse-to-client staffing ratios.

Review how client rights are defined by policies at the federal, state, and organizational levels in the following box.

32. American Nurses Association. (2021). *Nursing: Scope and standards of practice* (4th ed.). American Nurses Association.

Client's Rights Defined at Multiple Levels

In 1973 the American Hospital Association (AHA) adopted the Patient's Bill of Rights. The bill has since been updated and adapted for use throughout the world in all health care settings, but, in general, it safeguards a client's right to accurate and complete information, fair treatment, and self-determination when making health care decisions. In 2010 the Affordable Care Act was passed at the federal level. It included additional client rights and protections for health care consumers in the areas of preexisting conditions, choice of providers, and limited lifetime coverage limits imposed by insurance companies.

States further define client rights beyond federal regulations and provide specific rights of health care consumers in their state. For example, Wisconsin's Department of Health Services defines treatment rights, protections for records privacy and access, communication rights, personal rights, and privacy rights.

Read more about patient rights in the American health care system. Access supplementary digital content in the online book using this QR code.

Visit the CMS web page to read more about the Affordable Care Act and the revised Patient's Bill of Rights. Access supplementary digital content in the online book using this QR code.

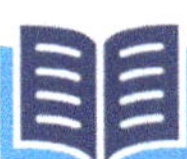

Research advocacy policies in your state. Here is Wisconsin's law regarding client rights. Access supplementary digital content in the online book using this QR code.

Nurses' Roles in Legislative Policies

With over four million registered nurses in the United States, nursing has a powerful voice that can significantly influence health care legislation. Nurses have been recognized as a major influence on health care policies related to client safety and quality care. They can become involved in policy making at the state and federal level by joining a professional nursing organization, communicating with their state representatives, or running for political office to take an active role in policy creation.

Most professional nursing organizations have a legislative policy committee that reviews proposed federal and state legislation and makes recommendations for change, endorses the legislation, or leads opposition. For example, organizations such as the American Nurses Association (ANA), National League of Nursing (NLN), and state nursing associations inform members of current legislative initiatives, provide comprehensive reviews, and encourage members to contact their representatives about pending legislation.

Read more about current advocacy efforts by the Wisconsin Nurses Association. Access supplementary digital content in the online book using this QR code.

Whistleblowing

Nurses are expected to follow federal, state, and agency policies and regulations, be proactive in policy development, and speak up when policies are not being followed. When regulations and policies are not being followed, nurses must advocate for public safety by reporting the problem to a higher authority. Whistleblowing refers to reporting a significant concern to your supervisor, the federal or state agency responsible for the regulation, or in the case of criminal activity, to law enforcement agencies. A **whistleblower** is a person who exposes any kind of information or activity that is deemed illegal, unethical, or not correct within an organization. See Figure 10.5[33] for federal instructions regarding whistleblowing.

Whistleblowing typically begins with reporting the wrongdoing to a supervisor and following the internal chain of command. This first step of reporting allows the organization to correct the issue internally. However, there may be situations where an individual may need to directly report to an external authority, such as a State Board of Nursing or another regulatory agency. For example, any person who has knowledge of conduct by a licensed nurse violating state or federal law may report the alleged violation to the State Board of Nursing where the conduct occurred.

Acting as a whistleblower can be a difficult decision because the individual may be labelled "disloyal" or potentially face retaliatory actions by the accused individual or organization. Although there are legal protections for whistleblowers, these types of actions may occur. Read important information from the ANA regarding whistleblowing in the following box.

33. "Whistleblowing.pdf" by United States Office of Special Counsel is in the Public Domain

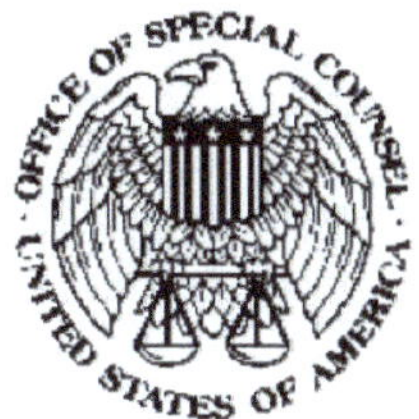

Whistleblowing

A "whistleblower" discloses information he or she reasonably believes evidences:

- A violation of any law, rule or regulation
- Gross mismanagement
- A gross waste of funds
- An abuse of authority
- A substantial and specific danger to public health
- A substantial and specific danger to public safety

The Office of Special Counsel (OSC) provides a secure channel through which current and former federal employees and applicants for federal employment may make confidential disclosures. OSC evaluates the disclosures to determine whether there is a substantial likelihood that one of the categories listed above has been disclosed. If such a determination is made, OSC has the authority to require the head of the agency to investigate the matter.

To make a disclosure contact:

U.S. OFFICE OF SPECIAL COUNSEL
1730 M STREET, N.W., SUITE 218
WASHINGTON, DC 20036-4505

PHONE: (202) 254-3640*   TOLL FREE: 1-800-572-2249*

***Hearing and Speech Disabled: Federal Relay Service 1-800-877-8339**

WWW.OSC.GOV

Rev. 12/05

FIGURE 10.5 Whistleblowing

ANA Information Regarding Whistleblowing[34]

- If you identify an illegal or unethical practice, reserve judgment until you have adequate documentation to establish wrongdoing.
- Do not expect those who are engaged in unethical or illegal conduct to welcome your questions or concerns about this practice.
- Seek the counsel of someone you trust outside of the situation to provide you with an objective perspective.
- Consult with your state nurses' association or legal counsel if possible before taking action to determine how best to document your concerns.
- Remember, you are not protected in a whistleblower situation from retaliation by your employer until you blow the whistle.
- Blowing the whistle means that you report your concern to the national and/or state agency responsible for regulation of the organization for which you work or, in the case of criminal activity, to law enforcement agencies as well.
- Private groups, such as The Joint Commission or the National Committee for Quality Assurance, do not confer protection. You must report to a state or national regulator.
- Although it is not required by every regulatory agency, it is a good rule of thumb to put your complaint in writing.
- Document all interactions related to the whistleblowing situation and keep copies for your personal file.
- Keep documentation and interactions objective.
- Remain calm and do not lose your temper, even if those who learn of your actions attempt to provoke you.
- Remember that blowing the whistle is a very serious matter. Do not blow the whistle frivolously. Make sure you have the facts straight before taking action.

10.6 STEPS TO BECOMING AN ADVOCATE

To become a nursing advocate, identify causes, issues, or needs where YOU can exert influence.

Steps to becoming an advocate include the following[35]:

1. **Identify a problem that interests you:** Start by pinpointing a specific issue or area within nursing that you are passionate about. This could range from client safety and quality of care to workplace conditions and professional development opportunities.
2. **Research the subject and select an evidence-based intervention:** Conduct thorough research on the identified issue. Look for evidence-based practices and interventions that have been proven to address

34. American Nurses Association. *Things to know about whistle blowing.* https://www.nursingworld.org/practice-policy/workforce/things-to-know-about-whistle-blowing/
35. Olson, K. (2020). *Influence through policy: Four steps you can take.* Nursing Centered. https://nursingcentered.sigmanursing.org/commentary/more-commentary/Vol42_2_influence-through-policy-four-steps-you-can-take

or mitigate the problem effectively. Gathering robust data will help you build a solid case for your advocacy efforts.

3. **Network with experts who are, or could be, involved in making the change:** Connect with professionals and experts who are either already involved in addressing the issue or who could play a crucial role in implementing changes. Building a network of like-minded individuals can provide support, resources, and additional perspectives.
4. **Work hard for change:** Advocacy requires dedication and persistence. Actively participate in efforts to bring about the desired change. This might include engaging in public speaking, writing articles or blogs, meeting with policymakers, or organizing community events to raise awareness.

Once you have identified a topic of interest, it's crucial to get involved in activities that can amplify your advocacy efforts:

- **Committees:** Volunteer to participate in committees that review and develop practice policies within your health care institution.
- **Professional Nursing Organizations:** Become a member of state and national nursing organizations. These groups often provide valuable resources, including access to current legislative and policy initiatives, public policy agendas, and ways to get involved.
- **Research and Review:** Stay informed by researching best practices and reviewing the health policy agendas of elected officials. Understanding the current landscape will help you identify opportunities to influence policy and practice.

Nurses hold a powerful position to be effective advocates due to their frontline role in health care delivery. Their unique insights into client care, the work environment, and health care systems make them valuable voices in policy discussions. As the largest sector of the health care workforce, nurses have significant potential to influence decisions at every level.

Advocating for change can lead to improved quality of care, better client outcomes, and safe work environments. By pushing for evidence-based practices and policies, nurses can help ensure that clients receive the best possible care. Advocacy efforts focused on client safety and quality can directly impact client health and recovery. Additionally, nurses can advocate for better working conditions, which can lead to a safer and more supportive environment for all healthcare workers.

Imagine the impact if every nurse actively engaged in advocacy. The collective efforts could drive substantial improvements in health care delivery and policy, leading to positive changes across the profession.

Review information about a new professional nursing association called the Nurse Advocacy Association. Access supplementary digital content in the online book using this QR code.

10.7 QSEN: ADVOCATING FOR PATIENT SAFETY AND QUALITY CARE IN NURSING EDUCATION

The Quality and Safety Education for Nurses (QSEN) project began advocating for safe, quality client care in 2005 by defining six competencies for nursing graduates. This initiative was created after a decade of review and investigation into the high number and high cost of medical errors in the United States. The goal of the QSEN initiative was to prepare future nurses with the knowledge, skills, and attitudes needed to improve the quality and safety of the health care system. Historically, nursing education focused on knowledge and skill acquisition, but did not address the attitudes and values of the nurse. The QSEN competencies are designed to train nursing students in prelicensure nursing programs. The six QSEN competencies, as shown in Figure 10.6,[36] are Patient-Centered Care, Teamwork and Collaboration, Evidence-Based Practice, Quality Improvement, Safety, and Informatics.[37]

Read the QSEN Prelicensure Table of Competencies. Access supplementary digital content in the online book using this QR code.

QSEN Competencies

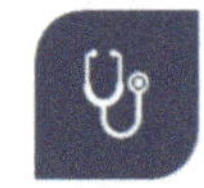

PATIENT-CENTERED CARE

TEAMWORK AND COLLABORATION

EVIDENCE-BASED PRACTICE

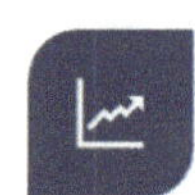

QUALITY IMPROVEMENT

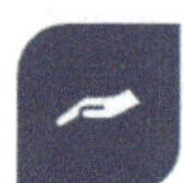

SAFETY

INFORMATICS

FIGURE 10.6 QSEN Competencies

36. "QSEN Competencies.png" by Chippewa Valley Technical College is licensed under CC BY 4.0
37. QSEN. (n.d.). *About.* https://qsen.org/about-qsen/

Patient-Centered Care

The **Patient-Centered Care** QSEN competency advocates for the client as "the source of control and full partner in providing compassionate and coordinated care based on respect for client's preferences, values, and needs."[38] This competency encourages nurses to consider clients' cultural traditions and personal beliefs while providing compassionate care. Client-centered care also includes the family in the care team. The goal of client-centered care is to improve the individual's health outcomes. Integration of this competency has led to improved client satisfaction scores, reduced expenses, and a positive care environment.[39]

Teamwork and Collaboration

The **Teamwork and Collaboration** QSEN competency focuses on functioning effectively within nursing and interprofessional teams and fostering open communication, mutual respect, and shared decision-making to achieve quality client care.[40] Effective communication has been proven to reduce errors and improve client safety.[41] The Joint Commission also includes improved communication as one of the National Patient Safety Goals, aligning with this QSEN competency. Collaboration requires information sharing across disciplines with respect for the knowledge, skills, and experience of each team member. Two examples of tools used to promote effective teamwork and collaboration are ISBARR and TeamSTEPPS®. Additionally, "principles of collaboration" have been established by the ANA.

ISBARR

Several communication tools have been developed to improve communication in various health care settings. ISBARR is an example of a well-established communication tool. As previously discussed in the "Collaboration Within the Interprofessional Team" chapter, **ISBARR** is a mnemonic for the components to include when communicating with other health care team members: **I**ntroduction, **S**ituation, **B**ackground, **A**ssessment, **R**equest/**R**ecommendations, and **R**epeat back.[42]

TeamSTEPPS®

As previously discussed in the "Collaboration Within the Interprofessional Team" chapter, TeamSTEPPS® (Team Strategies and Tools to Enhance Performance and Patient Safety) is a well-established framework to improve client safety through effective communication in health care environments. It consists of four core competencies: communication, leadership, situation monitoring, and mutual support.

---

38. QSEN. (n.d.). *About.* https://qsen.org/about-qsen/
39. Roseman, D., Osborne-Stafsnes, J., Amy, C. H., Boslaugh, S., & Slate-Miller, K. (2013). Early lessons from four 'aligning forces for quality' communities bolster the case for patient-centered care. *Health Affairs, 32*(2), 232-241. https://doi.org/10.1377/hlthaff.2012.1085
40. QSEN. (n.d.). *About.* https://qsen.org/about-qsen/
41. Burgener, A. M. (2020). Enhancing communication to improve patient safety and to increase patient satisfaction. *The Health Care Manager, 39*(3), 128-132. https://doi.org/10.1097/hcm.0000000000000298
42. Enlow, M., Shanks, L., Guhde, J., & Perkins, M. (2010). Incorporating interprofessional communication skills (ISBARR) into an undergraduate nursing curriculum. *Nurse Educator, 35*(4), 176-180. https://doi.org/10.1097/nne.0b013e3181e339ac

Principles of Collaboration

The American Nurses Association (ANA) and the American Organization of Nurse Executives (AONE) jointly created the "Principles of Collaboration" to guide nurses in creating, enhancing, and sustaining collaborative relationships. These principles include effective communication, authentic relationships, and a learning environment and culture. The principle of authentic relationships includes the following guidelines[43]:

- Be true to yourself – be sure your actions match your words and those around you are confident that what they see is what they get.
- Empower others to have ideas, to share those ideas, and to participate in projects that leverage or enact those ideas.
- Recognize and leverage each other's strengths.
- Be honest 100% of the time – with yourself and with others.
- Respect others' personalities, needs, and wants.
- Ask for what you want but stay open to negotiating the difference.
- Assume good intent from others' words and actions, and assume they are doing their best.

Read more about the "Principles of Collaboration" by the ANA and AONE. Access supplementary digital content in the online book using this QR code.

Evidence-Based Practice

The **Evidence-Based Practice** QSEN competency focuses on integrating scientific evidence with clinical expertise and client/family preferences and values for delivery of optimal health care.[44] See Figure 10.7[45] for an illustration of Evidence-Based Practices (EBP). Read more about EPB in the "Quality and Evidence-Based Practice" chapter. Read examples of evidence-based improvements in the following box.

Evidence-Based Practice

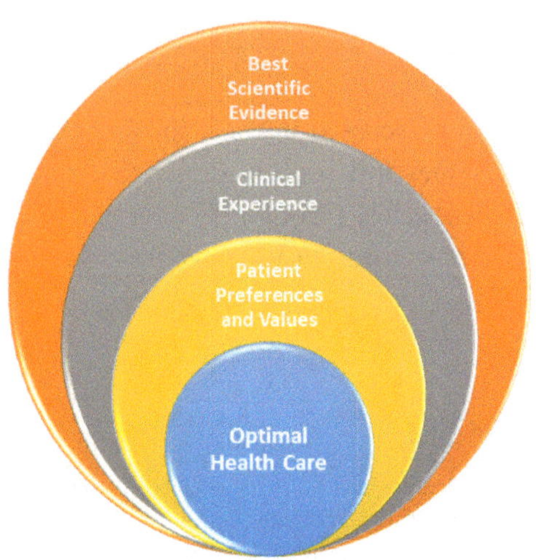

FIGURE 10.7 Evidence-Based Practice

43. American Nurses Association & American Organization of Nurses Executives. (n.d.). *ANA/AONE principles for collaborative relationships between clinical nurses and nurse managers.* https://www.nursingworld.org/~4af4f2/globalassets/docs/ana/ethics/principles-of-collaborative-relationships.pdf
44. QSEN. (n.d.). *About.* https://qsen.org/about-qsen/
45. "Evidence-Based Practice.jpg" by Kim Ernstmeyer for Chippewa Valley Technical College is licensed under CC BY 4.0

Read these examples of evidence-based practice improvements:

- Intravenous catheter sizes PDF
- Oxygen administration for COPD patients
- Recognizing alarm fatigue

Access supplementary digital content in the online book using this QR code.

Quality Improvement

The **Quality Improvement** QSEN competency focuses on using data to monitor the outcomes of care processes and using improvement methods to design and test changes to continuously improve the quality and safety of health care systems.[46] The goal of this competency is to improve processes, policies, and clinical decisions to improve client outcomes and system performance. As the pool of nursing literature grows and nursing practices have been updated to reflect current evidence, health care organizations have seen improvements in quality, safety, and experienced cost savings.[47] Read more about the quality improvement processes in the "Quality and Evidence-Based Practice" chapter.

Safety

The **Safety** QSEN competency focuses on minimizing "risk of harm to patients and providers through both system effectiveness and individual performance."[48] Although safety is embedded in all of the QSEN competencies, this competency specifically advocates for preventing client harm. Despite the health care industry's continued focus on process improvement and improving client outcomes, errors continue to occur, and nurses are often involved in these events as frontline caregivers. Safe nursing practice starts with an awareness of the potential risks for client harm in every situation.

Several initiatives have been adopted to reduce risk for client harm, such as double-checking high-risk medications and verifying a client's name and date of birth prior to every intervention. However, client safety is compromised when there are gaps in quality measures such as inadequate staff training, broken equipment, or an organizational culture that doesn't support best practices.

The "Safety" competency is best addressed by organizations establishing a safety culture where every worker commits to keeping client safety at the center of decision-making. An organization that has a culture of safety encourages reporting of unusual incidents, process failures, or other issues that could cause client harm, allowing the organization to investigate the event and take action to prevent the event from occurring in the future. Improvements are made as a result of a culture that questions attitudes, actions, and decisions in client care and recognizes threats to safety. Read more about safety culture in the "Legal Implications" chapter.

46. QSEN. (n.d.). *About.* https://qsen.org/about-qsen/
47. Cullen, L., Titler, M. G., & Rempel, G. (2011). An advanced educational program promoting evidence-based practice. *Western Journal of Nursing Research, 33*(3), 345-364. https://doi.org/10.1177/0193945910379218
48. QSEN. (n.d.). *About.* https://qsen.org/about-qsen/

Informatics

The **Informatics** QSEN competency focuses on using information and technology to communicate, manage knowledge, mitigate error, and support decision-making.[49] Health care is filled with various technologies used to promote a safe care environment, such as electronic medical records (EMRs), bedside medication administration devices, smart IV pumps, and medication distribution systems. These technologies provide safeguards and reminders to help prevent client harm, but the nurse must be knowledgeable in using technology, as well as understand how information obtained from technologies is used to improve client outcomes. As information related to technology continues to evolve, it is the responsibility of every nurse to participate in continued professional development related to informatics.

10.8 SPOTLIGHT APPLICATION

Case Study

An 85-year-old woman was admitted with sudden onset of dyspnea, pleuritic chest pain, and right upper arm edema. She had a peripherally inserted central catheter (PICC) placed three weeks previously for treatment of osteomyelitis of the left hand. A caretaker had been infusing her antibiotics and managing her PICC with the oversight of a home care nurse. A chest computerized tomography scan confirmed the presence of a pulmonary embolism. She was admitted to the inpatient floor at change of shift, and orders were received for a weight-based heparin bolus and infusion. The bolus was administered, and the infusion was initiated. During handoff report to the next shift, the pump alarm sounded. In responding to the alarm, the oncoming nurse discovered that the entire bag of heparin (25,000 units) had infused in less than 30 minutes. She discovered the rate on the pump was set by the previous nurse at 600 mL/hour rather than the weight-adjusted 600 units/hour.

The oncoming nurse who discovered the heparin error immediately disconnected the infusion, assessed the client for signs of bleeding, and notified the physician of the error. Appropriate precautions were initiated and an incident report was submitted. Subsequently, an investigation was conducted by the unit supervisor and the risk manager by interviewing involved staff. They found that the client's admitting nurse, who administered the heparin bolus and infusion, was a traveling nurse who had been in the organization for three weeks and had been floated to the telemetry unit for the first time. While the traveling nurse had been trained on an orthopedic unit, she had not initiated a heparin infusion at this facility. The facility used an infusion pump that included a drug library with medication-specific infusion limits for client safety. The nurse had been trained to use the infusion pump drug library in a brief orientation, but she had witnessed several nurses bypass this safety measure. In addition, although she had her heparin bolus and infusion calculations double-checked by another nurse, she was not aware that this double-check should include a review of pump settings.

Finally, because the change of shift handoff report was hurried, it did not include a bedside report to review infusions and client status with the oncoming nurse. What appeared to be a serious individual error was, in fact, a complex series of failures in the facility's safety culture that placed a nurse in the very difficult position

49. QSEN. (n.d.). *About.* https://qsen.org/about-qsen/

of making an error that placed a client at risk of harm. Fortunately, no significant bleeding events occurred as a result of the error.[50]

Reflective Questions

1. Create a list of safety failures in this example and categorize them based on the QSEN competencies.
2. Outline communication tools and best practices that could have prevented this error from occurring.

10.9 LEARNING ACTIVITIES

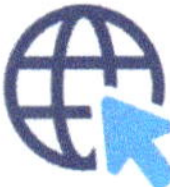

Interactive learning activities have been excluded from the print version of the text. Access free online learning activities in the online book using this QR code.

50. Sherwood, G., & Nickel, B. (2017). Integrating quality and safety competencies to improve outcomes: Application in infusion therapy practice. *Journal of Infusion Nursing, 40*(2), 116-122. https://doi.org/10.1097/NAN.0000000000000210

10.10 GLOSSARY

Advocacy: The act or process of pleading for, supporting, or recommending a cause of course of action for individuals, groups, organizations, communities, society, or policy issues.

Collective bargaining: Negotiation of wages and other conditions of employment by an organized body of employees.

Evidence-based practice: Integrating scientific evidence with clinical expertise and client/family preferences and values for delivery of optimal health care.[51]

Grievance process: A process for resolving disagreements between employees and management.

Informatics: Using information and technology to communicate, manage knowledge, mitigate error, and support decision-making.[52]

ISBARR: A mnemonic for the components to include when communicating with another health care team member: Introduction, Situation, Background, Assessment, Request/Recommendations, and Repeat back.

Magnet® Recognition Program: An organizational credential that recognizes quality client outcomes, nursing excellence, and innovations in professional nursing practice.

Patient-centered care: The client is the source of control and full partner in providing compassionate and coordinated care based on respect for client's preferences, values, and needs.[53]

Quality improvement: Using data to monitor the outcomes of care processes and using improvement methods to design and test changes to continuously improve the quality and safety of health care systems.[54]

Shared governance: A shared leadership model between management and employees working together to achieve common goals.

Social Determinants of Health (SDOH): The conditions in the environments where people live, learn, work, and play that affect a wide range of health, functioning, and quality of life outcomes and risks.

TeamSTEPPS® (Team Strategies and Tools to Enhance Performance and Patient Safety): An evidence-based framework to improve client safety through effective communication in health care environments consisting of four core competencies: communication, leadership, situation monitoring, and mutual support.

Teamwork and collaboration: Functioning effectively within nursing and interprofessional teams, fostering open communication, mutual respect, and shared decision-making to achieve quality client care.[55]

Whistleblower: A person who exposes any kind of information or activity that is deemed illegal, unethical, or not correct within an organization.

51. QSEN. (n.d.). *About.* https://qsen.org/about-qsen/
52. QSEN. (n.d.). *About.* https://qsen.org/about-qsen/
53. QSEN. (n.d.). *About.* https://qsen.org/about-qsen/
54. QSEN. (n.d.). *About.* https://qsen.org/about-qsen/
55. QSEN. (n.d.). *About.* https://qsen.org/about-qsen/

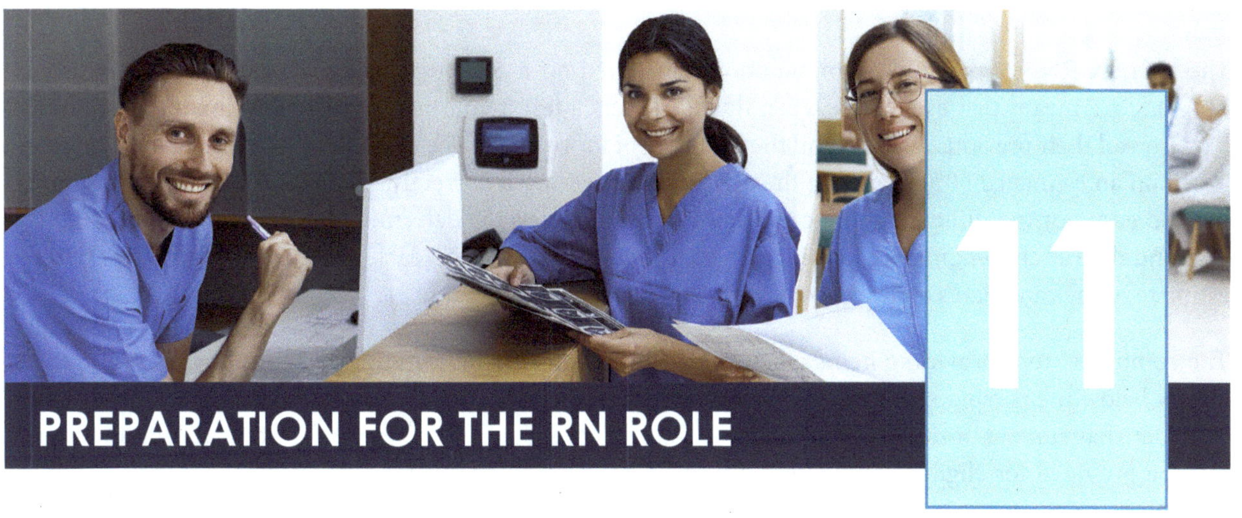

11.1 PREPARATION FOR THE RN ROLE INTRODUCTION

LEARNING OBJECTIVES

- Develop a current professional resume or portfolio
- Identify steps for preparing for the NCLEX-RN examination
- Identify actions for obtaining nursing credential
- Identify strategies for successful nursing interviews
- Develop goals for lifelong learning and professional development

Preparing to enter the workforce as a registered nurse (RN) can be a challenging but exciting time. Being aware of available resources to help navigate this process will decrease stress and make the process more manageable. This chapter will discuss how to prepare for the NCLEX-RN examination, obtain a nursing license, create a resume and portfolio, effectively participate in an interview, transition into the RN role, and become a lifelong learner.

11.2 PREPARING FOR THE NCLEX

The National Council Licensure Examination for Registered Nurses (**NCLEX-RN**) is the exam that nursing graduates must pass successfully to obtain their nursing license and become a registered nurse. The purpose of the NCLEX is to evaluate if a nursing graduate (i.e., candidate) is competent to provide safe, competent, entry-level nursing care. The NCLEX-RN is developed by the National Council of State Board of Nursing (NCSBN), an independent, nonprofit organization composed of the 50 state boards of nursing and other regulatory agencies.[1]

1. NCSBN. https://www.ncsbn.org/nclex.htm

The NCLEX-RN is a pass/fail examination administered on a computer using computer adaptive testing (CAT). CAT means that every time a candidate answers a test item, the computer reestimates their ability based on all their previous answers and the difficulty of those items. The computer then selects the next item based on an estimated 50% chance of the candidate answering it correctly. In this manner, the next item is not too easy nor too difficult, and a candidate's true ability level is determined. Each item is perceived by the candidate as challenging because it is targeted to their ability. With each item answered, the computer's estimate of the candidate's ability becomes more precise.

The computer stops providing items when it is 95% certain that the candidate's ability is clearly above or clearly below the passing standard, the candidate has received the maximum number of questions, or the candidate has run out of time without demonstrating a competence level to pass. Testing accommodations may be provided for eligible candidates with the authorization of the candidate's State Board of Nursing (SBON).[2,3]

See an image of a simulated graduate taking the NCLEX in Figure 11.1.[4]

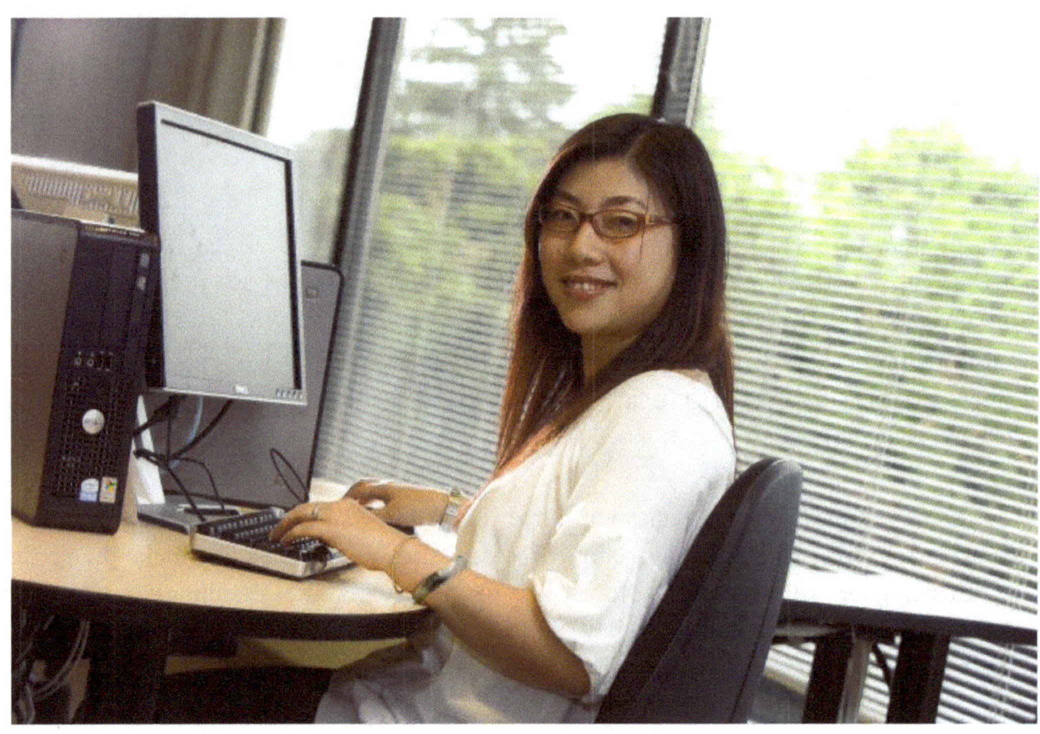

FIGURE 11.1 Simulated Graduate Taking the NCLEX

2. NCSBN. (2025). *NCLEX*. https://www.ncsbn.org/nclex.htm
3. NCSBN Examinations. (2024). *2024 NCLEX examination candidate bulletin*. https://www.nclex.com/files/2024_NCLEX_Candidate_Bulletin_English_FINAL.pdf
4. "Woman_with_computer.jpg" by Cumminsr at English Wikipedia is licensed under CC BY-SA 3.0

Read more about the NCLEX at https://www.ncsbn.org/nclex.htm. Access supplementary digital content in the online book using this QR code.

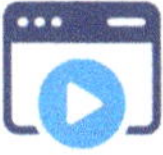

Watch a video about how the NCLEX uses computer assistive technology (CAT) at https://www.ncsbn.org/356.htm. Access supplementary digital content in the online book using this QR code.

Registering to Take the NCLEX

Before you can register to take the NCLEX, you will need an Authorization to Test (ATT). To receive an ATT, complete the following steps[5]:

- Apply for a nurse license from your State Board of Nursing (SBON) or other nursing regulatory body
- Register with Pearson VUE and pay the exam fee
- Wait to receive your ATT from Pearson Vue
- Schedule your exam with Pearson VUE

Be sure to start this process well in advance of your target date for taking the NCLEX.

Read specific instructions regarding registering and taking the NCLEX-RN by downloading the most current *NCLEX-Candidate Bulletin* from the NCSBN. The content includes the following:

- Registering for the exam
- Scheduling the exam
- Understanding test site rules and regulations
- Preparing for the day of the exam

Download the most current *NCLEX-Candidate Bulletin* from https://www.ncsbn.org/nclex.htm. Access supplementary digital content in the online book using this QR code.

5. NCSBN. (2025). *NCLEX*. https://www.ncsbn.org/nclex.htm

Next Generation NCLEX

A new edition of NCLEX was released in 2023 with "Next Generation" questions. The Next Generation NCLEX (Next Gen) uses evolving case studies and new types of test questions based on a new NCSBN Clinical Judgment Measurement Model (NCJMM) that assesses how well the candidate can think critically and use clinical judgment when providing nursing care. The NCJMM assess the candidate's ability to recognize cues, analyze cues, prioritize hypotheses, generate solutions, take actions, and evaluate outcomes.[6]

Five new Next Generation test item types are called extended multiple response, extended drag and drop, cloze (drop-down), extended hot spot (highlighting), and matrix-grid[7]:

- **Extended Multiple Response:** Extended Multiple Response items allow candidates to select one or more answer options at a time. This item type is similar to the current NCLEX multiple response item but has more options and uses partial credit scoring.
- **Extended Drag and Drop:** Extended Drag and Drop items allow candidates to move or place response options into answer spaces. This item type is like the current NCLEX ordered response items but not all of the response options may be required to answer the item. In some items, there may be more response options than answer spaces.
- **Cloze (Drop – Down):** Cloze (Drop – Down) items allow candidates to select one option from a drop-down list. There can be more than one drop-down list in a cloze item. These drop-down lists can be used as words or phrases within a sentence or within tables and charts.
- **Enhanced Hot Spot (Highlighting):** Enhanced Hot Spot items allow candidates to select their answer by highlighting predefined words or phrases. Candidates can select and deselect the highlighted parts by clicking on the words or phrases. These types of items allow an individual to read a portion of a client medical record (e.g., a nursing note, medical history, lab values, medication record, etc.), and then select the words or phrases that answer the item.
- **Matrix/Grid:** Matrix/Grid items allow the candidate to select one or more answer options for each row and/or column. This item type can be useful in measuring multiple aspects of the clinical scenario with a single item. In the example below, each of the eight rows will need to have one of the three answer choices selected.

View a NCSBN video on Next Generation test items. Access supplementary digital content in the online book using this QR code.

6. NCSBN. (2025). *NCLEX*. https://www.ncsbn.org/nclex.htm
7. NCSBN. (2025). *NCLEX*. https://www.ncsbn.org/nclex.htm

Participate in an NCLEX tutorial at https://www.ncsbn.org/nclex-tutorial.htm. Access supplementary digital content in the online book using this QR code.

Preparing for the Examination

Since the first day of nursing school, you have been working towards successfully passing the NCLEX-RN. After you graduate, it is important to implement strategies for success for taking the NCLEX, such as reviewing the NCLEX-RN Test Plan, setting up a dedicated review schedule based on your test date, and reviewing material you learned throughout nursing school.[8]

NCLEX Test Plan

The **NCLEX-RN Test Plan** provides a concise summary of the content and scope of the exam and serves as an excellent guide for preparation. NCLEX-RN test plans are updated every three years based on surveys of newly licensed registered nurses to ensure the NCLEX questions reflect fair, comprehensive, current, and entry-level nursing competency.[9]

The NCLEX Test Plan categorizes test questions based on categories and subcategories referred to as "Client Needs"[10]:

- Safe and Effective Care Environment
  - Management of Care
  - Safety and Infection Control
- Health Promotion and Maintenance
- Psychosocial Integrity
- Physiological Integrity
  - Basic Care and Comfort
  - Pharmacological and Parenteral Therapies
  - Reduction of Risk Potential
  - Physiological Adaptation

In addition, the following concepts are applied throughout the client needs categories[11]:

- Nursing Process
- Caring
- Communication and Documentation
- Teaching and Learning
- Culture and Spirituality

8. NCSBN. (2025). *NCLEX*. https://www.ncsbn.org/nclex.htm
9. NCSBN. (2025). *NCLEX*. https://www.ncsbn.org/nclex.htm
10. NCSBN. (2025). *NCLEX*. https://www.ncsbn.org/nclex.htm
11. NCSBN. (2025). *NCLEX*. https://www.ncsbn.org/nclex.htm

Download the current NCLEX-RN Test Plan from https://www.ncsbn.org/testplans.htm. Access supplementary digital content in the online book using this QR code.

Review Schedule

Many students find it helpful to create and follow a study calendar with topics to review based on the NCLEX Test Plan.

Reviewing Material

Some graduates prefer to attend an NCLEX review course to prepare for the examination whereas others prefer to review their notes from nursing school on their own. Be sure to review the NCLEX Candidate Rules before the day of the examination.[12,13]

Day of the Examination

On the day of the examination, it is normal to experience some anxiety. However, it is important to use techniques to manage anxiety, so it does not impact your ability to think through and answer the test questions. Use positive self-talk and remind yourself that you have been preparing for this examination since the first day of nursing school. Read additional tips for the day of the NCLEX and tips for testing in the following boxes.

Tips for the Day of the NCLEX[14]

- Locate the test center prior to the day of the exam, if possible.
- Get plenty of sleep the night before the exam.
- Eat prior to the examination.
- Dress comfortably.
- Bring your ID.
- Arrive early (30 minutes).
- All personal items must be placed in a sealable, plastic bag that is provided and placed in lockable storage. This includes electronic devices such as cell phones, tablets, smart watches, or other electronic devices.

12. NCSBN. (2025). *NCLEX*. https://www.ncsbn.org/nclex.htm
13. NCSBN Examinations. (2024). *2024 NCLEX examination candidate bulletin*. https://www.nclex.com/files/2024_NCLEX_Candidate_Bulletin_English_FINAL.pdf
14. NCSBN. (2025). *NCLEX*. https://www.ncsbn.org/nclex.htm

Tips for Testing[15]

- Perform relaxation breathing to stay calm and focused (take a few deep breaths in and out and remind yourself you are ready).
- Set your pace as you proceed through the questions based on the time limit for the exam.
- There are two optional breaks during the exam (the first break occurs two hours into testing, and the second break occurs after 3.5 hours of testing).
- Take time to analyze each question carefully—once you submit an answer, you can't return to that question.
- The exam ends with a short, computerized survey. Afterwards, raise your hand and wait for the testing administrator to dismiss you. The sealed bag that was placed in locked storage will be inspected.

After the Examination

If your State Board of Nursing (SBON) or nursing regulatory body (NRB) participates in the "Quick Results Service," you can receive your "unofficial" results two business days after the exam if you pay for this service. Official results are sent to you approximately six weeks after the exam.[16]

If you didn't pass the exam, you'll receive an NCLEX Candidate Performance Report (CPR). The CPR is an individualized document that shows how a candidate performed in each of the test plan content areas. Graduates who fail the exam can use the CPR as a guide to prepare them to retake the exam.[17]

If you need to retake the exam, you will need to wait a minimum of 45 days before you can retake the NCLEX per NCSBN policy. This length of time is determined by your SBON (or NRB) and will be reflected in your new ATT's validity dates. Read the steps for retaking the NCLEX in the following box.

Steps for Retaking the NCLEX

- Contact your State Board of Nursing (SBON) or nursing regulatory body (NRB) and notify them that you plan to retake the exam.
- Determine what fees or materials you need to submit to the SBON or NRB.
- Reregister with Pearson VUE and pay the fee.
- Wait to receive your new ATT.
- Schedule your new exam.
- Review your CPR and set up a review plan.

15. NCSBN. (2025). *NCLEX*. https://www.ncsbn.org/nclex.htm
16. NCSBN. (2025). *NCLEX*. https://www.ncsbn.org/nclex.htm
17. NCSBN. (2025). *NCLEX*. https://www.ncsbn.org/nclex.htm

11.3 OBTAINING YOUR NURSING LICENSE

Licensure is the process by which a State Board of Nursing (SBON) grants permission to an individual to engage in nursing practice after verifying the applicant has attained the competency necessary to perform the scope of practice of a registered nurse (RN).[18] The SBON verifies these three components:

- Verification of graduation from an approved prelicensure RN nursing education program
- Verification of successful completion of NCLEX-RN examination
- A criminal background check (in some states)[19]

In the United States there are three common types of prelicensure educational programs that prepare a student to become an RN, including a two-year associate degree of nursing (ADN), a hospital-based diploma program, or a four-year baccalaureate degree (BSN). Some universities offer an "Entry Level Master of Science in Nursing Track" for non-nurses holding a baccalaureate or master's degree in another field who wish to become a nurse. All graduates must pass the same NCLEX-RN to obtain their RN license from their SBON (or other nursing regulatory body).

Requirements for licensure renewal vary from state to state. Some states require continued education credits (CEUs), along with the payment of fees. In Wisconsin the nursing license is renewed every two years. See Figure 11.2[20] for an image of a simulated nursing license.

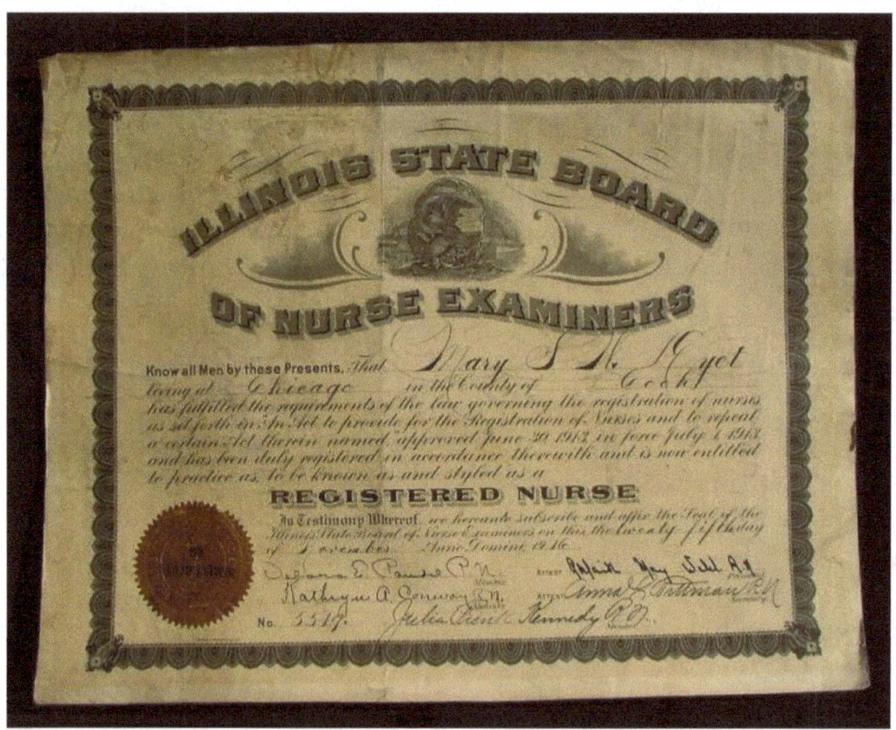

FIGURE 11.2 Simulated Nursing License

18. NCSBN. (2025). *NCLEX*. https://www.ncsbn.org/nclex.htm
19. NCSBN. (2025). *NCLEX*. https://www.ncsbn.org/nclex.htm
20. "3277658479_86d3d7d61c_o.jpg" by Vernon Dutton is licensed under CC BY-NC-SA 2.0

Use this map for contact information for the State Boards of Nursing.

Read more details on obtaining a Wisconsin RN license at https://dsps.wi.gov/Pages/Professions/RN/Default.aspx.

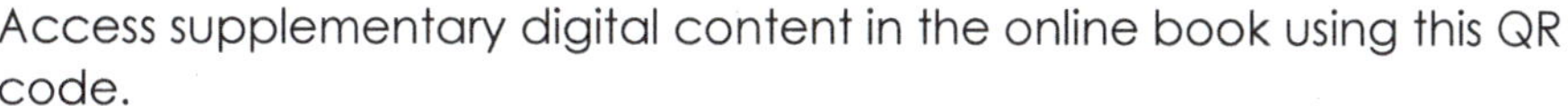

Access supplementary digital content in the online book using this QR code.

Nurse Licensure Compact

When applying for your nursing license from your State Board of Nursing (SBON), you may also be eligible to apply for a multistate license. The **Nurse Licensure Compact** (NLC) allows nurses to practice in other NLC states with their original state's nursing license without having to obtain additional licenses, contingent upon remaining a resident of that state. Currently, 38 states have enacted the NLC. Read more information about the NLC using the information in the following box.

View the current Nurse Licensure Compact Map.

Read this algorithm on how to Navigate the Nurse Licensure Compact.

Read more information about the Nurse Licensure Compact Rules.

Watch a video for nursing students on the Nurse Licensure Compact.

Access supplementary digital content in the online book using this QR code.

Temporary Permit

In some states before taking the NCLEX, an applicant may apply to receive a temporary permit from their State Board of Nursing (SBON). A **temporary permit** allows the applicant to practice practical nursing under the direct supervision of a registered nurse until the RN license is granted. A temporary permit is typically valid for a period of three months or until the holder receives failing NCLEX results, whichever is shorter.

Read about the temporary permit available in Wisconsin. Access supplementary digital content in the online book using this QR code.

11.4 APPLYING FOR A NURSING POSITION

Many students begin applying for their first nursing position before they graduate or take the NCLEX-RN. Read tips for employment in the following box.

Tips for Employment

- Reflect on previous clinical rotations and the experience. It is helpful to apply at agencies where you have had a positive learning experience.
- Obtain employment at a health care agency as a nursing assistant, licensed practical/vocational nurse (LPN/VN), or intern prior to graduation. This allows you to experience the workplace culture. Intern and extern roles allow the nursing student to perform nursing skills under the supervision of an RN, often with a temporary permit obtained from their State Board of Nursing (SBON). After receiving your RN license, it is often an easier transition into the nursing role. Working at the facility prior to graduation also increases familiarity with the environment, electronic health record, and health care team.

During your job-search process, it is helpful to begin by reviewing Medicare's quality ratings of health care agencies and providers. The "overall star rating" is based on how well the agency performs on various quality indicators and client satisfaction surveys.

Review Medicare ratings of hospitals, nursing homes, home health agencies, and providers at www.medicare.gov/care-compare. Access supplementary digital content in the online book using this QR code.

When applying for a job position, a resume and/or portfolio is typically included as part of the application process.

Resume

A **resume** is a document that highlights one's background, education, skills, and accomplishments to potential employers. There are many types of resume formats, and some individuals elect to use online services to create a professional resume.

A resume typically includes the following components:

- Personal contact information
- Professional objective statement/Goals
- Education
- Work experience
- Awards and achievements
- Community service
- Languages, hobbies, volunteer experiences (optional)

When creating a resume, it is helpful to highlight skills and experience that separate you from the other candidates applying for the position. It is also helpful to tailor your resume to the skills and experience expressed in the job description.

Read more details about what to put in a resume and nursing resumes and cover letters.

View a sample resume.

View a sample Online Resume Service.

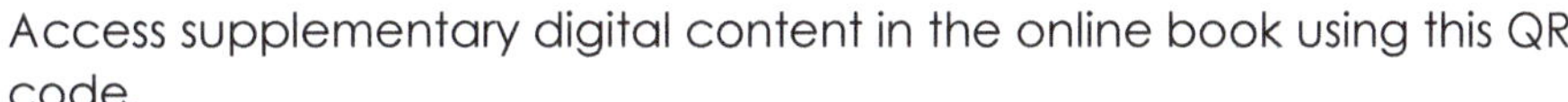
Access supplementary digital content in the online book using this QR code.

Portfolio

A **portfolio** is a compilation of materials showcasing examples of previous work demonstrating one's skills, qualifications, education, training, and experience. They can be submitted in electronic or paper form. See Figure 11.3[21] for an image of a sample electronic portfolio.

21. "4805383850_7385e60b6c_k.jpg" by Hung Le is licensed under CC BY 2.0

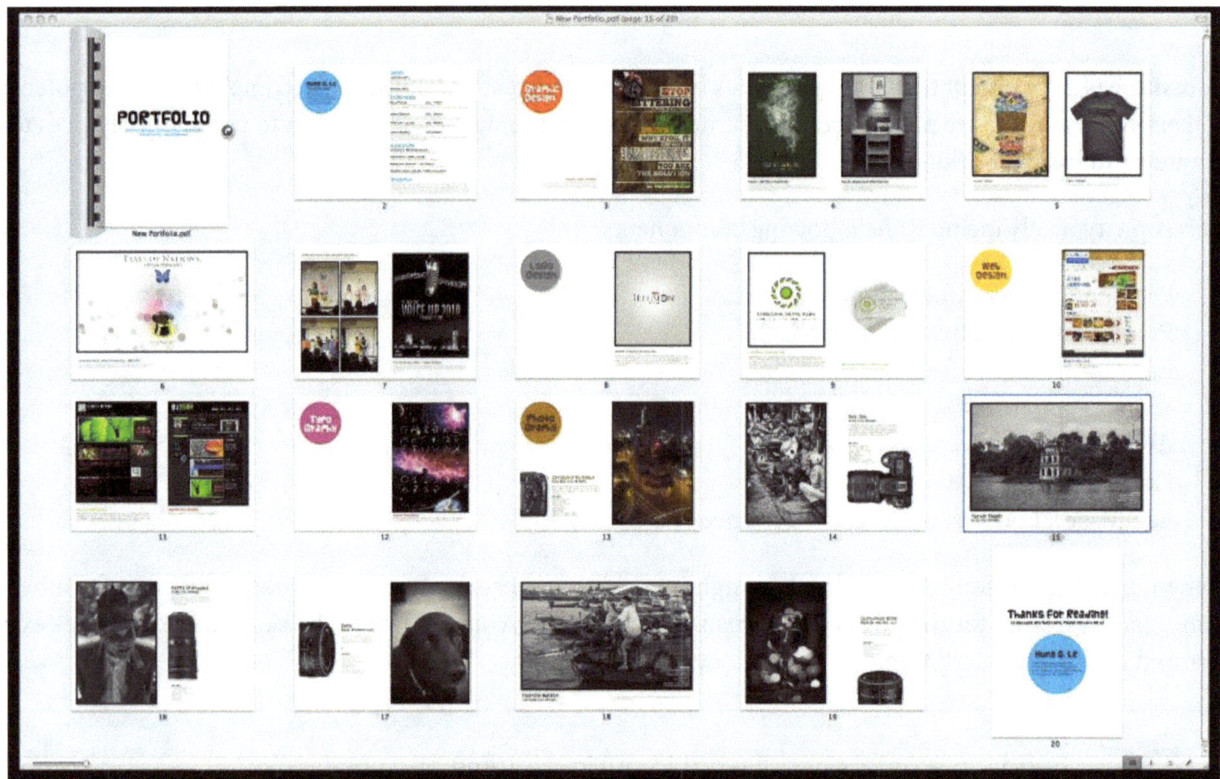

FIGURE 11.3 Sample Electronic Portfolio

Some schools of nursing require portfolios to be completed throughout the program. These portfolios are a representation of work demonstrating the student's accomplishments.

Portfolios typically include the following:

- Personal contact information
- Resume
- Professional goals
- Skilled work with examples (e.g., a nursing care plan, process recording, teaching plan, etc.)
- Accomplishments (e.g., dean's list)
- Degrees
- Certifications (e.g., CPR)
- Professional memberships (e.g., Student Nurse Association)
- Community service activities
- References (if requested)

 Read more about what to include in a portfolio.

 Visit an online portfolio service.

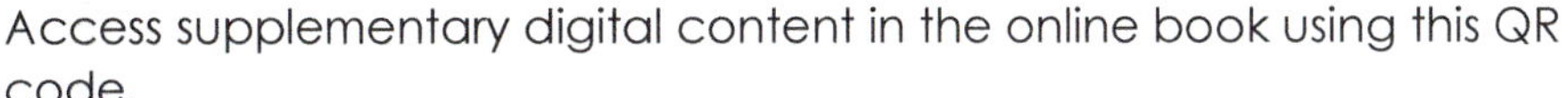

Access supplementary digital content in the online book using this QR code.

Interviewing

After applying for a position and submitting your resume and/or portfolio, you may be contacted to set up an interview. When you're interviewing for an RN position, you will be asked about your skills, experience, and your education. Some questions may be basic, such as, "Why did you become a nurse?" Other questions may be more difficult to answer, such as "Explain your strengths and weaknesses as an RN." See Figure 11.4[22] for a simulated interview.

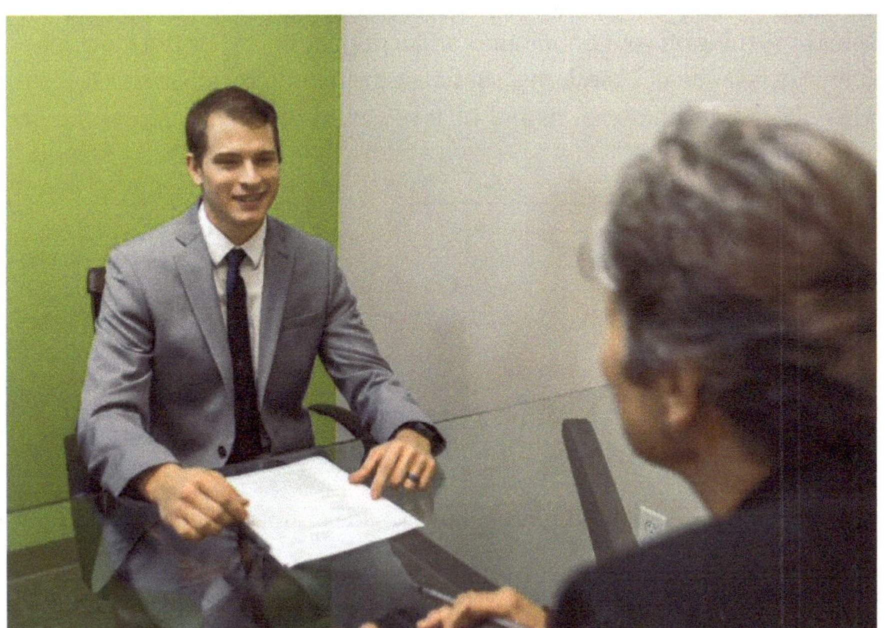

FIGURE 11.4 Simulated Interview

Interviewing for a new position can cause anxiety because you are required to answer questions and provide examples. A strategy to make the interview process easier and reduce anxiety is to prepare answers for commonly asked questions prior to the interview. Completing this task will help you prepare and increase your confidence. See common interview questions in the following box. It is helpful to tailor your answers to the skills and experience provided in the position description of the job you are seeking.

22. "24835247668_0828e986ad_k.jpg" by Amtec Photos is licensed under CC BY-SA 2.0

Common Questions During an Interview

- Tell me about yourself.
- Why did you become an RN?
- What is your educational background?
- What are your future goals?
- What are your strengths?
- What are your weaknesses?
- Give an example of how you were a good team player.
- Tell me about a time you cared for a challenging client and how you handled the situation.

Prior to your interview, research the organization's website. Be aware of their mission and vision statements and any "current events" in the news. Interviewers are impressed when an applicant has taken the time to learn about the organization and demonstrates interest.

Interviews may take place face-to-face, virtually on a computer, or over the phone. If you are interviewing face-to-face or virtually, dress for success in professional attire. If interviewing virtually, be sure to decrease distractions at home by turning off your phone and conducting the interview in a quiet space. Establish good eye contact with the interviewer and speak in a confident manner. Remember, this is the time to "sell your nursing self," so highlight your achievements and what you are proud of accomplishing. See additional tips for interviews in the following box.

Tips for Interviews

- Dress in business casual attire.
- Arrive ten minutes early for the interview.
- Bring copies of your resume or portfolio.
- Silence your cell phone.
- Do not chew gum.
- Answer all questions honestly and thoroughly. Provide examples when feasible.
- Ask questions.
- At the end, thank the interviewer and ask when you will be notified if you are offered the position.

The interview process is also an opportunity for you to determine if this position and agency is a good fit for you. Remember that it is important to select an agency that has good ratings for providing safe client care and client satisfaction. It is not worth taking a position that may place your nursing license at risk. Ask questions of the interviewer to clarify your understanding of the job position and expectations, agency policies, and workplace culture. Suggested interview questions are listed in the following box.

Questions for Interviewer

- How long is the orientation process?
- How long will I have access to a mentor?
- Do you have a nurse residency program?
- What system do you use for the electronic health record?
- What is the weekend rotation requirement?
- What are the holiday requirements?
- What are the staffing ratios?
- What are your policies regarding "mandatory overtime" and "off with benefits"?
- How long are the shifts?
- What is your policy for tuition reimbursement?
- What is the salary range?
- How does this organization handle error reporting?
- How has this organization adopted The Joint Commission's Culture of Safety, such as the Just Culture model?
- Do you have an ethics committee or other resources for nurses?

11.5 TRANSITIONING TO THE RN ROLE

Reality Shock

As a new graduate transitions into the role of being a registered nurse (RN), it is very common to experience something called "reality shock." Although Kramer's "Reality Shock" theory is several decades old, it continues to apply to new nurses transitioning to their new role through a process of learning and growing. Kramer's Reality Shock theory characterizes four phases of transitioning into a new role referred to as the honeymoon, shock, recovery, and resolution phases[23]:

- **Honeymoon phase:** The first phase occurs when the newly graduated RN is excited to join the nursing profession and it is everything they imagined. During this phase, the new nurse is typically paired up with a preceptor RN to orient them to the new role.
- **Shock phase:** The second phase is when the new RN is the most vulnerable. They are moved off orientation and independently perform tasks without the guidance of their preceptor. The RN role is often more difficult than the new nurse previously imagined. The new RN realizes their expectations associated with the nursing role may be inconsistent with the actual responsibilities. During this phase, negative feelings regarding their new profession may arise, and the new RN is at greatest risk for leaving the unit or quitting.
- **Recovery phase:** The third phase is when new RNs begin to have positive feelings towards their profession again. During this phase, the new RN is able to reflect on their experiences and develop a clear understanding of their responsibilities and role expectations. The novice RN typically experiences decreased tension and anxiety and begins to assist other RNs as needed.

23. Kramer, M. (1974). *Reality shock: Why nurses leave nursing*. C. V. Mosby Co.

- **Resolution phase:** The fourth and final phase is usually at the end of the first year of the new position. The new RN can visualize how the role contributes to the profession, and work expectations are easily met.

Transitioning Into Practice

Over the years, the National Council of State Boards of Nursing (NCSBN) has researched the complex issue of retaining new nursing graduates and found the inability of new nurses to properly transition into practice can have grave consequences. New nurses care for sicker clients in increasingly complex health settings and feel increased stress levels. As a result, new nurses are involved in more client safety and practice errors than experienced nurses. It has been reported by the NCSBN that within the first year of employment, 25% of novice RNs leave their nursing positions.[24]

There are several potential strategies for helping new nurses transition into practice. The first step of the transition is being aware of "reality shock" and the phases of the transition process. A thorough orientation process with an experienced preceptor is a traditional strategy for transitioning into a new nursing position. A newer strategy being implemented in some agencies is a nurse residency program.

Orientation may last anywhere from one to four months, but can be longer depending on the specialty (e.g., Intensive Care or Labor and Delivery). Orientation is based on the new nurse's demonstration and completion of competencies. During this time, the novice RN will work with a preceptor to experience all aspects of the role.

Preceptors are experienced and competent RNs who serve as a role model and a resource to a newly hired nurse. Preceptors have the knowledge, skills, and the ability to coach the new RN into the nursing role and answer their questions. The preceptor also evaluates a new hire's performance and provides feedback for improvement.

Nurse residency programs provide additional professional development support for all newly licensed nurses. Nurse residency programs vary from institution to institution, but many start around the time the new graduate ends their orientation with a preceptor and continue to provide routine support throughout the year. Residency programs are structured to provide a variety of learning opportunities, including nursing skill development, peer networking, and mentorship. The goal of nurse residency programs is to provide organizational support for newly licensed nurses during the critical phase of transitioning from student to professional nurse.[25] See Figure 11.5[26] for an image of new nurses participating in a nurse residency program.

---

24. NCSBN. (n.d.). *Transition to practice: Why transition to practice (TTP)?* http://www.ncsbn.org/transition-to-practice.htm
25. Ackerson, K., & Stiles, K. A. (2018). Value of nurse residency programs in retaining new graduate nurses and their potential effect on the nursing shortage. *The Journal of Continuing Education in Nursing, 49*(6). https://doi.org/10.3928/00220124-20180517-09
26. "1637163589.jpg" by Monkey Business Images is used under license from Shutterstock.com

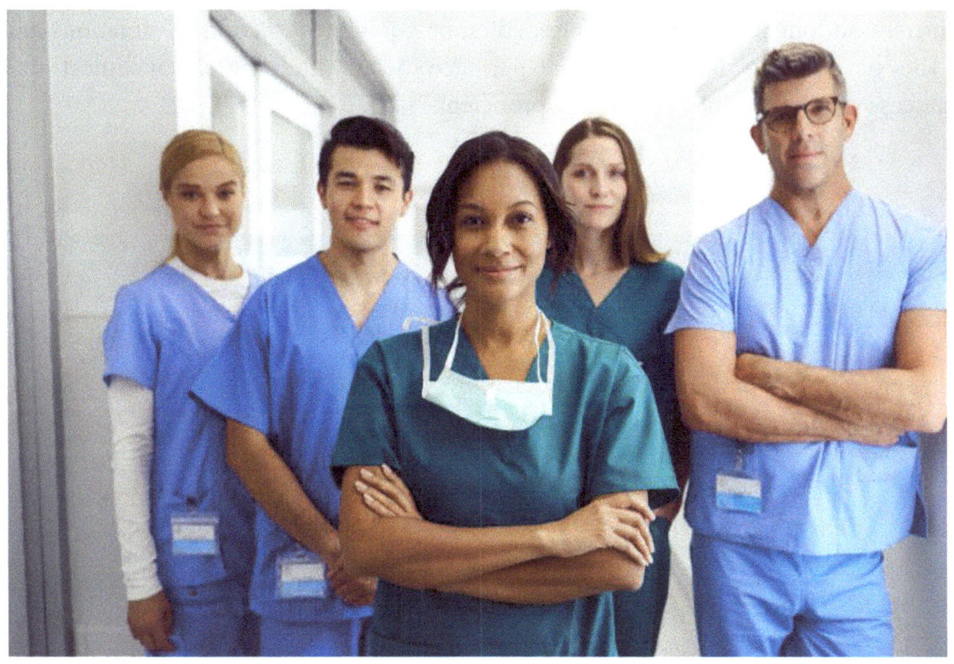

FIGURE 11.5 Nurse Residency Program

Benner's Novice to Expert Theory

As a nursing graduate transitions into a new nursing role, a well-known theory called "**Benner's Novice to Expert Theory**" explains how new hires develop skills and a holistic understanding of client care over time, resulting from a combination of a strong educational foundation and thorough clinical experiences. See Figure 11.6[27] for an illustration of Benner's Novice to Expert Theory. Benner's theory identifies five levels of nursing experience: novice, advanced beginner, competent, proficient, and expert.[28]

- A **novice** is a beginner with no clinical experience. They are taught general rules to help perform tasks, and their rule-governed behavior is limited and inflexible. In other words, they are told what to do and simply follow instructions.
- An **advanced beginner** shows acceptable performance and has gained prior experience in actual nursing situations. This experience helps the nurse recognize recurring patterns of client symptoms and behaviors. An advanced beginner begins to formulate strategies, based on their previous experiences, to guide actions.
- A **competent nurse** generally has two or three years' experience on the job in the same type of position that has similar day-to-day situations. Competent nurses become aware of long-term goals and gain perspective from planning their own actions. This helps them achieve greater efficiency and organization.
- A **proficient nurse** perceives and understands situations as whole parts, so they have a holistic understanding of nursing that improves their decision-making. Proficient nurses have learned what to expect in various client situations and how to modify plans as needed.

27. "Novice to Expert.png" by Meredith Pomietlo for Chippewa Valley Technical College is licensed under CC BY 4.0
28. Nursing Theory. (2020). *Dr. Patricia Benner novice to expert - nursing theorist.* https://nursing-theory.org/nursing-theorists/Patricia-Benner.php

- **Expert nurses** no longer rely on principles, rules, or guidelines to connect situations and determine actions. They have a deeper background of experience and an intuitive grasp of clinical situations. Their performances are fluid, flexible, and highly proficient.[29]

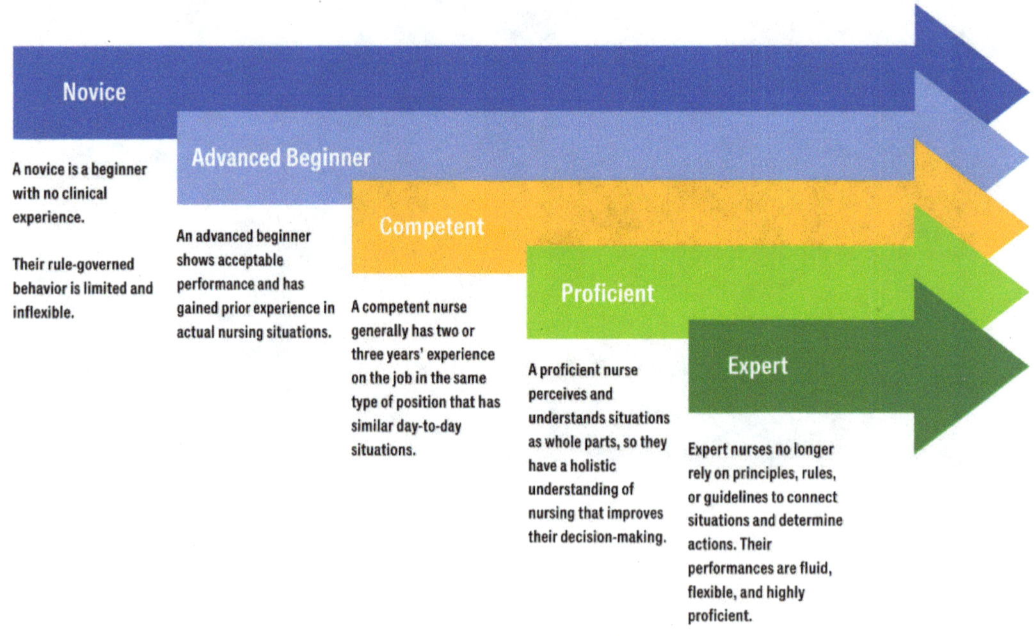

FIGURE 11.6 Novice to Expert Theory

Mentorship

The value of mentorship in the nursing profession is immense, impacting both the personal and professional development of nurses and the overall quality of client care. Mentorship involves experienced nurses providing guidance, support, and knowledge to less experienced or new nurses, fostering their growth and integration into the profession. This relationship is essential for building a competent, confident, and resilient nursing workforce.[30]

One of the primary benefits of mentorship is the enhancement of clinical skills and knowledge. Experienced mentors share their expertise, clinical insights, and practical tips with mentees, helping them develop critical thinking and problem-solving abilities. This hands-on learning experience is invaluable, as it bridges the gap between theoretical knowledge and practical application. Through mentorship, new nurses gain confidence in their clinical competencies, leading to improved client care and safety.[31]

29. Nursing Theory. (2020). *Dr. Patricia Benner novice to expert - nursing theorist.* https://nursing-theory.org/nursing-theorists/Patricia-Benner.php
30. ANA. (2024). *Mentorship in nursing: Benefits & why it's essential.* https://www.nursingworld.org/content-hub/resources/nursing-resources/benefits-of-mentorship-in-nursing/#:~:text=As%20a%20mentor%2C%20you'll,be%20conducted%20formally%20or%20informally.
31. ANA. (2024). *Mentorship in nursing: Benefits & why it's essential.* https://www.nursingworld.org/content-hub/resources/nursing-resources/benefits-of-mentorship-in-nursing/#:~:text=As%20a%20mentor%2C%20you'll,be%20conducted%20formally%20or%20informally.

Mentorship also plays a crucial role in professional development. Mentors guide mentees in setting career goals, navigating career paths, and pursuing continuing education opportunities. They offer advice on advancing in the profession, whether through specialization, leadership roles, or academic achievements. This guidance helps nurses achieve their professional aspirations and contribute more effectively to the health care system. Additionally, mentors often serve as role models, demonstrating the qualities and behaviors essential for success in nursing.[32]

The supportive nature of mentorship fosters emotional and psychological well-being. The transition from nursing school to clinical practice can be challenging and stressful. Having a mentor provides new nurses with a trusted confidant who offers encouragement, listens to concerns, and provides constructive feedback. This support system helps reduce feelings of isolation and burnout, promoting job satisfaction and retention. Mentors can also help new nurses develop coping strategies and resilience, which are critical for long-term success in the demanding field of health care.[33]

Mentorship contributes to the creation of a positive and collaborative workplace culture. By fostering strong relationships between experienced and novice nurses, mentorship programs encourage teamwork, mutual respect, and knowledge sharing. This collaborative environment enhances communication, reduces errors, and improves overall client outcomes. Furthermore, a culture of mentorship promotes lifelong learning and continuous improvement, essential elements for maintaining high standards of care in a rapidly evolving health care landscape. For mentors, the experience is also enriching and rewarding. Mentoring provides opportunities for professional growth, leadership development, and personal satisfaction. It allows experienced nurses to reflect on their own practices, stay current with new trends and technologies, and contribute to the future of the nursing profession. The act of mentoring fosters a sense of purpose and fulfillment, reinforcing the mentor's commitment to the profession and enhancing their own career satisfaction.[34]

Mentorship is a cornerstone of the nursing profession, offering substantial benefits to individual nurses, health care organizations, and clients. It enhances clinical skills, supports professional development, fosters emotional well-being, and promotes a positive workplace culture. By investing in mentorship programs, health care organizations can ensure the growth and success of their nursing staff, ultimately leading to higher quality care and better client outcomes.

11.6 LIFELONG LEARNER

After graduating, passing the NCLEX-RN, and obtaining your first nursing position, your learning as a nurse has just begun. The first year of your nursing career is a continual process of transitional stages and experiential learning and is the beginning of lifelong learning as a nurse. Lifelong learning can be achieved

32. ANA. (2024). *Mentorship in nursing: Benefits & why it's essential.* https://www.nursingworld.org/content-hub/resources/nursing-resources/benefits-of-mentorship-in-nursing/#:~:text=As%20a%20mentor%2C%20you'll,be%20conducted%20formally%20or%20informally.
33. ANA. (2024). *Mentorship in nursing: Benefits & why it's essential.* https://www.nursingworld.org/content-hub/resources/nursing-resources/benefits-of-mentorship-in-nursing/#:~:text=As%20a%20mentor%2C%20you'll,be%20conducted%20formally%20or%20informally.
34. ANA. (2024). *Mentorship in nursing: Benefits & why it's essential.* https://www.nursingworld.org/content-hub/resources/nursing-resources/benefits-of-mentorship-in-nursing/#:~:text=As%20a%20mentor%2C%20you'll,be%20conducted%20formally%20or%20informally.

through a variety of methods, such as obtaining additional nursing degrees, acquiring certifications, joining professional organizations, attending conferences and workshops, and staying up-to-date on current evidence-based practices by reading nursing literature and other research.

Advanced Nursing Degrees

After obtaining an RN license, there are many opportunities to advance your education through accredited schools of nursing. Many health care organizations encourage nurses to obtain higher degrees and provide tuition reimbursement for a BSN and other advanced degrees.

Baccalaureate Degree in Nursing

Many hospitals hire nurses with an Associate's Degree in Nursing (ADN) on a condition they complete their Baccalaureate Degree in Nursing (BSN) within a specific time frame.

Master's Degree in Nursing

A Master's of Science in Nursing Degree (MSN) requires additional credits and years of schooling beyond the BSN. There are a variety of degree options, including, but not limited to, Nurse Educator, Advanced Practice Nurse (APRN), Informatics, Leadership, and Clinical Educators.

Doctoral Degrees in Nursing

Doctoral nursing degrees include the Doctor of Philosophy in Nursing (PhD) and the Doctor of Nursing Practice (DNP). PhD-prepared nurses complete doctoral work that is focused on research. They often teach in a university setting and/or conduct research. DNP-prepared nurses complete doctoral work that is focused on clinical nursing practice. They typically have work roles in advanced nursing practice, clinical leadership, or academic settings.

Advanced Practice Nurses

Advanced Practice Nurses (APRN) are defined by the NCSBN as an RN who has a graduate degree and advanced knowledge. There are four categories of Advanced Practice Nurses: certified nurse-midwife (CNM), clinical nurse specialist (CNS), certified nurse practitioner (CNP), and certified registered nurse anesthetist (CRNA). APRNs can diagnose illnesses and prescribe treatments and medications. Additional information about advanced nursing degrees and roles is provided in the box below.[35]

35. Institute of Medicine. (2011). *The future of nursing: Leading change, advancing health.* National Academies Press. https://doi.org/10.17226/12956

Categories of Advanced Practice Nurses

Nurse Practitioners: Nurse practitioners (NPs) work in a variety of settings and complete physical examinations, diagnose and treat common acute illness, manage chronic illnesses, order laboratory and diagnostic tests, prescribe medications and other therapies, provide health teaching and supportive counseling with an emphasis on prevention of illness and health maintenance, and refer clients to other health professionals and specialists as needed. In many states, NPs can function independently and manage their own clinics, whereas in other states physician supervision is required. NP certifications include, but are not limited to, Family Practice, Adult-Gerontology Primary Care, Adult-Gerontology Acute Care, and Psychiatric/Mental Health.

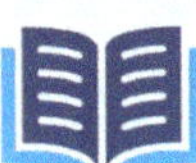

To read more about NP certification, visit Nursing World's Our Certifications web page. Access supplementary digital content in the online book using this QR code.

Clinical Nurse Specialists: Clinical Nurse Specialists (CNS) practice in a variety of health care environments and participate in mentoring other nurses, case management, research, designing and conducting quality improvement programs, and serving as educators and consultants. Specialty areas include, but are not limited to, Adult/Gerontology, Pediatrics, and Neonatal.

To read more about CNS certification, visit NACNS's What is a CNS? web page. Access supplementary digital content in the online book using this QR code.

Certified Registered Nurse Anesthetists: Certified Registered Nurse Anesthetists (CRNAs) administer anesthesia and related care before, during, and after surgical, therapeutic, diagnostic, and obstetrical procedures, as well as provide airway management during medical emergencies. CRNAs deliver more than 65 percent of all anesthetics to clients in the United States. Practice settings include operating rooms, dental offices, and outpatient surgical centers.

To read more about CRNA certification, visit NBCRNA's website. Access supplementary digital content in the online book using this QR code.

Certified Nurse Midwives: Certified Nurse Midwives (CNM) provide gynecological exams, family planning advice, prenatal care, management of low-risk labor and delivery, and neonatal care. Practice settings include hospitals, birthing centers, community clinics, and client homes.

To read more about CNM certification, visit AMCB Midwife's website. Access supplementary digital content in the online book using this QR code.

Specialty Certifications

Acquiring nursing specialty certification is a way to demonstrate expertise. National certifications have various requirements, but most require continuing education credits and successful completion of a national examination. After successfully obtaining a specialty certification, additional credentials are displayed after "RN" in a nurse's signature. See Table 11.6 for a list of common specialty certifications and their associated credentials.

TABLE 11.6 Nursing Specialty Certification

Certification	Credentials
Critical Care Nursing	CCRN
Certified Nurse Educator	CNE
Oncology Certified Nurse	ONC
Stroke Certified Registered Nurse	SCRN
Trauma Certified Registered Nurse	TCRN
Surgical Nurse	CORN
Nursing Professional Development	NPD-BC

Read more about specialty ANCC nursing certifications. Access supplementary digital content in the online book using this QR code.

Professional Organizations

Joining a local, state or national nursing organization is a way to connect with other RNs and promote continued professional growth. The largest national organization is the American Nurses Association (ANA). The ANA provides RN members with the following benefits:

- Advance your career with free development resources and webinars.
- Stay current with the most up-to-date nursing news.
- Save money with big discounts on continuing education (CE), certification, publications, and more.
- Network and connect with Registered Nurses (RN) for support and advice.
- Make your voice heard with opportunities to tell policymakers what you think.
- Receive state nurse association member benefits.

In addition to the ANA, each state has their own state nursing association.

Read more about joining the American Nurses Association and your state nursing association on the ANA website. Access supplementary digital content in the online book using this QR code.

Attending Conferences and Workshops

Regularly attending nursing conferences and workshops is an excellent way to maintain current, evidence-based knowledge and continue to provide safe, quality nursing care. Many opportunities exist for these types of experiences provided by local health care agencies, state nursing associations, or national conferences. Joining local, state, and national nursing organizations is the best way to be aware of upcoming conferences and workshops. See Figure 11.7[36] for an illustration of a lifelong learner and leader.

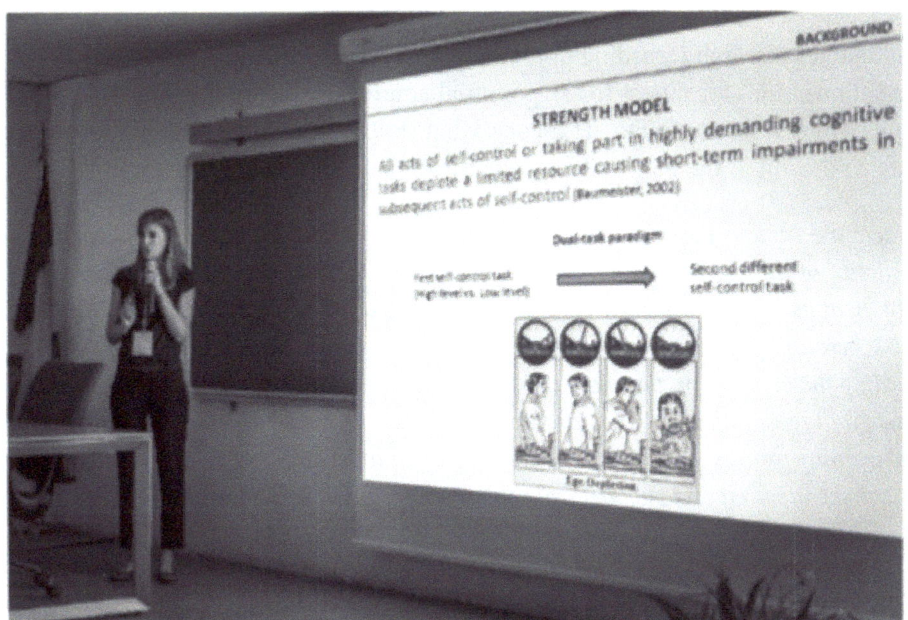

FIGURE 11.7 Lifelong Learner

36. "EFP_2015_speaker_II.jpg" by Adrian Soldati is licensed under CC BY-SA 4.0

Nursing Journals

There are many nursing journals that you can access electronically or have delivered to your home to read regularly. Read more about staying current on evidence-based practices in the "Quality and Evidence-Based Practice" chapter.

11.7 SPOTLIGHT APPLICATION

James is nearing the end of his associate degree nursing program and is interested in pursuing his first nursing employment opportunity within his community. He has a professional goal of becoming a nurse anesthetist and would like to start as a new graduate in the intensive care unit. He has interviews at three acute care organizations for various ICU positions.

Reflective Questions

1. Prior to the interview process, what employment elements should James consider in relation to each position?
2. What should James research regarding potential employers before his interviews?
3. List important questions for nurses to ask potential employers during the interview process?
4. Considering Benner's Novice to Expert theory, what skills sets might be helpful for James to obtain before starting a position in the ICU and working towards becoming a nurse anesthetist?

As James considers the various positions in each organization, he should take time to learn about the populations served and size of the organizations. Certain client populations may be more beneficial to James's professional development as he progresses in his goal of becoming a nurse anesthetist and, therefore, James should consider what background experience he will gain with each position. Additionally, James should ask potential employers regarding the orientation process within each organization. Intensive care positions can be challenging roles for new graduates, and it is important that James has an understanding of the method of orientation used in the ICU training process. James may also be interested in learning more about tuition reimbursement to facilitate his ongoing education and support from the organization for his continued education.

11.8 LEARNING ACTIVITIES

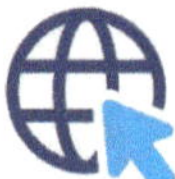

Interactive learning activities have been excluded from the print version of the text. Access free online learning activities in the online book using this QR code.

11.9 GLOSSARY

Benner's Novice to Expert Theory: A theory by Dr. Patricia Benner that explains how new hires develop skills and a holistic understanding of client care over time, resulting from a combination of a strong educational foundation and thorough clinical experiences. Benner's theory identifies five levels of nursing experience: novice, advanced beginner, competent, proficient, and expert.

Licensure: The process by which a State Board of Nursing (SBON) grants permission to an individual to engage in nursing practice after verifying the applicant has attained the competency necessary to perform the scope of practice of a registered nurse (RN). The SBON verifies three components:

- Verification of graduation from an approved prelicensure RN nursing education program
- Verification of successful completion of NCLEX-RN examination
- A criminal background check (in some states)[37]

NCLEX-RN: The exam that nursing graduates must pass successfully to obtain their nursing license and become a registered nurse.

NCLEX-RN Test Plan: A concise summary of the content and scope of the NCLEX that serves as an excellent guide for preparing for the exam. These plans are updated every three years based on surveys of newly licensed registered nurses to ensure the NCLEX questions reflect fair, comprehensive, current, and entry-level nursing competency.

Nurse Licensure Compact (NLC): State legislation that allows nurses to practice in other NLC states with their original state's nursing license without having to obtain additional licenses, contingent upon remaining a resident of that state.

Nurse residency programs: A transition process that provides additional professional development for newly licensed nurses. These programs vary from institution to institution, but many start around the time the new graduate ends their orientation with a preceptor and continue to provide routine support throughout the year.

Orientation: A structured transition process when hired into a new position that may last from one to four months but can be longer depending on the specialty (e.g., Intensive Care or Labor and Delivery). Orientation is based on the new nurse's demonstration and completion of competencies. During this time the novice RN will work with a preceptor to experience all the aspects of the role.

Portfolio: A compilation of materials showcasing examples of previous work demonstrating one's skills, qualifications, education, training, and experience.

Preceptors: Experienced and competent RNs who serve as a role model and a resource to a newly hired nurse. These nurses have the knowledge, skills, and the ability to coach the new RN into the nursing role and answer questions while also evaluating a new hire's performance and providing feedback for improvement.

Resume: A document that highlights one's background, education, skills, and accomplishments to potential employers.

37. NCSBN. (2025). *NCLEX*. https://www.ncsbn.org/nclex.htm

Temporary permit: A permit issued by the State Board of Nursing (SBON) that allows the applicant to practice practical nursing under the direct supervision of a registered nurse until their RN license is granted.

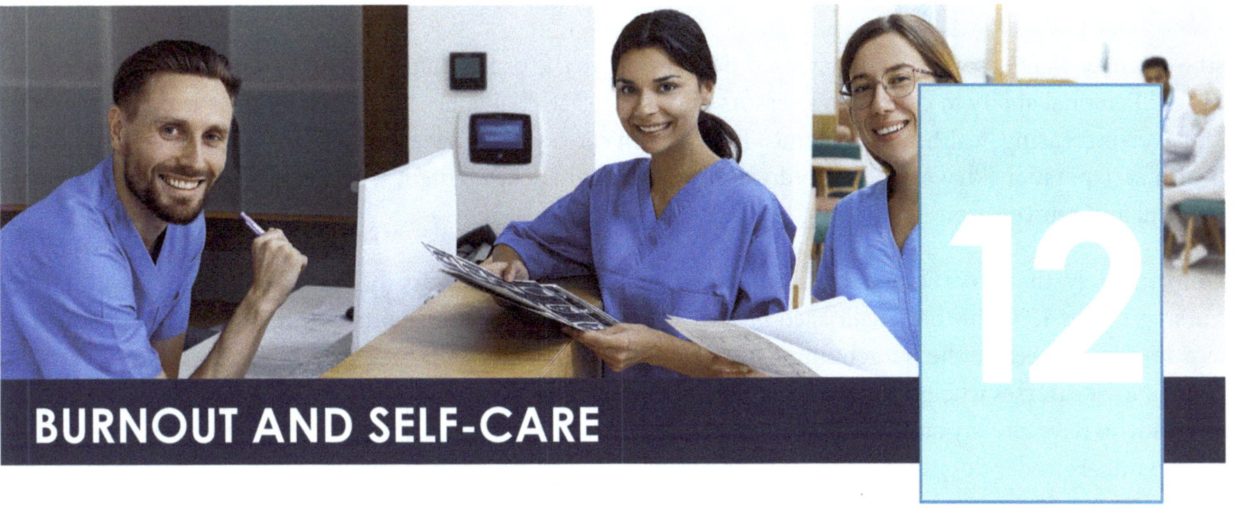

12.1 BURNOUT & SELF-CARE INTRODUCTION

LEARNING OBJECTIVES

- Identify the impact of situational stressors within the nursing profession
- Develop strategies to mitigate stress and burnout and maintain engagement in the profession

There is a continued demand for nurses due to complex health care issues facing our country and health care institutions across the world. Nursing is a challenging and demanding profession that requires rigorous educational preparation, clinical expertise, compassion, and the physical and mental capacity to meet a variety of health care needs. The complex demands of the profession can lead to professional burnout and workplace attrition as nurses struggle to balance the challenges of their daily work roles, manage personal and organizational stress, and maintain their health and well-being at home. Nurses are often accustomed to putting aside their own needs to provide care, yet a lack of attention to their personal needs can have significant negative professional consequences. In essence, care for others can easily become compromised when care for self is in jeopardy. Additionally, nurses who do not engage in self-care are more at risk for burnout and attrition from the profession, compounding issues associated with staffing shortages and personnel supply to meet health care demands.[1]

To fully consider the implications of stress management within the nursing profession, one must look no further than the challenges that have arisen as a result of the recent COVID-19 pandemic. Each day, news reports highlight the exhaustion being experienced by nurses across the world resulting from health care demands in acute inpatient care, long-term care, school nursing, and public health.[2] With increased job

1. Waddill-Goad, S. (2016). *Nurse burnout: Combating stress in nursing.* Sigma Theta Tau International.
2. Turale, S., & Nantsupawat, A. (2021). Clinician mental health, nursing shortages and the COVID-19 pandemic: Crises within crises. *International Nursing Review, 68*(1), 12-14. https://doi.org/10.1111/inr.12674

stress, nurses may experience an increased desire to leave the profession and look for other career opportunities.[3] Personal ability to cope with stressors and workplace challenges have been further taxed by ongoing and ever-increasing health care demands. Busy health care systems have struggled to meet care demands as health care personnel have experienced waning professional engagement with decreased time for personal renewal and rejuvenation.

Unfortunately, the COVID-19 pandemic has exacerbated many stressors that previously existed within the nursing profession. This has challenged nurses to find creative methods aimed at increasing self-resilience as a means of meeting the burgeoning health care demands and challenges arising during these uncertain times. Novice nurses who are entering the profession may feel these stressors more acutely than experienced nurses who have already cultivated personal resilience skills. As a result, attention must be given to assisting novice nurses in developing skills to address occupational stress as they navigate their way into the profession.[4] The nursing profession must acknowledge this new challenge for novice nurses and foster strategies and resources to provide additional emotional support for the unique needs of this group. Professional mentorship and support are even more important in times when many nurses may question their career choice and personally experience waning engagement with the profession.

Finally, it is important for the nursing profession to acknowledge that even outside of the pandemic environment there are unique challenges for long-term engagement. Nurses entering the profession should acknowledge the inherent nature of the work of nursing that can create measurable highs and lows as individuals provide the care and support needed to facilitate the health and well-being of others. Hours are long and care demands are high. Client care needs revolve around a cycle of illness and do not coincide with holidays, summer vacations, and weekend sports. As a result, many new nurses soon realize that job stress related to the schedule burden can become a challenge. It is one of the inherent job stressors that nurses must seek to resolve and manage. Additionally, nurses must recognize that stress management and personal wellness remain important aspects of professional growth throughout the various phases of their career.

12.2 STRESS IN THE HEALTH CARE SYSTEM

Stress within any health care profession occurs as a result of the challenging and dynamic conditions experienced in day-to-day work. See Figure 12.1[5] for an illustration of stress in a health care environment. Nurses and health care professionals are taxed with supporting clients and families in times of extensive life stress and change. Individuals who seek out care often experience rapid life changes as the result of a new diagnosis, altered body function, death of a family member, or significant mental distress. Nurses are frontline staff members who help clients and their families navigate these health stressors. It can be difficult to provide frontline support without taking on some of the stress encountered. As clients and families navigate their feelings of fear, frustration, anxiety, and anger, nurses are often the support members who first hear and react to these feelings. It is important to recognize the constant barrage of these emotions can take a toll, and it is challenging to not assume this emotional burden.

3. Maben, J., & Bridges, J. (2020). Covid-19: Supporting nurses' psychological and mental health. *Journal of Clinical Nursing, 29*(15-16), 2742-2750. https://doi.org/10.1111/jocn.15307

4. Horan, K. M., & Dimino, K. (2020). Supporting novice nurses during the COVID-19 pandemic. *AJN: American Journal of Nursing, 120*(12), 11. https://doi.org/10.1097/01.NAJ.0000724140.27953.d1

5. "Emergency_medicine_simulation_training_exercise_in_Balad%2C_Iraq.jpg" by Robert Couse-Baker is licensed under CC BY 2.0

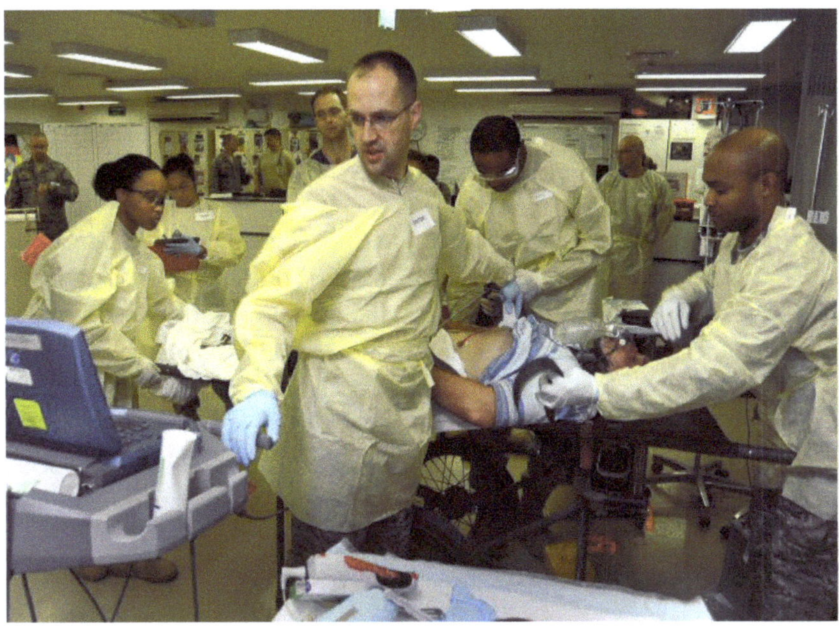

FIGURE 12.1 Stress in the Health Care Environment

In addition to the emotional burden of providing support for multiple clients and their family members, nurses experience a variety of other stressors inherent to the health care environment itself. These stressors include issues such as environmental stress, increased workload, changing practice conditions, lack of resources, communication barriers, unfavorable working conditions, frequency of engagement with a variety of personnel, challenges in care coordination, workplace violence, alarm fatigue, and staff turnover. Research has identified that the variety of stressors experienced by nursing staff result in inherently greater levels of stress than that experienced in the wider working population.[6] Therefore, nurses must acknowledge the variety of stressors they encounter within the profession and identify strategies to mitigate these forces.

Nursing is charged with emotional situations and topics even on days when no other situational stressors have significant impact. One cannot participate in the significant conversations that accompany health care decision-making, provide client education, and promote individual coping without acknowledging these conversations are more impactful than deciding, "What should we make for dinner?" By acknowledging this inherent job stress, nurses recognize that eliminating stress within the profession is not possible. There will always be a level of stress that accompanies the health care environment, and this underscores the importance of stress identification, mitigation, and incorporation of stress-reduction strategies.[7]

12.3 IDENTIFYING STRESS IN SELF

Health care professionals must recognize emerging signs of stress that may result from job demands and the nature of health care work. There are a variety of ways that stress can manifest itself. Taking action early can

6. Waddill-Goad, S. (2016). *Nurse burnout: Combating stress in nursing.* Sigma Theta Tau International.
7. Waddill-Goad, S. (2016). *Nurse burnout: Combating stress in nursing.* Sigma Theta Tau International.

help to prevent workplace burnout. **Burnout** can be manifested physically and psychologically with a loss of motivation for one's work. Nurses and other health care professionals must mitigate stress and burnout to sustain engagement with their profession. Failure to acknowledge the implications of professional burnout only exacerbates the cycle as stressors are transferred to remaining team members and colleagues, resulting in the potential for attrition and turnover.

Although the term "stress" often has negative connotations, it is important to remember that not all stress is considered harmful. **Normal stress,** also referred to as "eustress," does not have lasting consequences and is successfully managed by the individual who is experiencing it.[8] Normal stress, when successfully managed, can increase awareness and focus, resulting in feelings of motivation and competence in the individual who is experiencing it. For example, normal stress may be experienced by a nursing student as they organize their weekly planner specifying time for class, study time, work shifts, or meeting with friends. Although the calendar looks busy, the student can use the stress resulting from a "time-constrained schedule" to motivate oneself to be efficient in completing tasks. This student may feel great satisfaction as they cross off tasks on the "to-do" list. Hopefully, as task achievement occurs, the student transitions from feelings of stress to feelings of empowerment.

Conversely, harmful stress, also referred to as "distress," occurs when stress is not adequately self-managed. **Harmful stress** is reflected by physical, mental, and behavioral manifestations.[9] See Figure 12.2[10] for an illustration of an individual experiencing harmful stress. Harmful stress can lead to burnout and exhaustion, and if left unaddressed, it can have significant health implications for the individual experiencing it. Let's return to the example of the nursing student reviewing their busy schedule. Harmful stress can be experienced by a student looking at their busy weekly schedule and feeling overwhelmed and exhausted. Rather than focusing on manageable tasks and crossing items off the list, this student is reluctant to take action and feels distress regarding where to begin. The student demonstrating harmful stress may struggle with overwhelming fatigue, irritability, and may feel overwhelmed with feelings of inadequacy at one's ability to meet the task requirements.

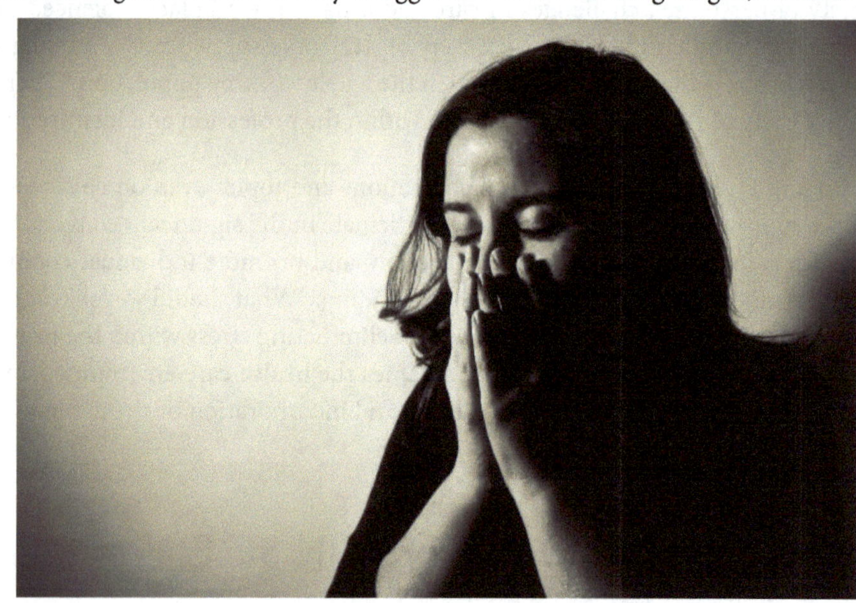

FIGURE 12.2 Harmful Stress

Harmful stress can impact the employment setting as well. It can damage staff engagement, cause significant physical manifestations, and impede the ability of the employee to safely perform work. Harmful stress can quickly result in the breakdown of collegial relationships and also influence the overall practice environment. Potential signs of harmful stress are described in Table 12.3.

8. Bamber, M. R. (2011). *Overcoming your workplace stress: A CBT-based self-help guide.* Routledge.
9. Bamber, M. R. (2011). *Overcoming your workplace stress: A CBT-based self-help guide.* Routledge.
10. "4347213145_bec129a6ae.jpg" by Michael Clesle is licensed under CC BY-NC 2.0

TABLE 12.3. Harmful Stress: Physical, Mental, & Behavioral Manifestations[11]

Physical	Headache Joint discomfort Sleep disturbance Cardiac abnormality (e.g., heart rate, rhythm changes) Increased blood pressure Dry mouth Indigestion Constipation or diarrhea Excessive sweating Dizziness Tremors
Mental	Anger Irritability Mood changes Depression Conflict with friends, family members, coworkers Isolation of self from others Reduced self-confidence
Behavioral	Increased alcohol consumption Smoking or drug use Overeating or loss of appetite Increased arguments with coworkers Increased errors in the workplace

Nurses and health care professionals should be mindful of the physical, mental, and behavioral manifestations of harmful stress so prompt action can be taken when signs begin to occur. Harmful stress must be addressed early so it does not continue to evolve and lead to career burnout. Additionally, stress can have significant implications beyond one's career. An individual's physical and emotional health and well-being are strongly aligned with positive stress management. Harmful stress that goes unaddressed can lead to unresolved physical ailments, deterioration in mental and physical well-being, and the breakdown of familial relationships. The negative impact of harmful stress can be difficult to overcome after it has taken hold of an individual.

It can be helpful to mindfully gauge how one is handling stress on a routine basis. See the link to the Perceived Stress Scale in the following box.

11. Bamber, M. R. (2011). *Overcoming your workplace stress: A CBT-based self-help guide.* Routledge.

Gauge your current level of stress using the State of New Hampshire's Perceived Stress Scale. Access supplementary digital content in the online book using this QR code.

Stressors Resulting From the COVID-19 Pandemic

In addition to the inherent stressors that can occur in health care settings as a result of normal job-related tasks and demands, unique challenges and stressors have occurred for nurses as a result of the COVID-19 pandemic. See Figure 12.3[12] for an image of a COVID care provider. *The Future of Nursing 2020-2030* highlights the impact of the COVID-19 pandemic on the profession. The COVID pandemic has placed extraordinary demands on nurses as they try to meet ever-expanding health care challenges placed on them. Hospitals are continuously overcrowded and needed medical equipment can be sparse.[13] Nurses are asked to provide frontline care to infectious clients with transmission-based precautions in isolation rooms.[14] These nurses then return to their home environments, hoping that they do not spread infection to their families while supporting the needs of the family unit. These continuous job and life stressors compound the physical and psychological demands on nurses. With little respite care for themselves, nurses are at risk for the impact of compounding stressors on their own health.

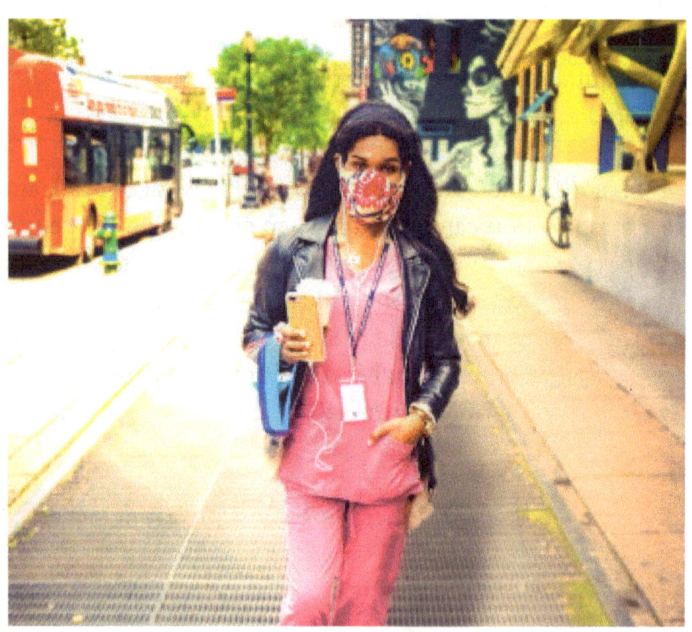

FIGURE 12.3 COVID Care Provider

12. "49855067292_d521d20931_o-e1626806176568.jpg" by Ted Eytan is licensed under CC BY-SA 4.0

13. National Academies of Sciences, Engineering, and Medicine. (2021). *The future of nursing 2020-2030: Charting a path to achieve health equity.* The National Academies Press. https://doi.org/10.17226/25982

14. National Academies of Sciences, Engineering, and Medicine. (2021). *The future of nursing 2020-2030: Charting a path to achieve health equity.* The National Academies Press. https://doi.org/10.17226/25982

Read a meta-analysis about interventions to support the resilience and mental health of frontline professionals during a pandemic. Access supplementary digital content in the online book using this QR code.

12.4 ACKNOWLEDGING STRESS IN OTHERS

In addition to recognizing stress manifestations in oneself, health care professionals must identify signs of stress in others. All members of the health care team experience stress, and effective coping can quickly turn into ineffective coping when manageable, normal stress shifts to harmful stress. Nurses should understand how stress may manifest in a colleague and how one can help and intervene if signs of harmful stress occur.

The signs of harmful stress in a colleague often manifest in a similar manner to what is seen in oneself, but certain signs may be more readily identified by an external source. It is not unusual to identify the mental or behavioral signs of harmful stress in a colleague more rapidly than the physical manifestations. Individuals should be mindful of signs of harmful stress in others, such as changes in mood, irritability, signs of fatigue, increased errors, and absenteeism.[15] Individuals exhibiting these signs may be signaling they are struggling to manage harmful stress. It is important to promptly address these signs with the individual. The tendency to assume one can self-manage or will "get over it" can lead to feelings of isolation that will only perpetuate the stress.

When observing potential signs of harmful stress in a colleague, providing an opportunity to discuss the stressors can be a valuable avenue for promoting effective coping. It is important to remember that the individual exhibiting signs of harmful stress may not recognize they are impacted by stress, but having a colleague acknowledge one's change in mood or attitude can open the opportunity for self-reflection. Although acknowledging signs of harmful stress in a colleague may feel awkward, asking if someone is okay and addressing signs of potential harmful stress can be a significant step in helping them cope. Acknowledgement can occur with statements such as, "I noticed that you seem more frustrated at work lately. Is everything okay?" or "You seem to be more quiet in the breakroom after our shifts. How are you feeling? I know the busy days can really add up." Simple statements and questions open opportunities to share feelings and frustrations and also demonstrate caring for team members.[16] This approach creates dialogue about stressful experiences and provides support needed to positively address harmful stress.

In addition to demonstrating care for one's colleague by inviting conversation about harmful stress, sharing resources is also helpful. It is important for nurses to know they are not alone in experiencing feelings of stress, and attention to these feelings can help one develop strategies to positively address them. Planning

15. Burton, A., Burgess, C., Dean, S., Koutsopoulou, G. Z., & Hugh-Jones, S. (2017). How effective are mindfulness-based interventions for reducing stress among healthcare professionals? A systematic review and meta-analysis. *Stress and Health, 33*(1), 3-13. https://doi.org/10.1002/smi.2673

16. Babore, A., Lombardi, L., Viceconti, M. L., Pignataro, S., Marino, V., Crudele, M., Candelori, C., Bramanti, S. M., & Trumello, C. (2020). Psychological effects of the COVID-2019 pandemic: Perceived stress and coping strategies among healthcare professionals. *Psychiatry Research, 293*, 113366. https://doi.org/10.1016/j.psychres.2020.113366

discussions with a trusted mentor or friend can be very helpful when exploring feelings related to stress. These discussions also provide an opportunity to share information regarding coping strategies such as mindfulness interventions, resiliency programs, or other formalized resources like employee assistance programs.[17] There are also routine workplace measures that significantly impact stress reduction. For example, many nurses do not take the time to ensure they are taking breaks, eating healthy meals, or simply removing themselves from the care environment for brief periods of time. Simple strategies that can dramatically reduce workplace stress include taking a brief walk outside during one's lunch break or taking a few deep breaths prior to the beginning of a work shift. Other simple measures such as daily exercise and meditation can reduce stress and increase confidence to address the tasks at hand.[18] Although experienced nurses may already be incorporating these strategies, it is important for novice nurses to understand the value of these strategies.

12.5 ORGANIZATIONAL STRESS & RETENTION CYCLE

The impact of inadequate stress management for health care personnel can greatly impact health care organizations. When harmful stress is not adequately addressed, burnout can rapidly become a burgeoning problem resulting in absenteeism, decreased productivity, decline in care quality, staff dissatisfaction, and employee turnover. Work environment and lack of workplace support often contribute to feelings of burnout and job attrition.[19] Organizations must recognize the significance of stress in regard to the cyclical nature it plays in the retention of employees. For example, if one employee experiences harmful stress resulting in depression and anxiety, this may influence their timeliness and attendance at work. If the employee begins to struggle, they may be more inclined to phone in as "sick time" for shifts or even be a "no show" for a scheduled shift. When this occurs, the burden of their absence is passed on to other employees on the unit. Calls for overtime, mandated stay, or increased client care assignments quickly increase the burden on the other members of the health care team. As a result, the team members experiencing increased workload feel an impact on their own job-related stress. The compounded stress can quickly overtax an individual who has been managing normal work-related stress. Many individuals who were previously self-managing stress may struggle under these increased role demands. When there is a decrease in an individual's "downtime," there is even less reprieve from the stressful work environment. As a result, the organization and health care system become even more overtaxed, and the cycle perpetuates itself among other staff.[20] Managers and directors often struggle with rehiring and orienting staff at a rate that is suitable to offset the stress cycle and decreased retention within the organization.

17. Dossett, M. L., Needles, E. W., Nittoli, C. E., & Mehta, D. H. (2021). Stress management and resiliency training for healthcare professionals. *Journal of Occupational and Environmental Medicine, 63*(1), 64-68. https://doi.org/10.1097/jom.0000000000002071
18. Perciavalle, V., Blandini, M., Fecarotta, P., Buscemi, A., Di Corrado, D., Bertolo, L., Fichera, F., & Coco, M. (2017). The role of deep breathing on stress. *Neurological Sciences, 38*, 451–458. https://doi.org/10.1007/s10072-016-2790-8
19. Mercado, M., Wachter, K., Schuster, R. C., Mathis, C. M., Johnson, E., & Davis, O. I. (2022). *A cross-sectional analysis of factors associated with stress, burnout and turnover intention among healthcare workers during the COVID-19 pandemic in the United States.* Health & Social Care in the Community. https://doi.org/10.1111/hsc.13712
20. Chegini, Z., Asghari Jafarabadi, M., & Kakemam, E. (2019). Occupational stress, quality of working life and turnover intention amongst nurses. *Nursing Critical Care, 24*, 283-289. https://doi-org.ezproxy.liberty.edu/10.1111/nicc.12419

Promoting Nurse Retention

Nurse leaders must be proactive in finding solutions to address clinical nurse and nursing faculty shortages and high nurse turnover rates. The *2018 National Healthcare Retention and RN Staffing Report* states the following data[21]:

- The U.S. Bureau of Labor Statistics reports that 233,000 new RN jobs will be created annually.
- Forty-five percent of hospitals anticipate increasing their RN staff.
- Hospital turnover is at 18.2%, an increase from previous years.
- RNs working in emergency care, step-down, and medical-surgical units experience high turnover rates, with the highest rate of turnover for certified nursing assistants.
- The average cost of each RN turnover is $49,500, resulting in an average hospital losing an estimated $4.4 to $7 million due to turnover.
- Each percent change in RN turnover will cost or save the average hospital $337,500.
- It takes approximately 2.5 months to recruit an experienced RN.
- More than half of hospitals would like to decrease reliance on supplemental staffing.
- For every 20 travel RNs eliminated, a hospital can save an average of $1,435,000.

Unfortunately, many nurse leaders struggle to receive organizational support for recruitment and hiring in a timely fashion. Demonstrating the need for staff replacement often cannot be established until a staff vacancy exists. As a result, the retention cycle is further compromised when workload is impacted due to staff vacancies during the recruitment and orientation process. Many frontline nursing staff may not be aware of the rigorous challenges that nurse leaders face when requesting administrative support for additional staff positions. Most organizations require executive-level approval for hiring, and unit productivity is examined for rationale that additional staff are needed. The time required for this investigation and executive-level approval can be very challenging for staff nurses who experience the workload burden during the vacancies. During this time frame, nurse leaders may struggle to maintain team morale while also acknowledging the organization's need to be financially responsible in staff hiring.

It is important for all parties to remain engaged in their current work roles during the recruitment, hiring, and orientation periods of new nurses. Trust in one another during this time is critical, and all parties must remember the needs of clients receive top priority. Providing optimal care to the best of one's ability is of the utmost importance even when experiencing staffing challenges. Additionally, staff, nursing leaders, and administrators within the organization must unite to find actionable solutions that acknowledge the impact of stress and reduce the impact of harmful stress contributing to the burnout of colleagues. There is no simple solution. All individuals must be united in exploring strategies to reduce the occurrence of burnout and seek to make change to enhance the health and well-being of all involved.

21. Kroning, M., & Hopkins, K. (2019). Healthcare organizations thrive with shared governance. *Nursing Management, 50*(5), 13-15. https://doi.org/10.1097/01.numa.0000557781.40049.2d

12.6 MITIGATING STRESS WITH SELF-CARE

As previously discussed, the action of providing nursing care can result in significant stress. The stress response is exacerbated when experiencing extreme or repeated stressors, such as client deaths. In some health care settings, nurses do not have time to resolve grief from one loss before another death occurs.

Compassion fatigue and burnout occur frequently with nurses and other health care professionals who experience cumulative deaths that are not addressed therapeutically. Compassion fatigue is a state of chronic and continuous self-sacrifice and/or prolonged exposure to difficult situations that affect a health care professional's physical, emotional, and spiritual well-being. This can lead to a person being unable to care for or empathize with someone's suffering. Additionally, many individuals who experience compassion fatigue may become detached from the emotions associated with the care experience or client needs. These individuals can often appear numb to the severity of the circumstance of the events that are occurring. **Burnout** can be manifested physically and psychologically with a loss of motivation. It can be triggered by workplace demands, lack of resources to perform work professionally and safely, interpersonal relationship stressors, or work policies that can lead to diminished caring and cynicism.[22] See Figure 12.4[23] for an image depicting a nurse at home experiencing burnout due to exposure to multiple competing demands of work, school, and family responsibilities.

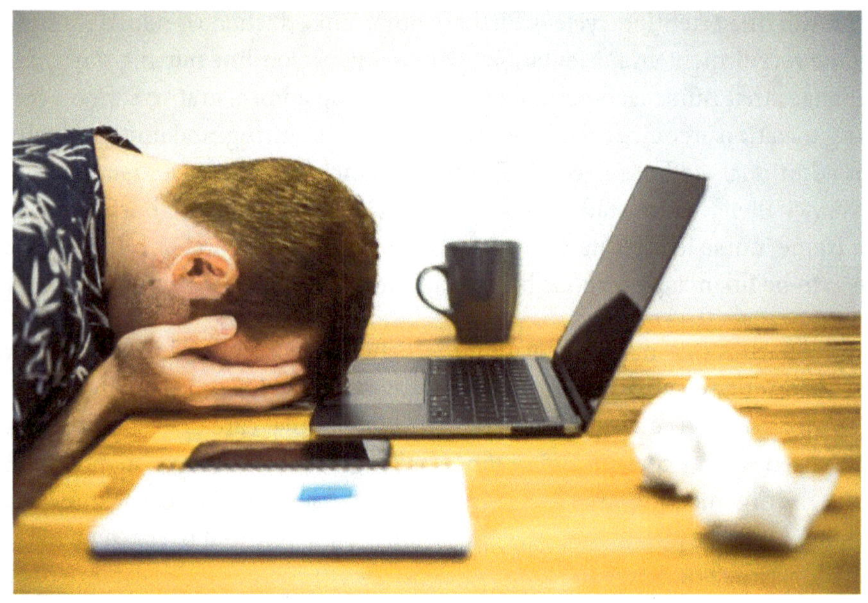

FIGURE 12.4 Burnout

With the significant dangers of burnout and compassion fatigue within the nursing profession, it is important to acknowledge actions and strategies to facilitate self-care. Self-care can occur in many actions that individuals take to maintain self-health and is critically important for preventing compassion fatigue and burnout.

22. Lowey, S. E. (2015). *Nursing care at the end of life.* Open Library. https://ecampusontario.pressbooks.pub/nursingcare/
23. "Burnout_At_Work_-_Occupational_Burnout.jpg" by Microbiz Mag is licensed under CC BY 2.0

To facilitate self-care, nurses must recognize the need to take time off, seek out individual healthy coping mechanisms, and voice concerns within their workplace. Prayer, meditation, exercise, art, and music are examples of healthy coping mechanisms that nurses can use for self-care. Nurses should reflect on what actions bring them personal satisfaction and rejuvenation. These strategies should then be purposefully included to help reduce the influence of work-related stressors. For example, perhaps you are a nurse working in a busy Level 1 trauma center and emergency department. You are nearing the end of your third 12-hour shift and have the following day off. The unit manager approaches you and states that there has been an ill call for tomorrow's evening shift. You are offered premium pay to come in and work. Although there is a part of you that is interested in receiving the premium pay, you also take a moment to think about your current situation. You are tired from working three 12-hour shifts the last three days and had plans to go to your child's baseball game tomorrow evening. Taking stock of these reflective thoughts, you politely decline the additional shift. Acknowledging your fatigue and the satisfaction that you will feel in attending your child's game are important parts of facilitating self-care. Although you could have chosen to work the shift, taking time to look inwardly on what will bring about the greatest rejuvenation and avoid burnout will help cultivate professional engagement.

Additionally, nurses must recognize when outside resources are needed to mitigate stress and facilitate self-care. Many organizations sponsor employee assistance programs that provide counseling services. These programs can be of great value and benefit in allowing individuals to share both individual and employment stressors. For example, employee assistance programs can address employment-related stressors, such as cumulative client deaths, as well as personal challenges impacting one's work role, such as a family illness. The support of an impartial, trained professional can be very helpful as individuals navigate through stressful stimuli.

There are specific stress stimuli that may require specialized intervention. For example, after a client death resulting from trauma, many organizations hold debriefing sessions to allow individuals who participated in care to come together to verbalize their feelings. These sessions are often held with the support of chaplains to facilitate individual coping and verbalization of feelings. Debriefing sessions can be very helpful as individuals experience collegial support in working through traumatic stress stimuli.

Read more about the role of chaplains in facilitating coping in the "Spirituality" chapter in Open RN *Nursing Fundamentals, 2e*. Access supplementary digital content in the online book using this QR code.

Reflective Questions

Throughout your nursing career, there will be times to stop and pay attention to warning signs of compassion fatigue and burnout. Here are some questions to consider:

- Has my behavior changed?
- Do I communicate differently with others?

- What destructive habits tempt me?
- Do I project my inner pain onto others?[24]

Strategies for Self-Care

By becoming self-aware regarding signs of stress, you can implement self-care strategies to prevent compassion fatigue and burnout. Use the following "A's" to assist in building resilience, connection, and compassion:

- **Attention:** Become aware of your physical, psychological, social, and spiritual health. For what are you grateful? What are your areas of improvement? This protects you from drifting through life on autopilot.
- **Acknowledgement:** Honestly look at all you have witnessed as a health care professional. What insight have you experienced? Acknowledging the pain of loss you have witnessed protects you from invalidating the experiences.
- **Affection:** Choose to look at yourself with kindness and warmth. Affection prevents you from becoming bitter and "being too hard" on yourself.
- **Acceptance:** Choose to be at peace and welcome all aspects of yourself. By accepting both your talents and imperfections, you can protect yourself from impatience, victim mentality, and blame.[25]

Cultivating Care of Self

Taking care of oneself can feel as if it goes against the nature of the nursing role, but it is a vital component for professional success. Provision 5 of the American Nurses Association Code of Ethics states, "The nurse owes the same duties to self as to others, including the responsibility to promote health and safety, preserve wholeness of character and integrity, maintain competence, and continue personal and professional growth."[26] In a profession where one spends most of their time thinking about the needs of others, it can be difficult to recognize when special care and attention is needed for one's own health. However, there are many strategies that nurses can use to help them navigate stress and prioritize their own health and wellness. Although not every strategy may be "right" for every nurse, it is critical for nurses to find actionable interventions to help them address their own stress.

Here are some examples of stress management strategies:

- **Meditation.** Meditation can induce feelings of calm and clear-headedness, improving concentration and attention. Research has shown that meditation increases the brain's gray matter density, which can reduce sensitivity to pain, enhance the immune system, help regulate difficult emotions, and relieve stress. Mindfulness meditation in particular has been proven helpful for people with depression and anxiety, cancer, fibromyalgia, chronic pain, rheumatoid arthritis, type 2 diabetes, chronic fatigue syndrome, and cardiovascular disease.[27] See Figure 12.5[28] for an image of an individual participating in meditation.

---

24. Lowey, S. E. (2015). *Nursing care at the end of life.* Open Library. https://ecampusontario.pressbooks.pub/nursingcare/
25. Lowey, S. E. (2015). *Nursing care at the end of life.* Open Library. https://ecampusontario.pressbooks.pub/nursingcare/
26. American Nurses Association. (2015). *Code of ethics for nurses with interpretive statements.* American Nurses Association. https://www.nursingworld.org/practice-policy/nursing-excellence/ethics/code-of-ethics-for-nurses/coe-view-only/
27. Delagran, L. (n.d.). *What is spirituality?* University of Minnesota. https://www.takingcharge.csh.umn.edu/what-spirituality
28. "yoga-class-a-cross-legged-palms-up-meditation-position-850x831.jpg" by Amanda Mills, USCDCP on Pixnio is licensed under CC0

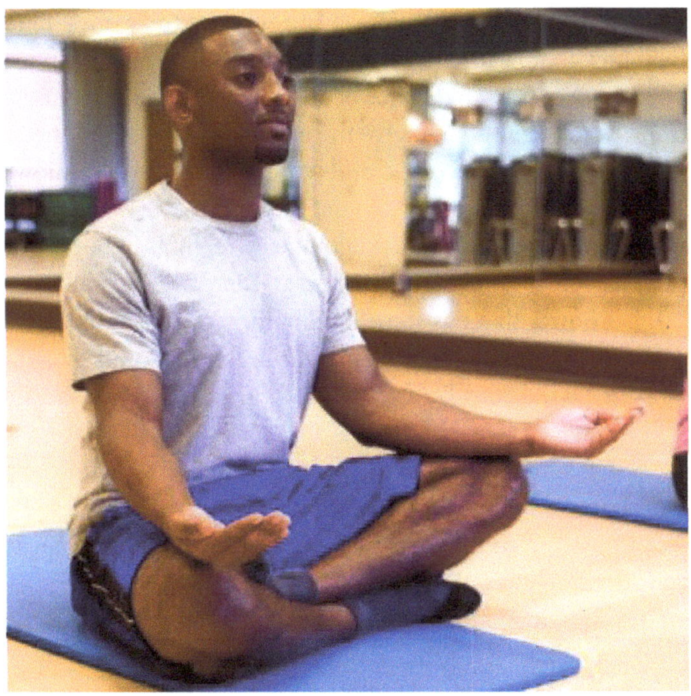

FIGURE 12.5 Meditation

- **Yoga.** Yoga is a centuries-old spiritual practice that creates a sense of union within the practitioner through physical postures, ethical behaviors, and breath expansion. The systematic practice of yoga has been found to reduce inflammation and stress, decrease depression and anxiety, lower blood pressure, and increase feelings of well-being.[29] See Figure 12.6[30] for an image of an individual participating in yoga.

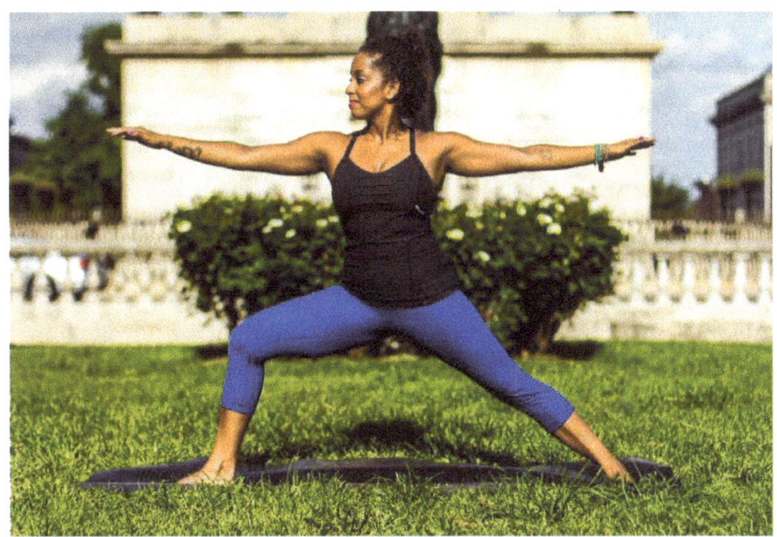

FIGURE 12.6 Yoga

29. Delagran, L. (n.d.). *What is spirituality?* University of Minnesota. https://www.takingcharge.csh.umn.edu/what-spirituality
30. "9707554768.jpg" by Dave Rosenblum is licensed under CC BY 2.0

- **Journaling.** Journaling can help a person become more aware of their inner life and feel more connected to experiences. Studies show that writing during difficult times may help a person find meaning in life's challenges and become more resilient in the face of obstacles. When journaling, it can be helpful to focus on three basic questions: What experiences give me energy? What experiences drain my energy? Were there any experiences today where I felt alive and experienced "flow"? Allow yourself to write freely, without stopping to edit or worry about spelling and grammar.[31]
- **Prayer.** Prayer can elicit the relaxation response, along with feelings of hope, gratitude, and compassion, all of which have a positive effect on overall well-being. There are several types of prayer rooted in the belief that there is a higher power that has some level of influence over one's life. This belief can provide a sense of comfort and support in difficult times. A recent study found that clinically depressed adults who believed their prayers were heard by a concerned presence responded much better to treatment than those who did not believe.[32]
- **Spiritual community.** Join a spiritual group, such as a church, synagogue, temple, mosque, meditation center, yoga class, or other local group that meets to discuss spiritual issues. The benefits of social support are well-documented, and having a spiritual community to turn to for fellowship can provide a sense of belonging and support.[33]
- **Nurturing relationships.** Relationships with family, significant others, and friends aren't static – they are living, dynamic aspects of our lives that require attention and care. To benefit from strong connections with others, you should take charge of your relationships and put in the time and energy you would any other aspect of your well-being. It can be helpful to create rituals together. With busy schedules and the presence of online social media that offer the façade of real contact, it's very easy to drift from friends. Research has found that people who deliberately make time for gatherings or trips enjoy stronger relationships and more positive energy. An easy way to do this is to create a standing ritual that you can share and that doesn't create more stress, such as talking on the telephone on Fridays or sharing a walk during lunch breaks.[34]
- **Mindfulness. Mindfulness** has been defined as, "Awareness that arises through paying attention, on purpose, in the present moment, and nonjudgmentally." Mindfulness has also been described as, "Non-elaborative, nonjudgmental, present-centered awareness in which each thought, feeling, and sensation that arises is acknowledged and accepted as it is." Mindfulness helps us be present in our lives and gives us some control over our reactions and repetitive thought patterns. It helps us pause, get a clearer picture of a situation, and respond more skillfully. Compare your default state to mindfulness when studying for an exam in a difficult course or preparing for a clinical experience. What do you do? Do you tell yourself, "I am not good at this" or "I am going to look stupid"? Does this distract you from paying attention to studying or preparing? How might it be different if you had an open attitude with no concern or judgment about your performance? What if you directly experienced the process as it unfolded, including the challenges, anxieties, insights, and accomplishments, while acknowledging each thought or feeling and accepting it without needing to figure it out or explore it further? If practiced regularly, mindfulness helps a person start to see the habitual patterns that lead to automatic negative reactions that create stress. By observing these thoughts and emotions instead of reacting to them, a person can develop a broader perspective and can choose a more effective response.[35]

---

31. Delagran, L. (n.d.). *What is spirituality?* University of Minnesota. https://www.takingcharge.csh.umn.edu/what-spirituality
32. Delagran, L. (n.d.). *What is spirituality?* University of Minnesota. https://www.takingcharge.csh.umn.edu/what-spirituality
33. Delagran, L. (n.d.). *What is spirituality?* University of Minnesota. https://www.takingcharge.csh.umn.edu/what-spirituality
34. Delagran, L. (n.d.). *What is spirituality?* University of Minnesota. https://www.takingcharge.csh.umn.edu/what-spirituality
35. Delagran, L. (n.d.). *What is spirituality?* University of Minnesota. https://www.takingcharge.csh.umn.edu/what-spirituality

- **Nature.** Spending time in nature is cited by many individuals as a spiritual practice that contributes to their mental health.[36]
- **Physical activity.** Regular physical activity, such as brisk walking, can relieve stress and tension.[37]

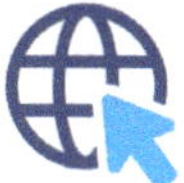

Explore additional free resources regarding well-being and resilience: American Nurses Association Healthy Nurse Healthy Nation. Access supplementary digital content in the online book using this QR code.

12.7 EMERGING MODELS

With the increased emphasis on the impact of stress for health care professionals, many organizations and nursing programs have identified resources for formal stress reduction and mitigation. See Figure 12.7[38] for an illustration of stress management. Many of these models and resources have emerged as a professional necessity to help facilitate coping for individuals encountering innumerable job-related stressors. The U.S. Department of Veterans Affairs developed a Stress First Aid (SFA) framework to improve stress management in oneself and in others.[39] Many organizations are moving to frameworks such as the Stress First Aid framework and other stress management programs to help provide health care professionals with the knowledge, skills, and resources to aid in stress management reduction.

The Stress First Aid (SFA) framework offers the health care professional an opportunity to examine stress along a continuum, from normal stress that allows for adaptive functioning to signs of harmful stress requiring intensive intervention. It provides health care professionals with core functions for progressing through stress identification and resolution. The seven core functions are: Check, Coordinate, Cover, Calm, Connect, Competence, and Confidence.[40] The SFA model encourages health care professionals to self-reflect on a stress experience and take action to facilitate self-resolution and resource identification.

---

36. Yamada, A., Lukoff, D., Lim, C., & Mancuso, L. (2020). Integrating spirituality and mental health: Perspectives of adults receiving public mental health services in California. *Psychology of Religion and Spirituality, 12*(3), 276–287. https://doi.org/10.1037/rel0000260
37. American Heart Association. (2024). *Working out to relieve stress.* https://www.heart.org/en/healthy-living/healthy-lifestyle/stress-management/working-out-to-relieve-stress
38. "stress-management.html" by Nick Youngson is licensed under CC BY-SA 3.0
39. Watson, P., & Westphal, R.J. (2020). *Stress First Aid for Health Care Workers.* National Center for PTSD. https://www.ptsd.va.gov/disaster_events/for_providers/stress_first_aid.asp.
40. Watson, P., & Westphal, R.J. (2020). *Stress First Aid for Health Care Workers.* National Center for PTSD. https://www.ptsd.va.gov/disaster_events/for_providers/stress_first_aid.asp.

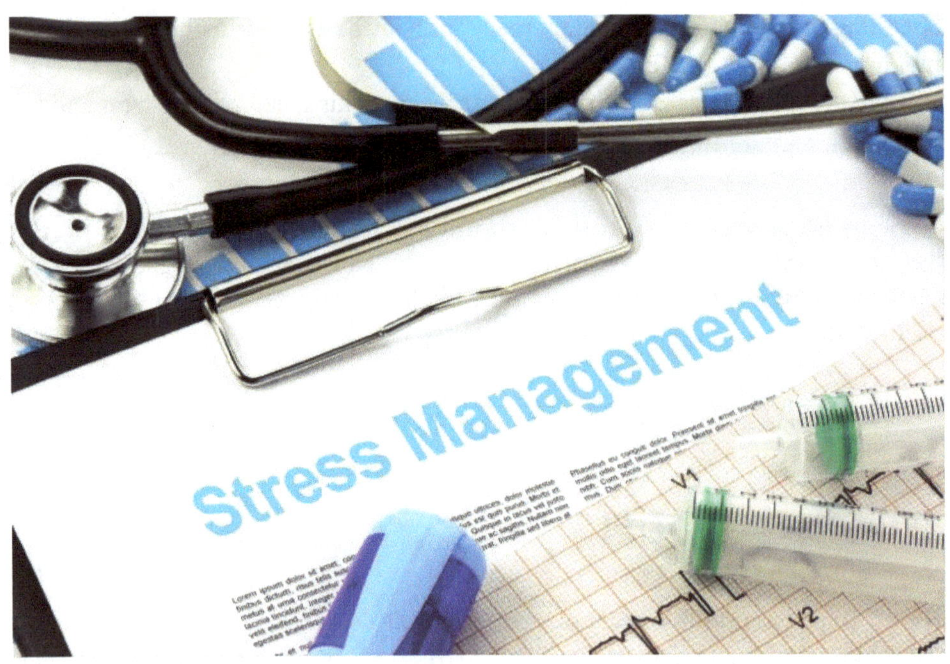

FIGURE 12.7 Stress Management

Many health care organizations embrace wellness as a foundational tenet of workplace culture. They have dedicated wellness committees or wellness champions who promote initiatives aimed at improving stress management among staff.[41] These formalized committees or positions reflect organizational commitment to the importance of self-care and personal wellness. When nursing graduates are interviewing for their first nursing positions, wellness initiatives may be a consideration when exploring professional employment benefits and organizational support structures.

The impact of wellness and stress-reduction strategies is often included in new hire orientation and nurse residency programs. Many nurse residency programs formally acknowledge in their curriculum that novice nurses must be educated about the signs of stress.[42] Novice nurses are particularly vulnerable to harmful stressors during their role transition. Many organizations provide training about strategies and resources to assist with coping and stress reduction, which is referred to as resiliency training programs.[43] **Resiliency training** fosters feelings of mindfulness, sensitivity to self, and professional development techniques that contribute to long-term engagement in the profession.

41. Mayzell, G. (2020). *The resilient healthcare organization: How to reduce physician and healthcare worker burnout* (1st ed.). Productivity Press. https://doi.org/10.4324/9780429286025
42. Chesak, S. S., Morin, K. H., Cutshall, S., Carlson, M., Joswiak, M. E., Ridgeway, J. L., Vickers, K. S., & Sood, A. (2019). Stress management and resiliency training in a nurse residency program: Findings from participant focus groups. *Journal for Nurses in Professional Development, 35*(6), 337-343. https://doi.org/10.1097/NND.0000000000000589
43. Chesak, S. S., Morin, K. H., Cutshall, S., Carlson, M., Joswiak, M. E., Ridgeway, J. L., Vickers, K. S., & Sood, A. (2019). Stress management and resiliency training in a nurse residency program: Findings from participant focus groups. *Journal for Nurses in Professional Development, 35*(6), 337-343. https://doi.org/10.1097/NND.0000000000000589

Read about ways to manage stress from the U.S. Department of Health and Human Services Office on Women's Health. Access supplementary digital content in the online book using this QR code.

12.8 SPOTLIGHT APPLICATION

You have been working for six months on a medical telemetry floor and notice a change in your colleague Allie. Allie has been showing up to work late for her shifts and recently made a medication error when drawing up insulin. She mentions to you in the break room that she is having trouble sleeping and has been struggling with migraine headaches. Her husband was recently laid off from his position with a local manufacturing company, so Allie has been volunteering for extra shifts and overtime. Allie is typically good-natured and has a great sense of humor, but lately she has been short-tempered and irritable. As her friend and colleague, you want to see if there is anything that you can do to help.

Reflective Questions

1. Using your own words, how would you address your concerns with Allie?
2. What strategies and assistance could you offer her?

As Allie's colleague, you note many signs of harmful stress beginning to manifest in Allie's physical, mental, and behavioral health. One of the first actions that you could take would be to invite Allie to discuss what you have noticed lately. Allie may not even realize that she has been exhibiting signs of ineffective coping and harmful stress. Opening the opportunity to discuss what you have seen and demonstrating that you acknowledge that she is in distress are important steps. Additionally, it is important to discuss with Allie what other resources are available to her. She may wish to reach out to the organization's employee assistance program for assistance, or there may be other organizational resources available to her. Allie should also be encouraged to reach out to her manager to discuss the challenges that she is currently experiencing. This is an important part of mobilizing the resources around her so that she can continue as a successful employee within the organization.

12.9 LEARNING ACTIVITIES

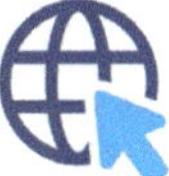

Interactive learning activities have been excluded from the print version of the text. Access free online learning activities in the online book using this QR code.

12.10 GLOSSARY

Burnout: A condition manifested physically and psychologically with a loss of motivation.

Compassion fatigue: A state of chronic and continuous self-sacrifice and/or prolonged exposure to difficult situations that affect a health care professional's physical, emotional, and spiritual well-being.

Harmful stress: Stress (also referred to as "distress") not adequately self-managed resulting in physical, mental, and behavioral consequences.[44]

Mindfulness: Awareness that arises through paying attention, being on purpose and in the present moment, and being nonjudgmental.

Normal stress: Stress (also referred to as "eustress") that does not have lasting consequences and is successfully managed by the individual who is experiencing it.[45]

Resiliency training: Educational sessions that foster feelings of mindfulness and sensitivity to self and cultivate professional development techniques that contribute to long-term engagement in the profession.

Self-care: Actions that individuals take to maintain health of oneself.

44. Bamber, M. R. (2011). *Overcoming your workplace stress: A CBT-based self-help guide.* Routledge.
45. Bamber, M. R. (2011). *Overcoming your workplace stress: A CBT-based self-help guide.* Routledge.

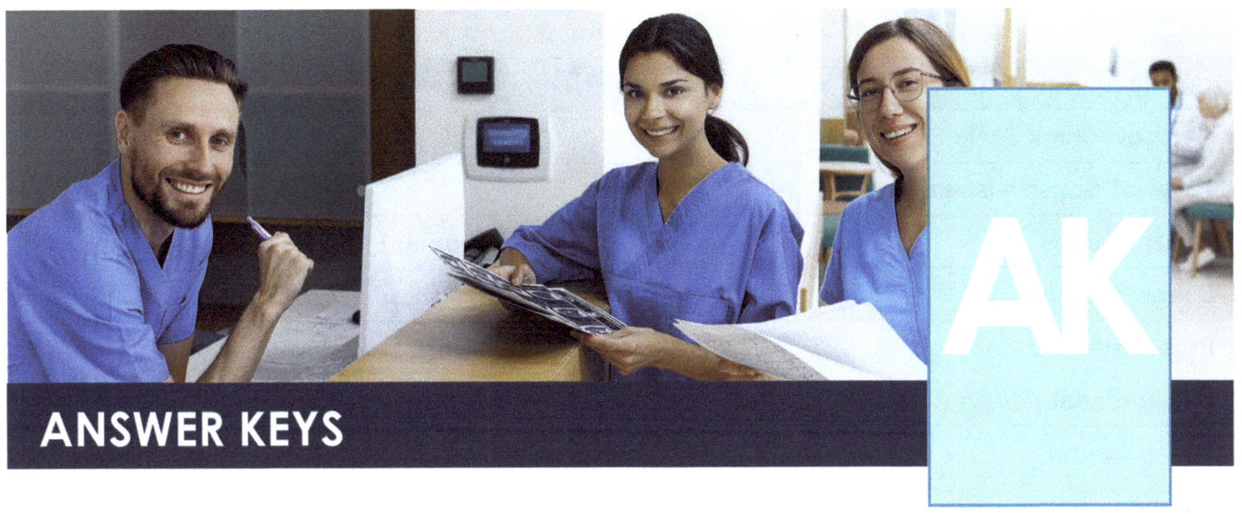

ANSWER KEYS

CHAPTER 1

This chapter is an overview and does not include accompanying learning activities.

CHAPTER 2

Answer Key to Chapter 2 Learning Activities

1. Select the assessment findings requiring immediate follow-up by the nurse.

Vital Signs	
Temperature	98.9 °F (37.2°C)
Heart Rate	***182 beats/min***
Respirations	***36 breaths/min***
Blood Pressure	152/90 mm Hg
Oxygen Saturation	***88% on room air***
Capillary Refill Time	*>3*
Pain	9/10 chest discomfort

Physical Assessment Findings	
Glasgow Coma Scale Score	14
Level of Consciousness	Alert
Heart Sounds	***Irregularly regular***
Lungs Sounds	Clear bilaterally anterior/posterior
Pulses-Radial	***Rapid/bounding***
Pulses-Pedal	***Weak***
Bowel Sounds	Present and active x 4
Edema	Trace bilateral lower extremities
Skin	Cool, clammy

2. Indicate whether the actions are "Indicated" (i.e., appropriate or necessary), "Contraindicated" (i.e., could be harmful), or "Nonessential" (i.e., makes no difference or are not necessary).

Nursing Action	Indicated	Contraindicated	Nonessential
Apply oxygen at 2 liters per nasal cannula.	X		
Call imagining for a STAT lung CT.			X
Perform the National Institutes of Health (NIH) Stroke Scale Neurologic Exam.			X
Obtain a comprehensive metabolic panel (CMP).	X		
Obtain a STAT EKG.	X		
Raise head-of-bed to less than 10 degrees.		X	
Establish patent IV access.	X		
Administer potassium 20 mEq IV push STAT.		X	

Answers to interactive elements are given within the interactive element.

CHAPTER 3

Answer Key to Chapter 3 Learning Activities

1. The answers to this activity are meant to elicit self-reflection in students as they consider the rights of delegation. Students should identify breach in right task, person, circumstance, communication, and supervision as they consider the errors in delegation within the case study scenarios.
2. The RN is delegating tasks to the LPN and UAP on a medical-surgical unit. Place an "X" in the appropriate column where an error in delegation occurred.

	Right Person	Right Task	Right Circumstances	Right Direction and Communication	Right Supervision and Evaluation
Directs the UAP to assess the pain level of a post op Day 3 hip replacement client and report back the finding.	x	x			
Directs the LPN to give 1 mg IV push morphine to a client who is 2-hours post total left knee replacement and ensure documentation.	x	x	x		
Assigns the UAP to collect blood pressures on all clients on the unit by 0800. Assumes the UAP will report back any abnormal blood pressures.				x	x
Directs a new UAP to ambulate a client who is post-op Day 2 from a shoulder replacement who needs the assistance of one person and an adaptive walker. The UAP voices concerns about never having used an adaptive walker before. The RN directs the UAP to get another UAP to help.					x

Answers to interactive elements are given within the interactive element.

CHAPTER 4

Answer Key to Chapter 4 Learning Activities

4.2 Leader vs. Manager Case Analysis

Case 1: Manager – Sima's tasks involve allocating resources, making assignments, and handling staffing needs, which are all core management functions related to budgeting and staffing.

Case 2: Leader – Juan focuses on establishing direction, identifying issues requiring change, and creating a shared vision, all of which are leadership functions. He also implements strategies and inspires his team, which further emphasizes his role as a leader.

Case 3: Manager – Maria's activities involve planning, organizing, and prioritizing, which are essential management functions. Setting goals, establishing time frames, and creating policies and procedures are typical responsibilities of a manager.

Case 4: Manager – Emily's responsibilities, such as budgeting, resource allocation, and managing staffing needs, are core management functions. These tasks involve planning and organizing to ensure operational efficiency.

Case 5: Leader – Rachel's focus on building effective teamwork, advocating for clients and the nursing profession, and open communication aligns with leadership functions. These activities emphasize influencing others and fostering a collaborative environment.

4.2 Just Culture Case Study

Case Investigation A

Classification of Error:

- Systemic Error (Design Flaw in Labeling)

Recommended Actions:

1. Report the Labeling Issue: Communicate with the insulin vial manufacturer about the confusing labeling and request a redesign to enhance clarity.
2. Labeling Review Committee: Establish a committee to review all medication labeling for potential confusion and initiate changes if necessary.
3. Training and Awareness: Conduct training sessions to educate nursing staff about the new labeling and interim measures to avoid confusion.
4. Double-Check Protocol Reinforcement: Reinforce the importance of adhering to double-check protocols, especially when using newly designed medication vials.
5. Incident Reporting System Enhancement: Enhance the incident reporting system to capture and analyze trends related to medication errors and implement preventive measures.

Case Investigation B

Classification of Error:

- Human Error (Due to Time Pressure and High Workload)

Recommended Actions:

1. Workload Assessment: Conduct a thorough assessment of the nursing workload and staffing levels to ensure they are adequate for safe client care.
2. Time Management Training: Provide training for nursing staff on time management strategies to handle high client loads without compromising safety protocols.
3. Staffing Solutions: Explore staffing solutions such as hiring additional staff, using float pools, or employing temporary nurses during peak times.
4. Protocol Reinforcement: Reinforce the importance of following safety protocols regardless of time pressures and workloads.
5. Supportive Environment: Create a supportive environment that encourages nurses to follow protocols without fear of repercussions for taking necessary time to ensure client safety.

Case Investigation C

Classification of Error:

- Reckless Behavior (Intentional Bypassing of Safety Protocols)

Recommended Actions:

1. Disciplinary Action: Take appropriate disciplinary action against the nurse for knowingly disregarding safety protocols, which may include suspension, retraining, or termination depending on the severity and frequency of the behavior.
2. Behavior Monitoring: Implement a system to monitor and review the behavior of nurses to ensure adherence to safety protocols.
3. Retraining Program: Mandate a retraining program for the nurse to emphasize the importance of safety protocols and the consequences of non-compliance.
4. Culture of Safety: Foster a culture of safety within the hospital where following protocols is non-negotiable and staff feel accountable for their actions.
5. Counseling and Support: Provide counseling and support for the nurse to address any underlying issues contributing to the reckless behavior.

4.5 Learning Activity Sample Scenario

1-3. This learning activity is meant to elicit students' reflection on leadership styles, coaching, and change theory. Responses and application will vary.

Answers to interactive elements are given within the interactive element.

CHAPTER 5

Answer Key to Chapter 5 Learning Activities

Section 5.4 Professional Misconduct Case Study

1. Identify the ethical and legal issues present in this case.

Ethical Issues:

- Non-maleficence: Sarah's primary duty is to do no harm to her clients. Administering the wrong medication dosage directly violated this principle.
- Fidelity: By not reporting the error and altering the medical records, Sarah violated the principle of fidelity, which emphasizes honesty and integrity in professional practice.
- Accountability: Nurses are ethically required to be accountable for their actions. Failing to report the medication error and falsifying records shows a lack of accountability.

Legal Issues:

- Negligence/Malpractice: Administering the wrong dosage of medication constitutes negligence, which can lead to malpractice claims.
- Falsification of Records: Altering medical records is a serious legal violation that can result in criminal charges and civil liabilities.
- Failure to Report: Not reporting a medication error is a breach of legal and professional duties, potentially leading to disciplinary actions by regulatory bodies.

2. How does Sarah's behavior constitute professional misconduct?

- She failed to adhere to established medication administration protocols by not double-checking the doctor's orders.
- She compromised client safety by administering the wrong medication dosage.
- She attempted to cover up her mistake by falsifying medical records, which is a severe breach of ethical and legal standards.
- She failed to report the medication error, preventing appropriate corrective actions from being taken and further endangering the client.

3. What are the potential consequences for Sarah, both professionally and legally?

Professional Consequences: Sarah could face disciplinary measures from the nursing board, including suspension or revocation of her nursing license. She might be terminated from her job due to her actions. Her professional reputation could be severely damaged, making it difficult to find future employment in the healthcare field.

Legal Consequences: Mr. Thompson or his family could file a malpractice lawsuit against Sarah, seeking compensation for the harm caused. Altering medical records is a criminal offense that could result in charges, leading to fines or imprisonment. Sarah could face civil penalties for her negligence and falsification of records.

4. How might the lack of adequate staffing and supervision have contributed to this incident?

Understaffing led to Sarah handling multiple clients at once, increasing the likelihood of errors due to the high workload and stress. Lack of adequate supervision might have left Sarah without the necessary support and guidance, contributing to her mistake and poor decision-making. The urgent call to assist another critical client likely pressured Sarah to act hastily, bypassing essential safety checks.

5. What policies should the hospital have in place to prevent such errors and ensure proper reporting?

Ensure sufficient staffing levels to reduce workload and stress, allowing nurses to follow protocols without rushing. Implement and enforce strict protocols for medication administration, including mandatory double-checking and verification processes. Establish non-punitive error reporting systems that encourage staff to report mistakes without fear of retribution, promoting a culture of transparency and learning. Provide ongoing training for staff on medication safety, error prevention, and ethical practices. Ensure adequate supervision and support for nurses, especially during busy or understaffed shifts.

6. How did Sarah's actions affect Mr. Thompson's safety and overall outcome?

Mr. Thompson's condition worsened significantly due to the wrong medication dosage, directly affecting his health and requiring intensive care. The failure to report the error delayed appropriate medical intervention, further compromising Mr. Thompson's safety and overall outcome. The altered medical records could have led to further incorrect treatments or misdiagnoses, increasing the risk to Mr. Thompson's health.

7. What impact might this incident have on the trust between health care professionals and clients?

Clients rely on health care professionals to provide safe and honest care. Incidents like this erode client trust in their caregivers and the health care system as a whole. Clients might become reluctant to seek care or follow medical advice, fearing potential errors and lack of transparency. Such incidents can damage the trust and collaboration among health care professionals, leading to a less cohesive and effective team dynamic.

End of Chapter Learning Activities

1. This learning activity is meant to elicit students' reflection on legal implications of nursing practice. Students should identify issues related to nurse fatigue, client assignment, medication administration, staff education, etc., as areas of potential error. They should discuss the actions that were taken by the nurse in the case, different alternatives to the actions that were taken, reflection on how this case might impact their own nursing practice, and considerations regarding their belief of culpability of others (organization and other staff) in the case with supporting rationale.

Answers to interactive elements are given within the interactive element.

CHAPTER 6

Answer Key to Chapter 6 Learning Activities

Case A & B

These learning activity case studies are meant to elicit students' reflection on ethical implications of nursing practice and client care. Students and instructors should recognize that there are a wide variety of ethical considerations when examining the case studies. They are meant to invoke discussion and critical thought.

Answers to interactive elements are given within the interactive element.

CHAPTER 7

7.6 Team Qualities Case Application

Team Success Strategies:

Dr. Patel (Primary Physician): Dr. Patel consults with Chris (physical therapist) and Emily (speech therapist) before making any changes to Mary's medication that might affect her therapy sessions. This demonstrates collaboration and respect for other team members' expertise. Actively participates in scheduled interdisciplinary team meetings to discuss Mary's progress and adjust her care plan.

Chris (Physical Therapist) and Emily (Speech Therapist): Chris and Emily coordinate their therapy schedules to maximize Mary's participation and avoid conflicting sessions and fatigue. This shows effective teamwork and prioritization of client-centered care. Engage in interdisciplinary team meetings, contributing to discussions and adjustments in Mary's care plan.

Individuals Lacking Demonstration of Team Strategies:

Laura (Social Worker): Struggles to include Mary's family in discharge planning discussions but moves forward with client placement paperwork independently. How to Modify Approach: Make a concerted effort to involve Mary's family in discharge planning discussions, perhaps by scheduling family meetings or using video conferencing if the family cannot be present. Actively seek feedback from Mary and her family regarding their preferences and needs for discharge planning to ensure the chosen facility is acceptable to all parties. Share concerns and discuss discharge plans in interdisciplinary meetings to gather input and support from other team members.

Lisa (Dietician): Identifies a dietary plan that she believes will best meet Mary's nutritional needs but disregards Mary's dietary preferences. How to Modify Approach: Work to incorporate Mary's dietary preferences into the nutritional plan to ensure it is both effective and acceptable to Mary. Engage in discussions with Mary and her family about dietary preferences and restrictions, explaining the importance of certain nutritional choices while finding a balance that meets Mary's needs and preferences. Discuss the dietary plan and any challenges in interdisciplinary meetings to get insights and support from other team members who may offer additional strategies for addressing dietary concerns.

End of Chapter Learning Activities

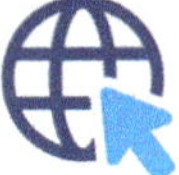

Please access the following link to explore the embedded TeamSTEPPS® activities: TeamSTEPPS® Instructor Manual: Specialty Scenarios.

Answers to interactive elements are given within the interactive element.

CHAPTER 8

8.2 Case Study Maria's Journey Through the Health Care System

1. Maria's financial stress can lead to poor medication adherence, unhealthy dietary choices, and infrequent medical visits. This results in poorly controlled diabetes and increased risk of complications. Additionally, the constant stress of managing her finances can raise cortisol levels, negatively impacting her blood sugar control.
2. Programs such as sliding scale fees at clinics, subsidies for medications, food assistance programs like SNAP, and community-based health initiatives could help reduce the financial burden on individuals like Maria. Expanding Medicaid and implementing prescription drug assistance programs are also effective measures.
3. Improved health literacy can empower Maria to understand her condition better, follow her treatment plan accurately, make healthier lifestyle choices, and seek timely medical help. This knowledge can lead to better diabetes control, fewer complications, and overall improved health outcomes.
4. Community health workshops, educational programs at local community centers, partnerships with local schools to provide health education, and accessible online resources can enhance health education. These programs should focus on diabetes self-management, nutrition, and general health literacy.
5. The lack of accessible health care services can lead to delayed treatment, worsening of Maria's condition, increased complications, and ultimately higher health care costs due to emergency care and hospitalizations. Poor access to health care also reduces preventive care opportunities, contributing to the progression of chronic diseases like diabetes.
6. Solutions include expanding community health centers, providing mobile health clinics, increasing funding for public health initiatives, and implementing telehealth services to reach underserved populations. Additionally, policies that incentivize health care providers to work in underserved areas and improving public transportation to healthcare facilities can help.
7. Living in a food desert forces Maria to consume high-calorie, low-nutrient foods, which can lead to poor diabetes control and increased complications. Limited access to healthy foods makes it challenging to follow dietary recommendations for managing diabetes.
8. Initiatives could include improving public transportation routes, providing subsidized transportation vouchers, partnering with ride-sharing services, and developing community-based transport programs.

Mobile clinics and telehealth services can also mitigate transportation barriers by bringing healthcare services directly to the community.

9. A lack of social support can lead to feelings of isolation, depression, and reduced motivation to adhere to treatment plans. Social support is crucial for emotional well-being and effective disease management. Without it, Maria may struggle more with managing her diabetes and overall health.
10. Community programs such as neighborhood watch groups, community centers offering social activities, mental health support groups, and safe spaces for exercise can enhance social support and safety. Initiatives to improve public safety, such as increased police presence and community policing, can also create a safer environment for residents to engage in outdoor activities and social interactions.

Answers to interactive elements are given within the interactive element.

CHAPTER 9

Answers to interactive elements are given within the interactive element.

CHAPTER 10

Answers to interactive elements are given within the interactive element.

CHAPTER 11

Answers to interactive elements are given within the interactive element.

CHAPTER 12

Answers to interactive elements are given within the interactive element

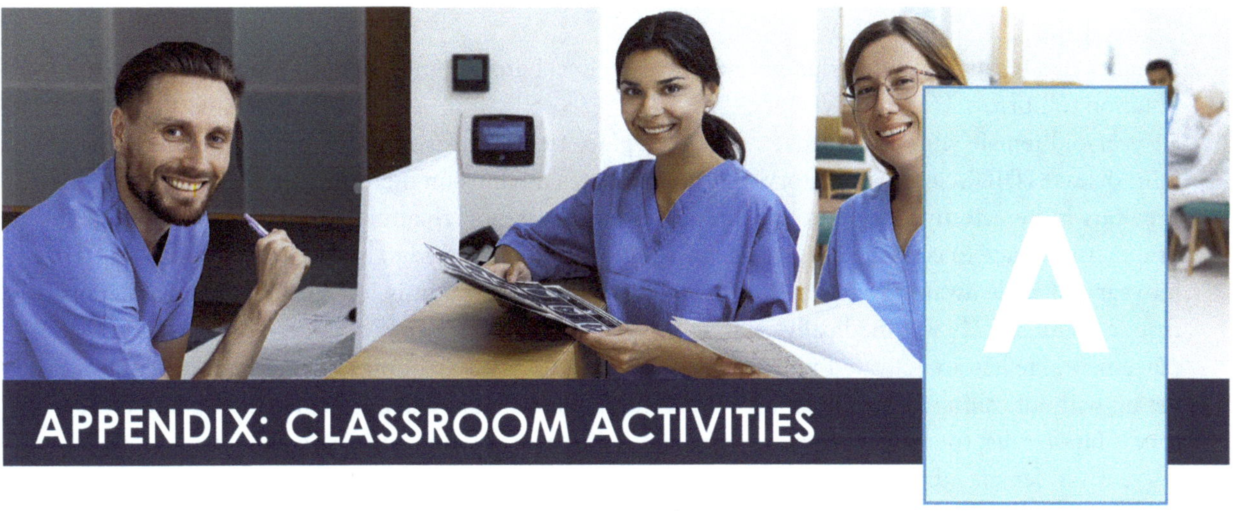

EXERCISES

Utilize the "Suite of Patients" and suggested prompt activities below to engage your students in knowledge application associated with the various learning units throughout the text.

Clients on the Inpatient Unit

1. 56-year-old female admitted yesterday afternoon with nausea/vomiting and right-sided upper abdominal pain that increases after eating. Has had two stools since admit and vomiting stopped after dose of Zofran in ER. Had ERCP yesterday afternoon for dilated biliary duct. She is scheduled for OR this morning for cholecystectomy. Only medical history is depression and surgical history of C-section x2. She does not take any medications routinely at home. She is accompanied by her 17-year-old daughter.
2. 65-year-old male hospitalized three days prior with malaise, cough, cachexia, and 30 pounds of unintentional weight loss over past six weeks. He has a remote history of alcohol and drug abuse but has been sober for more than 10 years. He was diagnosed with acquired immunodeficiency syndrome (AIDS), pneumocystis pneumonia (PCP), and oral candidiasis. He is being treated with IV fluids, IV Bactrim, and IV fluconazole. He is divorced and has one daughter. His ex-wife came to the hospital yesterday to visit. He has no visitors currently. The client is very quiet and withdrawn.
3. 32-year-old nonbinary person, who was transferred from the ICU this morning after being extubated. Client was admitted five days prior with COVID. Client cannot have visitors due to COVID status. Continues four liters nasal cannula oxygen.
4. 29-year-old female with cellulitis on right arm from infiltration from heroine injection. Her wife is present, along with their 4-year-old son. She had an I&D yesterday and may need to have repeat procedure tomorrow. Currently on IV antibiotics.
5. 52-year-old male with gangrene of fourth toe from having a nail through sole of shoe. Client has a history of uncontrolled diabetes, hypertension (HTN), peripheral vascular disease (PVD), chronic kidney

disease (CKD) stage 2, and peripheral neuropathy. Receiving IV antibiotics and scheduled for toe amputation tomorrow. He has no visitors.

6. 82-year-old female who had elective right hip replacement for uncontrolled hip pain and degenerative joint disease (DJD). She has a history of type 2 diabetes mellitus on metformin and dietary restrictions; previous hysterectomy, osteoporosis, carpal tunnel repair, and rheumatoid arthritis, which she takes oral methotrexate to control. She has a son who is visiting. Expected to be discharged today.
7. 68-year-old male awaiting nursing home placement following admission for hepatic encephalopathy from alcoholism. He was medically cleared last week but is a registered sex offender and has yet to find placement. He has an activated power of attorney, who is a state-appointed guardian. He continues to get up without calling, makes inappropriate remarks to staff, and had a fall three days prior. Other history is bipolar disorder, alcohol abuse, type 2 diabetic, chronic kidney disease stage 3, and hypertension.
8. 19-year-old female admitted for what is presumed Benadryl overdose last evening. On room air, needs to have 1:1 sitter present. Client is not responding to questions; does not know if this is accidental overdose or intentional. History of previous intentional overdose, depression, and anxiety. Dad is present and demanding to know if a toxicology screen was completed and what it showed.
9. 61-year-old male admitted six days prior with confusion. Was found by a neighbor wandering. Works at the local gas station. Initial work up shows what appears to be lung cancer with brain metastasis. Client does not have a power of attorney. He is not married and is estranged from his son. Neighbor who found him is a friend and is willing to become guardian. History from neighbor and review of medical records shows a history of smoking. Neighbor says it does appear he has lost weight recently but hadn't mentioned other concerns when he had talked to him about two weeks ago. In the process of paperwork to be completed for guardianship. Client had been aspirating when eating; decision to start nasal gastric feed was made yesterday by ethics committee. Awaiting guardianship for further decision on biopsy for confirmed diagnoses and decision to proceed with treatment or switch to hospice care.
10. 45-year-old female admitted last evening who is short of breath, dizzy, light-headed, and gastrointestinal bleed. Esophagogastroduodenoscopy (EGD) scheduled for this morning. If negative, will need prep for colonoscopy and then colonoscopy tomorrow. Client has little medical history except had recently returned from an overseas trip and had chest and back pain about two days after returning. Had been found to have a saddle PE and was hospitalized for five days on heparin drip and discharged home with coumadin about a week prior. Client continued to have back and intermittent chest pain and had been taking ibuprofen 1-2 times daily since discharge. Husband brought her in last night when she was found to have a Hgb of 6.2. Husband is furious that no one told them she should not be taking ibuprofen on previous discharge.
11. 64-year-old male with BKA for nonhealing diabetic ulcer; scheduled to go to rehab today if bed becomes available. Lives alone in a second floor, low-income apartment without an elevator. Does not have any visitors.
12. 32-year-old male admitted 15 days prior for newly diagnosed AML. Received induction therapy starting 13 days ago. Client is at nadir, will need 1 unit of PRBCs for a Hgb of 6.2 today and a unit of platelets for a platelet count of 8. Client has had fevers for the past two days and is currently receiving vancomycin and cefepime. Also, on prophylactic acyclovir and fluconazole. Client has mucositis and is on PCA pump and receiving TPN and diet as tolerated (magic mouthwash before meals).
13. Cachexic 25-year-old female with history of cystic fibrosis. Admitted for CF exacerbation overnight. Eats during the day and is tube fed overnight. Admitted for extensive pulmonary toileting, IV antibiotics (tobramycin and cefuroxime), continued home respiratory treatments. Client also needs to have

nutrition recommendations reviewed during this hospitalization. She is here with her boyfriend. The boyfriend also has two school-aged children who would like to visit.

14. 78-year-old male with a history of HTN and hypothyroid. Admitted two days prior to abdominal pain and nausea/vomiting. Had a colectomy yesterday for perforated diverticulitis. Client is NPO and has NG tube in place. Had nausea overnight. His wife is expected to visit later today; she went home after return from OR yesterday.
15. 89-year-old female admitted from nursing home yesterday with increased confusion. Has a history of dementia, HTN, type 2 diabetes, and dysphagia. Was found to have a UTI. Started on IV Levaquin; awaiting urine cultures. Expected discharge tomorrow. She has been trying to get up frequently overnight. No family present. Needs 1:1 supervision for all feedings.
16. 82-year-old man admitted with COPD exacerbation and is on 2 L of home oxygen baseline. Oxygen saturation was 78% on arrival and has not been able to do ADLs because of shortness of breath. Has CAD, HTN, and PAD. Lives in a duplex with his granddaughter who lives on the other side. His granddaughter called yesterday.
17. 68-year-old male who is morbidly obese and admitted two days prior for shortness of breath with CHF. Client is on IV bumex and is down 25 pounds since admit. He has a history of HTN, CAD, post CABG, and CKD stage 2. Expected discharge today.
18. 36-year-old female admitted for excessive uterine bleeding four days prior. Newly diagnosed with uterine cancer. Client had open hysterectomy, oophorectomy, salpingotomy, and lymph node biopsy. Had diagnostics, port placement, and staging over the past three days. Expected discharge today. Her husband is here with their 16-month-old daughter. The husband has been very inattentive during this hospitalization and has expected her to watch their daughter over the last couple days and even left to go for lunch yesterday while leaving the daughter in the room.
19. 68-year-old male with history of stage 3 CKD and admitted with AKI on CKD yesterday. Client has had nausea and vomiting for past 36 hours; baseline creatinine of 1.8 and was 4.6 on admit. Has been given fluid hydration and is down to 3.2 this morning.
20. Bed open.
21. It is "ortho day" in the OR. There are three clients scheduled. 1 is a 54-year-old male with bilateral knee replacement (0800 surgery time) and scheduled for observation admit. 68-year-old women with right knee (1100 surgery time) and expected to be discharged. 78-year-old male with hip replacement (1300 OR time) and scheduled for observation admit.
22. 72-year-old female waiting for a bed in the emergency room. Arrived overnight with hypoxia, cough, SOB. Positive for influenza.

Classroom Activity Ideas:

Prioritization

Put students in groups and a client assignment (4-5 clients). Have them identify whom they would see first, second, etc. Why?

Students will review all of the clients on the unit. Have them identify those who are most critical and why.

Add in "changes of conditions" – Client with AKI on CKD morning labs showed a K of 7.2 and Na of 118. AML spikes temp of 103.6 and develops hives and chest tightness when PRBCs are infusing. Client with newly diagnosed uterine cancer states she is concerned going home with her husband because she feels the abuse is going to get worse now that she is sick.

Classroom Activity Ideas:

Delegation/Supervision

Different staffing assignments: 5 RNs/2 CNAs; 4 RNS, 2 LPNs, 2 CNAs; charge nurse/no change nurse. Have students identify appropriate assignments, tasks for delegation, etc.

Consider different types of acute care units – would you organize assignments differently?

Classroom Activity Ideas:

Legal

Develop a scenario in which one client is upset about not being taught about ibuprofen. Consider the legal implications associated with the lack of education.

How would a student address the father who wants to get information on daughter who overdosed?

Can a 17-year-old daughter be at the hospital without another guardian?

Classroom Activity Ideas:

Economics

Talk about isolation/PPE use and staffing ratios.

Have students utilize a couple different staffing tools to see acuity score.

Classroom Activity Ideas:

Quality/Evidence-Based Practice

Have students look up EBP guideline on one of their clients in their assignment (e.g., when to transfuse with blood and platelets for AML client, ERCP prior to cholecystectomy, etc.).

Classroom Activity Ideas:

Ethical Practice

Client who is waiting guardianship placement – diagnosed with new brain tumor.

Classroom Activity Ideas:

Managing the Nursing Team

Talk about the ways a charge nurse, nurse manager, and RN work with these clients.

Have each team assigned a new client (post op, one in ED) with different methods of assigning – choosing who the new client for the day would be, assigning at start of shift, and during the day.

Have one of the nurses refuse a new client.

Classroom Activity Ideas:

Collaborating with Multidisciplinary Team

With your assigned clients, whom would you interact with during the day (e.g., PT, OT, ST, provider, lab, case management)?

Classroom Activity Ideas:

Advocacy

What community agencies might you recommend to the clients with whom you are working?

How would you work with a client (e.g., the hip client #6) who doesn't feel comfortable being discharged today?

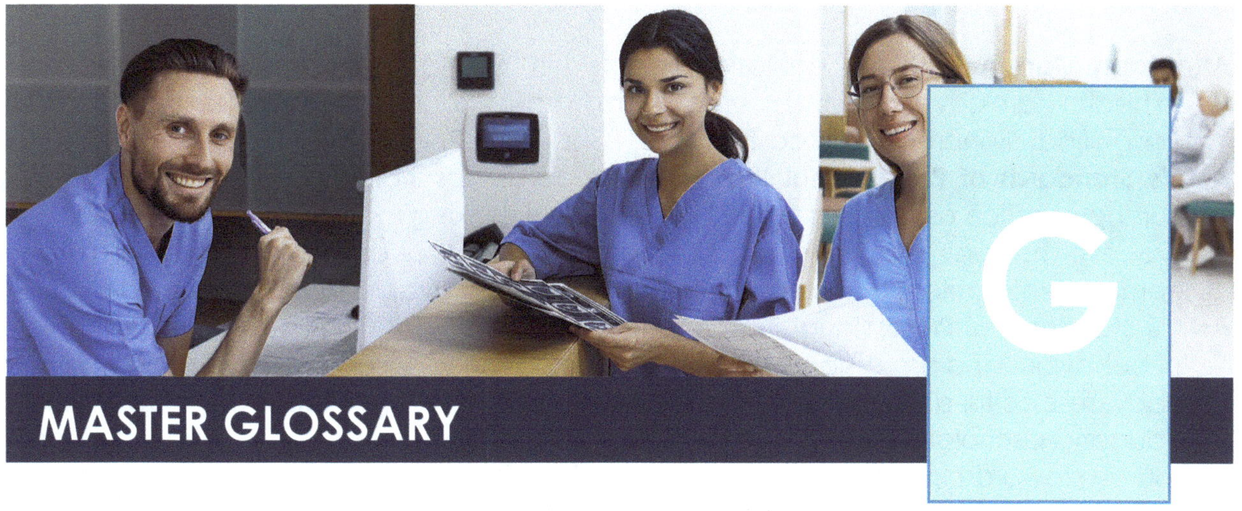

A

ABCs: Airway, breathing, and circulation. (Chapter 2.3)

Accountability: Being answerable to oneself and others for one's own choices, decisions, and actions as measured against a standard. (Chapter 3.4)

Accreditation: A review process to determine if an agency meets the defined standards of quality determined by the accrediting body. (Chapter 9.2)

Actual problems: Nursing problems currently occurring with the client. (Chapter 2.3)

Acuity: The level of client care that is required based on the severity of a client's illness or condition. (Chapter 2.3)

Acuity-based staffing: A client assignment model that takes into account the level of client care required based on the severity of a client's illness or condition. (Chapter 8.5)

Acuity-rating staffing models: A staffing model used to make client assignments that reflects the individualized nursing care required for different types of clients. (Chapter 2.3)

Acute conditions: Conditions having a sudden onset. (Chapter 2.3)

Administrative law: Law made by government agencies that have been granted the authority to pass rules and regulations. For example, each state's Board of Nursing is an example of administrative law. (Chapter 5.2)

Admission: Refers to an initial visit or contact with a client. (Chapter 7.8)

Advanced directives: Written instruction, such as a living will or durable power of attorney for health care, recognized under state law, relating to the provision of health care when the individual is incapacitated. (Chapter 5.6)

Advocacy: The act or process of pleading for, supporting, or recommending a cause or course of action. Advocacy may be for persons (whether an individual, group, population, or society) or for an issue, such as potable water or global health. (Chapter 6.2, Chapter 10.2)

Affordable Care Act (ACA): Legislation enacted in 2010 to increase consumers' access to health care coverage and protect them from insurance practices that restrict care or significantly increase the cost of care. (Chapter 8.2)

ANA's Standards of Professional Practice: Standards describing a competent level of nursing practice as demonstrated by the critical thinking model known as the nursing process. The nursing process includes the components of assessment, diagnosis, outcomes identification, planning, implementation, and evaluation. (Chapter 1.1)

ANA's Standards of Professional Performance: Standards describing a competent level of behavior in the professional nursing role, including activities related to ethics, advocacy, respectful and equitable practice, communication, collaboration, leadership, education, scholarly inquiry, quality of practice, professional practice evaluation, resource stewardship, and environmental health. (Chapter 1.1, Chapter 9.2)

Assault: Intentionally putting another person in reasonable apprehension of an imminent harmful or offensive contact. (Chapter 5.2)

Assignment: Routine care, activities, and procedures that are within the authorized scope of practice of the RN, LPN/VN, or routine functions of the assistive personnel. (Chapter 3.3)

Autonomy: The capacity to determine one's own actions through independent choice, including demonstration of competence. (Chapter 6.2)

B

Battery: Intentional causation of harmful or offensive contact with another's person without that person's consent. (Chapter 5.2)

Beneficence: The bioethical principle of benefiting others by preventing harm, removing harmful conditions, or affirmatively acting to benefit another or others, often going beyond what is required by law. (Chapter 6.2)

Benner's Novice to Expert Theory: A theory by Dr. Patricia Benner that explains how new hires develop skills and a holistic understanding of client care over time, resulting from a combination of a strong educational foundation and thorough clinical experiences. Benner's theory identifies five levels of nursing experience: novice, advanced beginner, competent, proficient, and expert. (Chapter 11.5)

Board of Nursing: The state-specific licensing and regulatory body that sets standards for safe nursing care and issues nursing licenses to qualified candidates, based on the Nurse Practice Act. (Chapter 1.1)

Brief: A short session to share a plan, discuss team formation, assign roles and responsibilities, establish expectations and climate, and anticipate outcomes and contingencies. (Chapter 7.6)

Budget: An estimate of revenue and expenses over a specified period of time, usually over a year. (Chapter 8.5)

Burnout: A condition manifested physically and psychologically with a loss of motivation. (Chapter 12.6)

C

Capacity: A functional determination that an individual is or is not capable of making a medical decision within a given situation. (Chapter 5.6)

Capital budgets: Budgets used to plan investments and upgrades to tangible assets that lose or gain value over time. Capital is something that can be touched, such as buildings or computers. (Chapter 8.5)

Change: The process of altering or replacing existing knowledge, skills, attitudes, systems, policies, or procedures. (Chapter 4.3)

Change agent: Anyone who has the skill and power to stimulate, facilitate, and coordinate the change effort. (Chapter 4.3)

Change management: Process of making changes in a deliberate, planned, and systematic manner. (Chapter 4.3)

Chronic conditions: Conditions that have a slow onset and may gradually worsen over time. (Chapter 2.3)

Civil law: Law focusing on the rights, responsibilities, and legal relationships between private citizens. (Chapter 5.2)

Clinical reasoning: "A complex cognitive process that uses formal and informal thinking strategies to gather and analyze client information, evaluate the significance of this information, and weigh alternative actions." (Chapter 2.4)

Closed-loop communication: A communication strategy used to ensure that information conveyed by the sender is heard by the receiver and completed. (Chapter 3.2, Chapter 7.5)

Code of ethics: A set of ethical principles established by a profession that is designed to govern decision-making and assist individuals to distinguish right from wrong. (Chapter 6.2)

Collective bargaining: Negotiation of wages and other conditions of employment by an organized body of employees. (Chapter 10.4)

Commission: Doing something a reasonable nurse would not have done. (Chapter 5.2)

Communication conflict: Occurs when there is a failure in the exchange of information. (Chapter 7.7)

Compassion fatigue: A state of chronic and continuous self-sacrifice and/or prolonged exposure to difficult situations that affect a health care professional's physical, emotional, and spiritual well-being. (Chapter 12.6)

Competence: In a legal sense, the ability of an individual to participate in legal proceedings. A judge decides if an individual is "competent" or "incompetent." (Chapter 5.6)

Confidentiality: The right of an individual to have personal, identifiable medical information kept private. (Chapter 5.2)

Consequentialism: An ethical theory used to determine whether or not an action is right by the consequences of the action. For example, most people agree that lying is wrong, but if telling a lie would help save a person's life, consequentialism says it's the right thing to do. (Chapter 6.2)

Constitutional law: The rights, privileges, and responsibilities established by the U.S. Constitution. For example, the right to privacy is a right established by the constitution. (Chapter 5.2)

Constructive feedback: Supportive feedback that offers solutions to areas of weakness. (Chapter 3.5)

Continuity of care: The use of information on past events and personal circumstances to make current care appropriate for each individual. (Chapter 7.8)

Contracts: Binding written, verbal, or implied agreements. (Chapter 5.2)

Co-pay: A flat fee the consumer pays at the time of receiving a health care service as a part of their health care plan. (Chapter 8.3)

Core measures: National standards of care and treatment processes for common conditions. These processes are proven to reduce complications and lead to better client outcomes. (Chapter 9.2)

Core values: The foundational ideals that guide the organization's actions and decision-making processes. (Chapter 4.2)

Crime: A type of behavior defined by Congress or state legislature as deserving of punishment. (Chapter 5.2)

Criminal law: A system of laws concerned with punishment of individuals who commit crimes. (Chapter 5.2)

Critical thinking: A broad term used in nursing that includes "reasoning about clinical issues such as teamwork, collaboration, and streamlining workflow." (Chapter 2.4)

Cultural diversity: A term used to describe cultural differences among clients, family members, and health care team members. (Chapter 7.3)

Cultural humility: A humble and respectful attitude toward individuals of other cultures that pushes one to challenge their own cultural biases, realize they cannot possibly know everything about other cultures, and approach learning about other cultures as a lifelong goal and process. (Chapter 6.2, Chapter 7.3)

Culture of safety: Organizational culture that embraces error reporting by employees with the goal of identifying systemic causes of problems that can be addressed to improve client safety. Just Culture is a component of a culture of safety. (Chapter 4.2, Chapter 5.5))

CURE hierarchy: A strategy for prioritization based on identifying "critical" needs, "urgent" needs, "routine" needs, and "extras." (Chapter 2.3)

CUS statements: Assertive statements that are well-recognized by all staff across a health care agency as implementation of the two-challenge rule. These assertive statements are "I am Concerned – I am Uncomfortable – This is a Safety issue!" (Chapter 7.6)

D

Data cues: Pieces of significant clinical information that direct the nurse toward a potential clinical concern or a change in condition. (Chapter 2.3)

Debrief: An informal information exchange session designed to improve team performance and effectiveness through reinforcement of positive behaviors and reflecting on lessons learned after a significant event occurs. (Chapter 7.6)

Deductible: The amount of money a consumer pays for health care before their insurance plan pays anything. These amounts generally apply per person per calendar year. (Chapter 8.3)

Defamation of character: An act of making negative, malicious, and false remarks about another person to damage their reputation. Slander is spoken defamation and libel is written defamation. (Chapter 5.2)

Defendants: The parties named in a lawsuit. (Chapter 5.2)

Delegated responsibility: A nursing activity, skill, or procedure that is transferred from a license nurse to a delegatee. (Chapter 3.4)

Delegatee: An RN, LPN/VN, or AP who is delegated a nursing responsibility by either an APRN, RN, or LPN/VN who is competent to perform the task and verbally accepts the responsibility. (Chapter 3.4)

Delegation: Allowing a delegatee to perform a specific nursing activity, skill, or procedure that is beyond the delegatee's traditional role but in which they have received additional training. (Chapter 3.4)

Delegator: An APRN, RN, or LPN/VN who requests a specially trained delegatee to perform a specific nursing activity, skill, or procedure that is beyond the delegatee's traditional role. (Chapter 3.4)

Deontology: An ethical theory based on rules that distinguish right from wrong. (Chapter 6.2)

DESC: A tool used to help resolve conflict. DESC is a mnemonic that stands for Describe the specific situation or behavior and provide concrete data, Express how the situation makes you feel/what your concerns are using "I" messages, Suggest other alternatives and seek agreement, and Consequences are stated in terms of impact on established team goals while striving for consensus. (Chapter 7.6)

Discharge: The completion of care and services in a health care facility and the client is sent home (or to another health care facility). (Chapter 7.8)

Durable power of attorney for healthcare (DPOAHC): Person chosen to speak on one's behalf if one becomes incapacitated. (Chapter 5.6)

Duty of reasonable care: Legal obligations nurses have to their clients to adhere to current standards of practice. (Chapter 5.2)

E

Economics: The study of how society makes decisions about its limited resources. (Chapter 8.1)

Ethical conflict: Occurs when individuals or groups have fundamentally different beliefs and values. (Chapter 7.7)

Ethical dilemma: Conflict resulting from competing values that requires a decision to be made from equally desirable or undesirable options. (Chapter 6.3)

Ethical principles: Principles used to define nurses' moral duties and aid in ethical analysis and decision-making. Foundational ethical principles include autonomy (self-determination), beneficence (do good), nonmaleficence (do no harm), justice (fairness), and veracity (tell the truth). (Chapter 6.2)

Ethics: A system of moral principles that a society uses to identify right from wrong. (Chapter 6.2)

Ethics committee: A formal committee established by a health care organization to problem-solve ethical dilemmas. (Chapter 6.4)

Evidence-Based Practice (EBP): A lifelong problem-solving approach that integrates the best evidence from well-designed research studies and evidence-based theories; clinical expertise and evidence from assessment of the health care consumer's history and condition, as well as health care resources; and client, family, group, community, and population preferences and values. (Chapter 8.4, Chapter 9.4, Chapter 10.7)

Expected conditions: Conditions that are likely to occur or anticipated in the course of an illness, disease, or injury. (Chapter 2.3)

Extrinsic factors: External elements that impact health care costs. (Chapter 8.2)

F

False imprisonment: An act of restraining another person causing that person to be confined in a bounded area. Restraints can be physical, verbal, or chemical. (Chapter 5.2)

Feedback: Information is provided to a team member for the purpose of improving team performance. Feedback should be timely, respectful, specific, directed towards improvement, and considerate. (Chapter 7.6)

Felonies: Serious crimes that cause the perpetrator to be imprisoned for greater than one year. (Chapter 5.2)

Fidelity: An ethical principle meaning keeping promises. (Chapter 6.2)

Five rights of delegation: Right task, right circumstance, right person, right directions and communication, and right supervision and evaluation. (Chapter 3.4)

Floating: An agency strategy that asks nurses to temporarily work on a different unit to help cover a short-staffed shift. (Chapter 8.5)

Followership: The upward influence of individuals on their leaders and their teams. (Chapter 4.2)

Fraud: An act of deceiving an individual for personal gain. (Chapter 5.2)

G

Goal conflict: Happens when the objectives of individuals or groups are incompatible. (Chapter 7.7)

Good Samaritan Law: State law providing protections against negligence claims to individuals who render aid to people experiencing medical emergencies outside of clinical environments. (Chapter 5.2)

Grievance process: A process for resolving disagreements between employees and management. (Chapter 10.4)

H

Handoff reports: A transfer and acceptance of client care responsibility achieved through effective communication. It is a real-time process of passing client specific information from one caregiver to another, or from one team of caregivers to another, for the purpose of ensuring the continuity and safety of the client's care. (Chapter 7.5)

Harmful stress: Stress (also referred to as "distress") not adequately self-managed resulting in physical, mental, and behavioral consequences. (Chapter 12.3)

Health care disparity: Differences in access to health care and insurance coverage. (Chapter 8.4)

Health disparities: Differences in health outcomes that result from social determinants of health (SDOH). (Chapter 8.4)

Horizontal aggression: Hostile behavior among one's peers. (Chapter 7.7)

Huddle: A brief meeting during a shift to reestablish situational awareness, reinforce plans already in place, and adjust the teamwork plan as needed. (Chapter 7.6)

I

I'M SAFE: A tool used to assess one's own safety status, as well as that of other team members in their ability to provide safe client care. It is a mnemonic standing for personal safety risks as a result of Illness, Medication, Stress, Alcohol and Drugs, Fatigue, and Eating and Elimination. (Chapter 7.6)

Informatics: Using information and technology to communicate, manage knowledge, mitigate error, and support decision-making. This allows members of the health care team to share, store, and analyze health-related information. (Chapter 9.3, Chapter 10.7)

Informed consent: The fundamental right of a client to accept or reject health care. (Chapter 5.6)

Infractions: Minor offenses, such as speeding tickets, that result in fines but not jail time. (Chapter 5.2)

Institutional liability: When the health care institution (e.g., hospital, clinic) is held responsible for the actions of its employees or for failing to implement adequate policies and procedures to prevent harm. (Chapter 5.3)

Institutional Review Board (IRB): A group that has been formally designated to review and monitor biomedical research involving human subjects. (Chapter 6.4)

Intentional tort: An act of commission with the intent of harming or causing damage to another person. Examples of intentional torts include assault, battery, false imprisonment, slander, libel, and breach of privacy or client confidentiality. (Chapter 5.2)

Interdisciplinary care conferences: Meetings where interprofessional team members professionally collaborate, share their expertise, and plan collaborative interventions to meet client needs. (Chapter 7.8)

Interprofessional collaborative practice: Multiple health workers from different professional backgrounds working together with clients, families, caregivers, and communities to deliver the highest quality of care. (Chapter 7.1)

Intrinsic factors: Factors that are inherent to the characteristics and needs of the population. (Chapter 8.2)

I-PASS: A mnemonic used as a structured communication tool among interprofessional team members. I-PASS stands for Illness severity, Patient summary, Action list, Situation awareness, and Synthesis by the receiver. (Chapter 7.5)

ISBARR: A mnemonic for the components to include when communicating with another health care team member: Introduction, Situation, Background, Assessment, Request/Recommendations, and Repeat back. (Chapter 7.5, Chapter 10.7)

J

Just Culture: A culture where people feel safe raising questions and concerns and report safety events in an environment that emphasizes a nonpunitive response to errors and near misses. Clear lines are drawn between human error, at-risk, and reckless employee behaviors. (Chapter 4.2)

Justice: A moral obligation to act on the basis of equality and equity and a standard linked to fairness for all in society. (Chapter 6.2)

L

Laws: Rules and regulations created by society and enforced by courts, statutes, and/or professional licensure boards. (Chapter 5.2)

Leadership: The art of establishing direction and influencing and motivating others to achieve their maximum potential to accomplish tasks, objectives, or projects. (Chapter 4.2)

Libel: Written defamation. (Chapter 5.2)

Licensure: The process by which a State Board of Nursing (SBON) grants permission to an individual to engage in nursing practice after verifying the applicant has attained the competency necessary to perform the scope of practice of a registered nurse (RN). The SBON verifies three components:

- Verification of graduation from an approved prelicensure RN nursing education program
- Verification of successful completion of NCLEX-RN examination
- A criminal background check (in some states) (Chapter 11.3)

Living will: A type of advance directive in which an individual identifies what treatments they would like to receive or refuse if they become incapacitated and unable to make decisions.

M

Magnet® Recognition Program: An organizational credential that recognizes quality client outcomes, nursing excellence, and innovations in professional nursing practice. (Chapter 10.4)

Malpractice: A specific term used for negligence committed by a professional with a license. (Chapter 5.2)

Management: Roles that focus on tasks such as planning, organizing, prioritizing, budgeting, staffing, coordinating, and reporting. (Chapter 4.2)

Mandatory overtime: A requirement by agencies for nurses to stay and care for clients beyond their scheduled shift when short staffing occurs. (Chapter 8.5)

Maslow's Hierarchy of Needs: Prioritization strategies often reflect the foundational elements of physiological needs and safety and progress toward higher levels. (Chapter 2.3)

Medicaid: A joint federal and state program covering groups of eligible individuals, such as low-income families, qualified pregnant women and children, and individuals receiving Supplemental Security Income (SSI). States may choose to cover additional groups, such as individuals receiving home and community-based services and children in foster care who are not otherwise eligible. (Chapter 8.3)

Medicare: A federal health insurance program used by people aged 65 and older, younger individuals with permanent disabilities, and people with end-stage renal disease requiring dialysis or a kidney transplant. (Chapter 8.3)

Meta-analysis: A type of nursing research (also referred to as a "systematic review") that compares the results of independent research studies asking similar research questions. This research often collects both quantitative and qualitative data to provide a well-rounded evaluation by providing both objective and subjective outcomes. (Chapter 9.4)

Mindfulness: Awareness that arises through paying attention, being on purpose and in the present moment, and being nonjudgmental. (Chapter 12.6)

Misdemeanors: Less serious crimes resulting in fines and/or imprisonment for less than one year. (Chapter 5.2)

Mission statement: An organization's statement that describes how the organization will fulfill its vision and establishes a common course of action for future endeavors. (Chapter 4.2)

Moral conflict: Feelings occurring when an individual is uncertain about what values or principles should be applied to an ethical issue. (Chapter 6.3)

Moral courage: The willingness of an individual to speak out and do what is right in the face of forces that would lead us to act in some other way. (Chapter 6.3)

Moral distress: Feelings occurring when correct ethical action is identified but the individual feels constrained by competing values of an organization or other individuals. (Chapter 6.3)

Moral injury: The distressing psychological, behavioral, social, and sometimes spiritual aftermath of exposure to events that contradict deeply held moral beliefs and expectations. (Chapter 6.3)

Morality: Personal values, character, or conduct of individuals or groups within communities and societies. (Chapter 6.2)

Moral outrage: Feelings occurring when an individual witnesses immoral acts or practices they feel powerless to change. (Chapter 6.3)

Morals: The prevailing standards of behavior of a society that enable people to live cooperatively in groups. (Chapter 6.2)

Mutual support: The ability to anticipate and support team members' needs through accurate knowledge about their responsibilities and workload. (Chapter 7.6)

N

National Patient Safety Goals: Guidelines specific to organizations accredited by The Joint Commission that focus on problems in health care safety and ways to solve them. (Chapter 9.2)

NCLEX-RN: The exam that nursing graduates must pass successfully to obtain their nursing license and become a registered nurse. (Chapter 11.2)

NCLEX-RN Test Plan: A concise summary of the content and scope of the NCLEX that serves as an excellent guide for preparing for the exam. These plans are updated every three years based on surveys of newly licensed registered nurses to ensure the NCLEX questions reflect fair, comprehensive, current, and entry-level nursing competency. (Chapter 11.2)

Negligence: The failure to exercise the ordinary care a reasonable person would use in similar circumstances. Wisconsin civil jury instruction states, "A person is not using ordinary care and is negligent, if the person, without intending to do harm, does something (or fails to do something) that a reasonable person would recognize as creating an unreasonable risk of injury or damage to a person or property." (Chapter 5.2)

Nonmaleficence: The bioethical principle that specifies a duty to do no harm and balances avoidable harm with benefits of good achieved. (Chapter 6.2)

Normal stress: Stress (also referred to as "eustress") that does not have lasting consequences and is successfully managed by the individual who is experiencing it. (Chapter 12.3)

Nurse Licensure Compact (NLC): State legislation that allows nurses to practice in other NLC states with their original state's nursing license without having to obtain additional licenses, contingent upon remaining a resident of that state. (Chapter 11.3)

Nurse Practice Act: Law enacted by a state's legislature that defines the scope of nursing practice and establishes regulations for nursing practice within that state. (Chapter 1.1)

Nurse residency programs: A transition process that provides additional professional development for newly licensed nurses. These programs vary from institution to institution, but many start around the time the new graduate ends their orientation with a preceptor and continue to provide routine support throughout the year. (Chapter 11.5)

Nursing: Integrates the art and science of caring and focuses on the protection, promotion, and optimization of health and human functioning; prevention of illness and injury; facilitation of healing; and alleviation of suffering through compassionate presence. Nursing is the diagnosis and treatment of human responses and advocacy in the care of individuals, families, groups, communities, and populations in recognition of the connection of all humanity." (Chapter 1.1)

Nursing informatics: The science and practice integrating nursing, its information and knowledge, with information and communication technologies to promote the health of people, families, and communities worldwide. (Chapter 9.3)

Nursing process: Includes the components of assessment, diagnosis, outcomes identification, planning, implementation, and evaluation. (Chapter 1.1)

Nursing research: The systematic inquiry designed to develop knowledge about issues of importance to the nursing profession. The purpose of nursing research is to advance nursing practice through the discovery of new information. It is also used to provide scholarly evidence regarding improved client outcomes resulting from nursing interventions. (Chapter 9.4)

Nursing team members: Advanced practice registered nurses (APRN), registered nurses (RN), licensed practical/vocational nurses (LPN/VN), and assistive personnel (AP). (Chapter 3.1)

O

Off with benefits: An agency staffing strategy when a nurse is not needed for their scheduled shift. The nurse does not typically receive an hourly wage and is not expected to report to work, but they still accrue benefits such as insurance and paid time off. (Chapter 8.5)

Omission: Not doing something a reasonable nurse would have done. (Chapter 5.2)

On call: An agency staffing strategy when a nurse is not immediately needed for their scheduled shift. They may have options to stay at work and complete work-related education or stay home. (Chapter 8.5)

Operating budgets: Budgets including personnel costs and annual facility operating costs. (Chapter 8.5)

Organizational culture: The implicit values and beliefs that reflect the norms and traditions of an organization. An organization's vision, mission, and values statements are the foundation of organizational culture. (Chapter 4.2)

Orientation: A structured transition process when hired into a new position that may last from one to four months but can be longer depending on the specialty (e.g., Intensive Care or Labor and Delivery). Orientation is based on the new nurse's demonstration and completion of competencies. During this time the novice RN will work with a preceptor to experience all the aspects of the role. (Chapter 11.5)

P

Paternalism: The interference by the state or an individual with another person, defended by the claim that the person interfered with will be better off or protected from harm. (Chapter 6.2)

Patient-centered care: The client is the source of control and full partner in providing compassionate and coordinated care based on respect for clients preferences, values, and needs. (Chapter 10.7)

Pay for Performance: A reimbursement model, also known as value-based payment, that attaches financial incentives based on the performance of health care agencies and providers. (Chapter 8.4)

Peer-reviewed: Scholarly journal articles that have been reviewed independently by at least two other academic experts in the same field as the author(s) to ensure accuracy and quality. (Chapter 9.4)

Personality conflict: Arises from differences in individual temperaments, attitudes, and behaviors. (Chapter 7.7)

Plaintiff: The person bringing the lawsuit. (Chapter 5.2)

Policy: An expected course of action set by an agency. (Chapter 1.1)

Portfolio: A compilation of materials showcasing examples of previous work demonstrating one's skills, qualifications, education, training, and experience. (Chapter 11.4)

Preceptors: Experienced and competent RNs who serve as a role model and a resource to a newly hired nurse. These nurses have the knowledge, skills, and the ability to coach the new RN into the nursing role and answer questions while also evaluating a new hire's performance and providing feedback for improvement. (Chapter 11.5)

Primary source: An original study or report of an experiment or clinical problem. The evidence is typically written and published by the individual(s) conducting the research and includes a literature review, description of the research design, statistical analysis of the data, and discussion regarding the implications of the results. (Chapter 9.4)

Private law: Laws that govern the relationships between private entities. (Chapter 5.2)

Procedure: An official way of completing a task. (Chapter 1.1)

Protected Health Information (PHI): Individually identifiable health information and includes demographic data related to the individual's past, present, or future physical or mental health or condition; the provision of health care to the individual; and the past, present, or future payment for the provision of health care to the individual. (Chapter 5.2)

Protocol: A detailed, written plan for performing a regimen of therapy. (Chapter 1.1)

Public law: Law regulating relations of individuals with the government or institutions. (Chapter 5.2)

Q

Qualitative studies: A type of study that provides subjective data, often focusing on the perception or experience of the participants. Data is collected through observations and open-ended questions and often referred to as experimental data. Data is interpreted by developing themes in participants' views and observations. (Chapter 9.4)

Quality: The degree to which nursing services for health care consumers, families, groups, communities, and populations increase the likelihood of desirable outcomes and are consistent with evolving nursing knowledge. (Chapter 9.2)

Quality Improvement (QI): A systematic process using measurable data to improve health care services and the overall health status of clients. The QI process includes the steps of Plan, Do, Study, and Act. (Chapter 9.3, Chapter 10.7)

Quantitative studies: A type of study that provides objective data by using number values to explain outcomes. Researchers can use statistical analysis to determine strength of the findings, as well as identify correlations. (Chapter 9.4)

R

Ratio-based staffing models: A staffing model used to make client assignments in terms of one nurse caring for a set number of clients. (Chapter 2.3)

Resiliency training: Educational sessions that foster feelings of mindfulness and sensitivity to self and cultivate professional development techniques that contribute to long-term engagement in the profession. (Chapter 12.7)

Resource stewardship: Using appropriate resources to plan, provide, and sustain evidence-based nursing services that are safe, effective, financially responsible, and used judiciously. (Chapter 8.6)

Resume: A document that highlights one's background, education, skills, and accomplishments to potential employers. (Chapter 11.4)

Risk problem: A nursing problem that reflects that a client may experience a problem but does not currently have signs reflecting the problem is actively occurring. (Chapter 2.3)

Role conflict: Arises when individuals have multiple, often conflicting, expectations associated with their roles. (Chapter 7.7)

S

Scope of practice: Procedures, actions, and processes that a health care practitioner is permitted to undertake in keeping with the terms of their professional license. (Chapter 3.3)

Secondary source: Evidence is written by an author who gathers existing data provided from research completed by another individual. This type of source analyzes and reports on findings from other research projects and may interpret findings or draw conclusions. In nursing research these sources are typically published as a systematic review and meta-analysis. (Chapter 9.4)

Self-care: Actions that individuals take to maintain health of oneself. (Chapter 12.6)

Shared governance: A shared leadership model between management and employees working together to achieve common goals. (Chapter 10.4)

Shared mental model: The actions of a team leader that ensure all team members have situation awareness and are "on the same page" as situations evolve on the unit. (Chapter 7.6)

Situation awareness: The awareness of a team member knowing what is going on around them. (Chapter 7.6)

Situation monitoring: The process of continually scanning and assessing the situation to gain and maintain an understanding of what is going on around you. (Chapter 7.6)

Slander: Spoken defamation. (Chapter 5.2)

Social Determinants of Health (SDOH): Conditions in the places where people live, learn, work, and play, such as unstable housing, low-income areas, unsafe neighborhoods, or substandard education that affect a wide range of health risks and outcomes. (Chapter 8.2, Chapter 8.4, Chapter 10.4)

Standards of Professional Nursing Practice: Authoritative statements of the actions and behaviors that all registered nurses, regardless of role, population, specialty, and setting, are expected to perform competently. (Chapter 1.1)

Statutory law: Written laws enacted by the federal or state legislature. For example, the Nurse Practice Act in each state is an example of statutory law that is enacted by the state government. (Chapter 5.2)

STEP tool: A situation monitoring tool used to know what is going on with you, your clients, your team, and your environment. STEP stands for Status of the clients, Team members, Environment, and Progress Toward Goal. (Chapter 7.6)

Student liability: When the student nurse is held responsible for their own actions that cause harm to clients or violate protocols. (Chapter 5.3)

Supervision: Appropriate monitoring of the delegated activity, evaluation of client outcomes, and follow-up with the delegatee at the completion of the activity. (Chapter 3.4)

Supervisory liability: When a clinical supervisor or preceptor is held responsible for the actions of the student nurse or for failing to properly supervise them. (Chapter 5.3)

Systems leadership: A set of skills used to catalyze, enable, and support the process of systems-level change that focuses on the individual, the community, and the system. (Chapter 4.2)

Systems theory: The concept that systems do not function in isolation but rather there is an interdependence that exists between their parts. Systems theory assumes that most individuals strive to do good work but are affected by diverse influences within the system. (Chapter 4.2)

T

Team nursing: A common staffing pattern that uses a combination of Registered Nurses (RNs), Licensed Practical/Vocational Nurses (LPN/VNs), and Assistive Personnel (AP) to care for a group of clients. (Chapter 8.5)

TeamSTEPPS® (Team Strategies and Tools to Enhance Performance and Patient Safety): An evidence-based framework to improve client safety through effective communication in health care environments consisting of four core competencies: communication, leadership, situation monitoring, and mutual support. (Chapter 7.6, Chapter 10.7)

Teamwork and collaboration: Functioning effectively within nursing and interprofessional teams, fostering open communication, mutual respect, and shared decision-making to achieve quality client care. (Chapter 10.7)

Temporary permit: A permit issued by the State Board of Nursing (SBON) that allows the applicant to practice practical nursing under the direct supervision of a registered nurse until their RN license is granted. (Chapter 11.3)

Time estimation: A prioritization strategy, including the review of planned tasks and allocation of time believed to be required to complete each task. (Chapter 2.5)

Time scarcity: A feeling of racing against a clock that is continually working against you. (Chapter 2.2)

Titrate: Making adjustments to medication dosage per an established protocol to obtain a desired therapeutic outcome. (Chapter 3.3)

Tort: An act of commission or omission that causes injury or harm to another person for which the courts impose liability. In the context of torts, "injury" describes the invasion of any legal right, whereas "harm" describes a loss or detriment the individual suffers. Torts are classified as intentional or unintentional. (Chapter 5.2)

Two-challenge rule: A strategy for advocating for client safety that includes a team member assertively voicing their concern at least two times to ensure that it has been heard by the decision-maker. (Chapter 7.6)

U

Unexpected conditions: Conditions that are not likely to occur in the normal progression of an illness, disease, or injury. (Chapter 2.3)

Unintentional tort: Acts of omission (not doing something a person has a responsibility to do) or inadvertently doing something causing unintended accidents leading to injury, property damage, or financial loss. Examples of unintentional torts impacting nurses include negligence and malpractice. (Chapter 5.2)

Unlicensed Assistive personnel (UAP): Any assistive personnel trained to function in a supportive role, regardless of title, to whom a nursing responsibility may be delegated. This includes, but is not limited to, certified nursing assistants or aides (CNAs), patient-care technicians (PCTs), certified medical assistants (CMAs), certified medication aides, and home health aides. (Chapter 3.1)

Utilitarianism: A type of consequentialism that determines whether or not actions are right based on their consequences, with the standard being achieving the greatest good for the greatest number of people. (Chapter 6.2)

Utilization review: An investigation by insurance agencies and other health care funders on services performed by doctors, nurses, and other health care team members to ensure money is not wasted covering things that are unnecessary for proper treatment or are inefficient. This review also allows organizations to objectively measure how effectively health care services and resources are being used to best meet their clients' needs. (Chapter 9.3)

V

Values: Individual beliefs that motivate people to act one way or another and serve as a guide for behavior. (Chapter 6.2)

Values statement: The organization's established values that support its vision and mission and provide strategic guidelines for decision-making, both internally and externally, by members of the organization. (Chapter 4.2)

Veracity: An ethical principle meaning telling the truth. (Chapter 6.2)

Vision statement: An organization's statement that defines why the organization exists, describes how the organization is unique and different from similar organizations, and specifies what the organization is striving to be. (Chapter 4.2)

W

Whistleblower: A person who exposes any kind of information or activity that is deemed illegal, unethical, or not correct within an organization. (Chapter 10.5)